Jason E. Squire is an independent producer who has over twelve years experience in the movie business. As a creative executive in feature films, he has worked in New York and Los Angeles for United Artists, Avco Embassy, Italian producer Alberto Grimaldi, and in Movies for Television at Twentieth Century-Fox. In the recording industry, he served as executive producer of the soundtrack album for *Conan the Barbarian.* Mr. Squire is a consultant for the USA Film Festival in Dallas and has served on conference panels for the Aspen Institute, the American Film Institute, the Beverly Hills Bar Association, UCLA, and the Audio Engineering Society. His writings include the screenplay for *Red Harvest,* an Italian-Spanish coproduction, a stage play *Waiting Room,* and working as co-editor of the pioneering textbook *The Movie Business: American Film Industry Practice.* A graduate of Syracuse University and UCLA, Mr. Squire has taught media writing and production, and lectured widely at colleges around the country. He is currently developing movie, record, theatre and book projects, and is based in the Westwood section of Los Angeles.

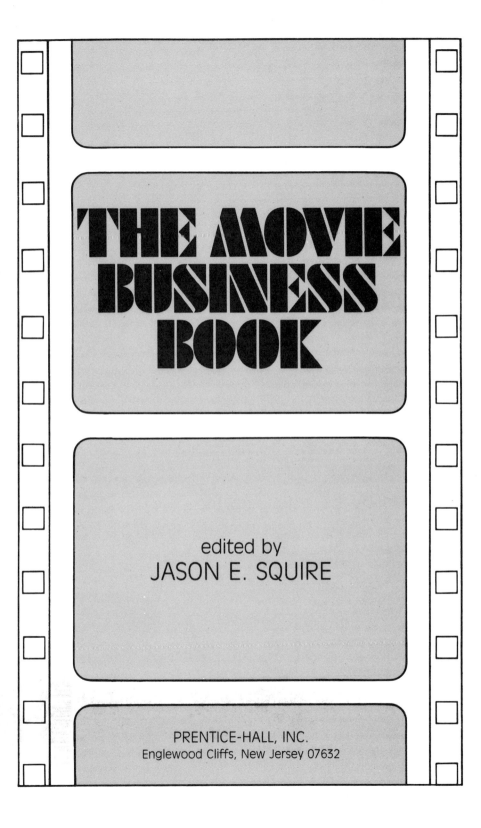

THE MOVIE BUSINESS BOOK

edited by
JASON E. SQUIRE

PRENTICE-HALL, INC.
Englewood Cliffs, New Jersey 07632

Library of Congress Cataloging in Publication Data

Main entry under title:

The Movie business book.

 Includes index.
 1. Moving-picture industry—United States—Addresses, essays, lectures.
I. Squire, Jason E.
PN1993.5.U6M666 1983   384'.8'0973   82-16126
ISBN 0-13-604603-7
ISBN 0-13-604595-2 (pbk.)

10 9 8 7 6 5

Printed in the United States of America

ISBN 0-13-604603-7

ISBN 0-13-604595-2 {A REWARD BOOK : PBK.}

Editorial and production supervision and
 interior design by Cyndy Lyle Rymer
Manufacturing buyer Pat Mahoney
Cover design © 1983 by Jeannette Jacobs

Prentice-Hall International, Inc., *London*
Prentice-Hall of Australia Pty. Limited, *Sydney*
Prentice-Hall of Canada Inc., *Toronto*
Prentice-Hall of India Private Limited, *New Delhi*
Prentice-Hall of Japan, Inc., *Tokyo*
Prentice-Hall of Southeast Asia Pte. Ltd., *Singapore*
Whitehall Books Limited, *Wellington, New Zealand*
Editora Prentice Hall do Brasil Ltda., *Rio de Janeiro*

WITH LOVE, FOR DAD, MOM, AND WALTER

Contents

I
THE CREATORS

CONTENTS

II
THE PROPERTY

CONTENTS

III
THE MONEY

IV
THE MANAGEMENT

CONTENTS

IX
THE EXHIBITORS

X
THE AUDIENCE

CONTENTS

XI
THE FUTURE

For moviegoers and movie makers,
and to everyone who has two businesses—
their own and the movie business.

Thank Yous

There are lots of nice people who touch the life of an enterprise such as this. Professor A. William Bluem asked me to be his co-editor on *The Movie Business* in 1970. That two-year, cross-country collaboration was a vivid education and delight. Bill died in 1974, but he lives on in his books and in the memories of his loved ones and of his thousands of Syracuse University students. If there is a guiding spirit behind this effort, it is Bill's. I miss him.

The spotlight of gratitude shines on the contributors to this text. It's their book. These gifted ladies and gentlemen, who daily practice the business on its highest levels, sensed a responsibility to join in and share their expertise and gave their time in an effort to create a legacy for the future. It's been a massive collaboration, just as movies are. Because these participants care about the spreading of understanding about the movie industry, they deserve all the credit. It was a pleasure working with them.

Columbia Pictures was generous with permission to reprint paper work examples from the production of *The China Syndrome*, arranged through the aid of Michael Douglas, Bruce Gilbert, and Jane Fonda, co-producers, and compiled with great care and skill by Debbie Getlin. The screenplay excerpt is included through the courtesy of writers Mike Gray, T.S. Cook, and James Bridges.

Twentieth Century–Fox kindly allowed their budget top sheet and exhibition contract to be used as illustrations, and the excerpt from the *Butch Cassidy and the Sundance Kid* screenplay is used thanks to Fox and writer William Goldman.

Syd Silverman, publisher of *Variety* and *Daily Variety*, extended the courtesy of allowing excerpts from the journalism of A. D. Murphy to be included.

Many people responded generously when I called on them for help and suggestions during the preparation and editing of the manuscript: William E. Bernstein, Charles B. Bloch, Robert Breech, Leonard Chassman, Kenneth Clark, Stuart Cornfeld, Joe Davis, Stephen M. Kravit, Sidney Landau, Judd Z. Magilnick, Francis McCarthy, James R. Miller, Marc Pevers, Thomas P. Pollock, James Powers, and Steven J. Schmidt.

A warm thank you goes to Thomas D. Selz of the law firm of Frankfurt, Garbus, Klein & Selz, New York, who rescued the ambition of this book by organizing an effort to allow me to pursue a broader, more thorough approach to the entire subject. Richard B. Heller of the same firm has also been an effective advocate. Joan Brandt of the Sterling Lord Agency in New York was instrumental in placing the completed manuscript. John G. Kirk of Prentice-Hall has provided much-appreciated enthusiasm and support for the book.

During the tough days when all this work was just beginning, my family overflowed with love and encouragement. Good friends who especially helped include Steve Alpern, Sheldon Finkelstein, Sam L. Grogg (who named the book), Robert L. Kravitz, Perry Oretzky, Basil Poledouris, and Martin Polon.

Warm thanks and love are saved for Beverly Canning Bluem, a source of inspiration.

Three teachers who care about movies and who made a difference along the way are Richard Averson, Norman O. Keim, and Howard Suber.

Much helpful typing was done by Margie Bresnahan, who always did a terrific job, usually under tight deadlines. And for providing sustenance, there was "The Apple Pan" on Pico Boulevard in Los Angeles, serving "quality forever" all hours of the day and night. Closed Mondays.

Finally, special gratitude is reserved for my brother, Walter C. Squire, who possesses an intuitive sense about the movie business, and who was my sounding board from start to finish. He is always there with good counsel and criticism, and for that he deserves more credit than he knows.

J.E.S.

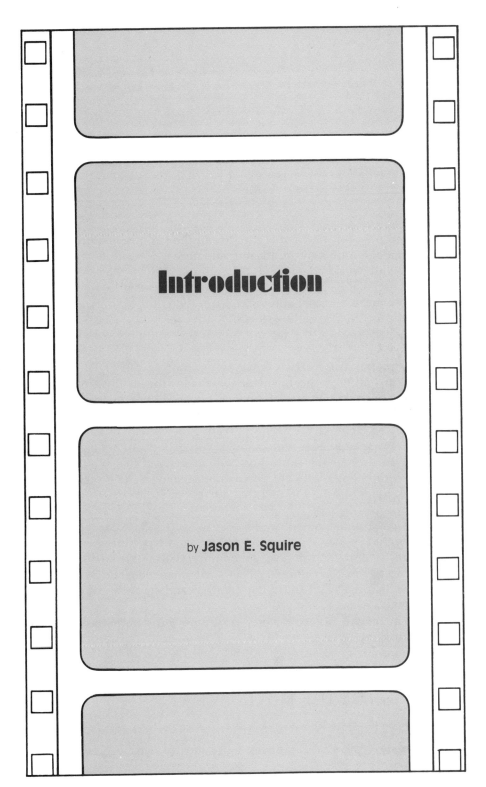

Introduction

by Jason E. Squire

This book is all about the business side of movies. The American motion picture, spawned at the turn of the century, matured in one generation into a mixture of art and commerce. It continues to have a profound and worldwide effect on culture, politics, and economics. The international language of film has been embraced by new generations as a natural form of expression, even though it is very costly compared with its artistic predecessors.

At its simplest, the feature film is the shuffling of light images to win hearts in dark rooms. At its most complex, it is a massive venture of commerce, a vast creative enterprise requiring the logistical discipline of the military, the financial foreshadowing of the Federal Reserve, and the psychological tolerance of the clergy, all harnessed in private hands on behalf of the telling of a story.

In the commercial movie industry, the idea is to make movies that attract vast audiences who cumulatively pay enough money for the privilege so that all the costs involved in making that movie are recouped, with enough left over to make more movies. The profit motive is at work here, but the formula that attracts audiences is as elusive as can be.

A note about business. The very word puts some people off. When applied to movies, it conjures up conflicts pitting west coast against east coast, the creative community against the business community, art against commerce. That's all changed. The responsible filmmaker learns early to mix the creative and business sense out of self-defense.

The movie industry works on money. It's important to know how the money is arranged for, spent, protected, and returned. This work is an effort to organize, simplify, and examine all that.

THE MOVIE BUSINESS

Like all businesses, the theatrical motion picture business exists to make money. That's the only way more movies can be produced and an on-going network of production, distribution, and exhibition can be fed. Comparisons can be loosely made to other industries: Production encompasses research, development, and manufacturing; distribution can be compared to wholesaling; and exhibition to retailing. But there the comparison ends because the public's demand and use of entertainment products such as motion pictures are unlike the demand and use of any other product. In no other business is a single example of product fully created at an investment of millions of dollars with no real assurance that the public will buy it. In no other business does the public "use" the product and then take away with them (as Samuel Marx observed in *Mayer and Thalberg*) merely the memory of it. In the truest sense, it's an industry based on dreams.

The movie industry defies strict analysis from a traditional business point of view. Any profiling of the business points to certain concepts not characteristic of other industries. These concepts can prevail only in an industry whose product is creative.

What are the hallmarks of the movie *business*? That movies are a collaborative medium; every picture-making experience is different; financing movies is an enormous crapshoot; there are no hard and fast rules; many of the essential decisions and choices spring from intuitive leaps; most successful practitioners possess a personal mix of creative and business sense; creative and business decisions often rely on relationships and personalities; an entire investment is made before anyone knows if the product is marketable; and as far as profits are concerned, the sky's the limit.

These elements focus on a cyclical industry, difficult to chart, rooted in creativity and intuition, capable of dismal losses and euphoric profits, engaged in an on-going seduction of the paying audience. At the retail level, there is the significant act of motivating people to leave their homes to go to see a specific movie. The single universally acknowledged marketing tool for this product—favorable audience word-of-mouth—can perhaps be influenced but it cannot be controlled. The success of the product cannot be predicted, but only tested (as Peter Myers notes) by the democratic means of people putting down hard cash to enjoy an entertainment first-hand.

All this points to why conservative capital has historically shied away from motion picture investments although control of motion picture companies has always been attractive to a broad spectrum of players. The early 1980s saw five major transactions involving changes of ownership in as many companies. In 1981, Denver businessman Marvin Davis bought Twentieth Century-Fox Film Corporation for an estimated $725-million, making it the only major studio in private hands; MGM Film Company (controlled by Kirk Kerkorian) purchased United Artists Corporation from Transamerica Corporation for an estimated

$380-million, becoming MGM/UA Entertainment Company; and entre-
preneurs A. Jerrold Perenchio and Norman Lear bought Avco Embassy
Pictures from Avco Corporation for $25-million, dropping Avco from
the company name. In 1982, Coca-Cola Company acquired Columbia
Pictures Industries, Inc. for an estimated $750-million and the princi-
pals of Orion Pictures Company, who had established Orion after de-
parting top management ranks at United Artists in 1978, joined with
other investors to take over Filmways (formerly American International
Pictures) in a deal involving a capital investment approximating $26-
million, then renamed it Orion Pictures Corporation. Industry observers often insist that "it's not a business . . ." while movies continue to
attract creative businessmen and artists who are devoted to the production and dissemination of this most valuable and influential national re-
source and export.

At its core, the whole industry is devoted to competing for the
work of creators in a limited talent pool which shifts each year based
on the strength of specific works and audience acceptance. But the list
of directors, for example, who can govern a feature-size budget averaging $10-million, or a two-hour television movie budget averaging
$2-million, is limited. Nevertheless, energies are intensely spent daily
to compete for this talent pool and to create new entries into it.

What has happened in the movie industry to warrant such in-
tensity? As a business, there recently have been far-reaching economic
changes. There is no longer a ceiling on box-office potential and there
are new, varied sources of revenue as well as financing. *Star Wars* was
the landmark picture that broke through the higher limits of traditional
revenue potential in 1977. Through the phenomenon of repeat business, coupled with easy access to the public because of the widest possible distribution, *Star Wars* redefined worldwide income potential at
the box office, and in merchandising, book and record sales, having a
great impact on the perception of movie economics. A carefully marketed picture such as *Saturday Night Fever* in 1977 proved that a movie
can generate revenue in other media, such as recordings, that can
match and then exceed box-office gross. *The Empire Strikes Back* during its 1980 release echoed the extraordinary success of *Star Wars* and
E.T. The Extra-Terrestrial in 1982–83 will most likely exceed *Star Wars*
business.

The long-awaited video revolution, bringing new home patrons
to the movies through pay-TV channels, video cassettes, discs and
other technologies can now have an impact on a theatrical feature before and after it is made. These markets can provide money to help finance the picture in advance of production and then generate revenue
potential second only to the first-run play-off of the picture in theatres.
Ten years ago, a theatrical feature would play itself out in a pattern

from first-run to neighborhood houses, and next appear on network television before it would be included in TV syndication packages for local station film libraries. Today, there are more exploitable steps in the life-cycle of a movie. After a broad, national release in theatres, the picture is next available in neighborhood stores on videodisc and videocassette. Later, the picture is featured on pay-TV services, followed by showings on network television, and finally put into TV syndication. Variations on this distribution pattern and time frames involved are being tested to garner the most revenue from different pictures.

Synergy between media has resulted in new sources of revenue, financing, and marketing for a picture if strategy is carefully choreographed. A book publisher can finance the writing of a screenplay in advance of the author's turning it into a novel; a movie company can finance the writing of a novel or a stage play prior to the development of a screenplay. The value of book tie-ins has made publication rights another negotiable point; merchandising of artwork from a movie to adorn t-shirts and accessories has also become a lucrative area.

Although pictures can lose more money than ever, they can also make more money than ever. This has attracted not only new investors to the business, but new financier-distributors as well. "Mini-majors" such as Orion have entered the marketplace in competition with the traditional majors for artists, product, and screens worldwide. The three American television networks distribute over 250 first-run movies and mini-series to their stations annually, and pay-TV systems are beginning to finance original movies themselves.

From the American standpoint, a graphic result of new money sources has been the growth of the Canadian film industry, which emerged on the strength of government-regulated tax incentives attracting Canadian investors. It would be useful domestically if American investors similarly enjoyed incentives to support American independent (non-studio initiated) feature filmmaking.

Through all of this financial, marketing and technological change, the essence of the movie business has remained the same. Pictures are a gamble, and businessmen work to apply formulas and intuition to reduce odds. Exhibitors remain suspicious of distributors and distributors are leery of exhibitors. Because the product requires the spending of money, it is up to the lawyers, accountants, and agents to construct some framework of responsibility and recourse to support the creators and businessmen. They deal in the movie *business* that operates under rules and procedures, however changeable and resistant to categories they may be.

Perhaps the hallmarks of the movie business appear risky to the traditional observer. But each year the motion picture community produces about 250 theatrical features and over 250 movies for television

5

and mini-series to compete for the worldwide leisure dollar. Because people literally line up around the block for specific pictures, passing the word that they like certain ones and returning to them at theatres or at home, the economic potential of this entertainment form is unlimited.

HISTORY

This book is a direct descendent of the pioneering text *The Movie Business: American Film Industry Practice,* published by Hastings House in 1972. It was my privilege to work on that project with Professor A. William Bluem, serving as his co-editor.

We began work in 1970 and it was pretty discouraging at first. Early efforts to enlist knowledgeable industry members to discuss the business side of their work were unsuccessful. One prominent lawyer wrote back that he was unwilling to share "industry secrets" and suggested that was why there was no book on the movie business around. But there were enough forthright professionals sensitive to the need for such a book, and their involvement and expertise made *The Movie Business* an industry standard, the primary text in the field adopted at schools all over the country.

The warm reception of that first work coincided with the growth and recognition of film study on campuses around the country. Institutions rich in courses in movie production, history, and aesthetics began to broaden their curricula to introduce the business of motion pictures as an inter-disciplinary study often coordinated with business and law schools as part of a well-rounded treatment of mass entertainment and popular culture.

FORMAT

To accurately cover the detail and scope of *The Movie Business Book,* the idea was to go to the source: industry specialists with specific expertise. If there is one point of view imposed upon the reader, it is that of the film producer who, more than anyone, must harness the variety of elements involved in making and marketing a picture. (A note on style: The contributors will often use terms that are interchangeable in the industry jargon. For example, a picture is a movie or a film, and a studio is a financier-distributor or a major.)

The sequence of chapters is organized to cover the lifespan of a movie, with each section building upon the succeeding one. After an orientation in Part One, *The Creators,* each chapter follows the process from writing, financing, dealmaking, and production through distribution to theatres and subsequent exposures. The format breaks down as follows:

I. *The Creators:* An orientation, this section focuses on the most visible of movie makers. The producer, represented by Robert Evans, often chooses the story, does the hiring, is responsible for the money spent, and is the chief executive on a picture. The director, personified by Sydney Pollack, is the captain on the set, working closely with the producer on most decisions which precede and follow production. The director is usually the single creator most closely identified with the finished picture. The range of creators includes a comic genius, Mel Brooks, a sensitive writer-director, Joan Micklin Silver, and a filmmaker who wears several hats on a production, Russ Meyer.

II. *The Property:* Following the overview of Part One, we return to the beginning of a movie's life, the word. The work of the writer, discussed by William Goldman, is represented in the marketplace by a literary agent, such as Lee G. Rosenberg and Lew Weitzman, whose job it is to sell the work so that it becomes property. This process usually involves submission to a buyer, perhaps through the story editor (Eleanor Breese of Lorimar). Such a purchase might increase the property's value in published form, as described by Roberta Kent of the Ufland Agency in Beverly Hills.

III. *The Money:* Money spent for services rendered is the key to most all activity in the business. In this section, the practices of the movie marketplace are examined, as buyers and sellers trade off. The diversity of types of financing available, detailed by Norman H. Garey, varies from the major financier-distributor's dealings with banks, covered by Peter W. Geiger, vice-president of Bank of America, to foreign governments making certain incentives available, described by Gary O. Concoff (of the law firm of Sidley & Austin in Los Angeles), to producers partially financing pictures through pre-sales to foreign distributors, as reviewed by journalists Sylvie Schneble and Tristine Rainer.

IV. *The Management:* The collective expertise responsible for key decision making is covered next. Movie executive philosophy has its own unique priorities, as interpreted by industry consultant Richard Lederer, molded on an individual basis by the personalities in the seats of power, such as Gordon Stulberg, president of Polygram Corporation, producer David V. Picker and Roger L. Mayer, vice-president of MGM/UA.

V. *The Deal:* A fundamental truth of the business is that all major transactions are structured to be set down in written agreements. These agreements are key reference documents. The basic elements of every deal are: what is the property or service; who is providing it to whom; what is the time frame; and what is the compensation. A chief architect for many deals is the entertainment lawyer, represented herein by Norman H. Garey, who negotiates the picture deal on behalf of his producer-client with the financier-distributor's business affairs chief executive, such as Richard Zimbert of Paramount. The producer would probably have to secure over-budget protection, as described by Norman G. Rudman (of the Los Angeles law firm of Slaff, Mosk & Rudman) and, in pursuit of specific performers and other creative people, will have countless dealings with talent agents, as detailed by producer Barry Weitz.

VI. *The Shooting:* All the complex preparation and military-style logistical planning is played out during shooting. Strictest compliance with the budget and shooting schedule is the daily responsibility of the line producer, personified by Paul Maslansky, the nuts-and-bolts executive on the set. This frees the director, represented here by James Bridges, to create with the other artists the necessary illusions amid the pervading pressures of time and money.

VII. *The Selling:* Getting the picture on film is only half the battle. The entire enterprise is in financial peril unless the audience can be convinced to pay for experiencing it. The critical relationship between distribution and exhibition is analyzed by long-time *Daily Variety* financial editor A. D. Murphy. Maneuvering the paying audience to the point of sale—the theatre—is enhanced by new techniques in motion picture marketing, described by Richard Kahn, executive vice-president of MGM/UA.

VIII. *The Distributors:* The distributors are the vital link to the public. Part salesmen and part magicians, distribution executives carry on a love/hate relationship with exhibitors to get the product into theatres, while weighing the outlay of advertising dollars against the income of box-office gross. Distribution companies range from the studio financier-distributor exemplified by Peter S. Myers, senior vice-president of Twentieth Century-Fox, to the smaller independents, represented by Barbara D. Boyle, writing as executive vice-president of New World Pictures in Los Angeles and Raphael D. Silver, president of Midwest Films in New York. Whatever their product slate or strength in the marketplace, distributors share certain problems in common, as detailed by industry veteran Paul N. Lazarus.

IX. *The Exhibitors:* The theatre owner is the retailer in the movie business, the only person in daily contact with the consumer. The exhibitor, as covered by Nat D. Fellman, founder of Exhibitor Relations Company, Los Angeles, is at once the consummate showman and the pragmatic businessman. At the point of sale he handles the cash. What binds the theatre owner and distributor is their need for each other, governed by the exhibition contract, as capsuled by Richard P. May, branch operations manager of Twentieth Century-Fox. Similar business problems are shared by large theatre chains, as represented by Stanley H. Durwood (president) and Joel H. Resnick (executive vice-president) of American Multi-Cinema, based in Kansas City, and independent exhibitors such as Robert Laemmle of Laemmle Theatres in Los Angeles. The exhibition segment of the industry is evolving, as viewed by Michael F. Mayer (of the New York law firm of Mayer & Bucher), to the point where refreshment sales have become a critical part of their balance-sheet profit, as detailed by Boston-based exhibitor Philip M. Lowe, past president of the National Association of Concessionaires.

X. *The Audience:* All of the energy and money described up to now has been applied to create a product and an atmosphere around it which will attract the paying audience. The moviegoer will make a conscious decision to go out of the house to see a specific movie. There is enormous competition for that share of the recreational dollar that people spend on movies. This decision to see a certain picture may be influenced by the rating, part of an industry support system described by Jack Valenti, president of the Motion Picture Association of America based in Washington, D.C., or the advertising campaign and its fixtures, as detailed by Martin Michel of National Screen Service, New York. A related industry has recently grown out of lucrative merchandising rights, covered by Stanford Blum (of Stanford Blum Enterprises in Sherman Oaks), which finds customers buying tie-in products associated with a picture.

XI. *The Future:* An industry that does not prepare for the future is destined to live in the past. Futurist Martin Polon, based in Los Angeles, projects the effect of research on production techniques and theatre enhancement. The greatest impact on the audience and product is taking place within the burgeoning home entertainment market in the form of pay-TV and other service subscriptions and video cassette/disc purchases. This will ultimately free the home viewer from the tyranny of passive television, making the viewer an active, selective programmer. The home entertainment revolution also promises more and diverse product, which means more movies and more jobs.

GOALS

This work sets out to shed light on the entire spectrum of feature movie making, covering the creation, financing, production, marketing, distribution, and exhibition of movies to paying audiences at box offices and beyond, throughout their exploitable lives. The idea is to cover this territory from the first-hand vantage points of industry specialists, as a service to movie goers and movie makers.

From this flow other purposes:

• to provide the movie audience with an exposure to the pressures and priorities of business decisions that affect, on multiple levels, the final product unspooling at the local theatre;

• to sensitize new filmmakers to the business procedures they will confront as they practice their craft;

• to acquaint people in production, distribution, and exhibition with how their jobs relate to the entire motion picture process;

• to remove misconceptions or resistance about the money side of movies and to make the concepts involved clearer and more accessible;

• to act as a record of current industry attitudes and styles of business that may take on new interest with the passage of time.

If the reader gains a basic understanding of how the movie business works, and comes away with a deeper fascination for the movie process and product, then the goals will have been fulfilled.

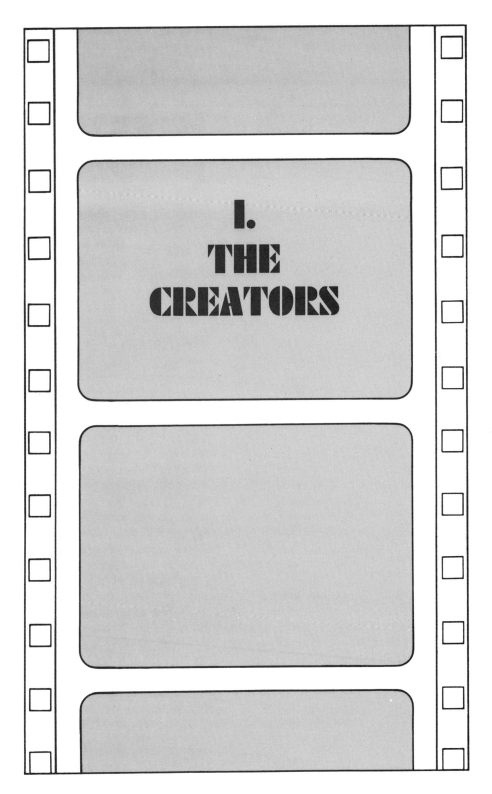

I.
THE
CREATORS

The Producer

by **Robert Evans,** chief of worldwide production for Paramount Pictures from 1966–1976, a tenure that was the longest of any studio head since World War II. Under his aegis, the studio released such landmark hits as *Rosemary's Baby, Love Story, Play It Again, Sam, True Grit, The Godfather*, and *The Godfather, Part II*. He is now a producer under an exclusive, long-term contract with Paramount and has produced such pictures as *Chinatown, Marathon Man, Black Sunday, Urban Cowboy*, and *Popeye*.

I'd rather have the next five films of Robert Towne than Robert Redford because extraordinary writing is a film-maker's greatest magnet. . . .

There's an ambiguity about the term *producer* because that screen credit can go to a lawyer, agent, deal maker, actor, or writer who produces pictures. Of the pure producers, there are those who make one picture in five years, and those who package six pictures in one year. I fall somewhere in between. Although the packaging producer makes a lot of money from development and producing fees, I can't work that way. As a working producer, I get involved in each minute detail on a picture to the point of obsession. As a result, I work from two to three years on a single picture. Frankly, I have been criticized by the studio and others for spending too much time on the post-production and minutiae of a film, but that's the only way I can work. I give the same amount of time and passion to a failure as to a success. There's no right or wrong way among the various styles of producing, and I am basing my comments on my own style.

The "independent producer" is a fallacy, unless he is putting up his own money to make a picture. I am a dependent producer under exclusive contract to Paramount. The studio finances my pictures and is very generous and supportive. There hasn't been a picture I've wanted to make that the studio has turned down. On a daily basis, this puts me in contact with Paramount's business affairs and creative staff.

Let me review the anatomy of a picture and discuss the five stages of picture making: research & development, pre-production, production, post-production, and marketing. For most producers, the search for material (research & development) is an ongoing venture. Naturally, film projects come from all possible sources. *Urban Cowboy* was originally an article in *Esquire* magazine; *Popeye* came from the cartoon character; *Black Sunday* and *Marathon Man* were novels; *Chinatown* was an original screenplay. I want to emphasize that best sellers don't make the best movies. I've taken *The New York Times* best-seller lists for the last ten years and found many novels that were made into unsuccessful movies and many that were purchased but never made into movies at all. There are two reasons for this. First, a best-selling novel may simply not have a cinematic story; that's subjective. Second, the book-reading audience is not the movie-going audience; that's objective. The book-reading audience consists mostly of adults over 35, while the majority of the frequent movie-going audience ranges in age from 12 to 30 and does not buy books avidly. Although a successful book doesn't guarantee a big film, it does guarantee a big purchase price for movie rights. This makes agents very happy but often leaves studios heavily inventoried in fashionable but unmakable material.

The process of submitting material to a financier-distributor is difficult, especially for an unknown producer, writer, or director. The only guidance I can give is to persevere. If six readers at Paramount each judge a piece of material as excellent, it still may never be read by the two or three people who make the decisions. A bare script with no "elements" usually remains on the shelf. It must be accompanied by an element—a director, star, or one of a handful of producers—for attention to be paid. Otherwise, the studio executive, whose job is usually to say no, will do just that.

In development, the all-important art of collaboration begins. The producer—if he really is a producer—usually works on a picture longer than anyone else. During the development stage, he starts to take on his creative team. A motion picture is a collaborative art form. Throughout film history, with rare exceptions, the best work done by directors has been done in collaboration with strong producers. It is the producer who hires the director, not the other way around. Pictures with runaway costs can be traced to negligent producers or financing sources. In an effective collaborative mix, which has to do with personality as well as creativity, one must be inquisitive and have a challenging attitude. This sometimes leads to very heated arguments. But pictures have a better chance of turning out well when they are born of conviction and passion.

In hiring a writer, the first requirement is to know the work of many writers in order to make an intelligent choice. Some writers are very good at structure; others, at dialogue. Usually, screenplays are rewritten, rewritten, and rewritten. If a writer feels he's "written out" after one draft, he must still be given every chance before another writer is taken on. To me, it's important to be irreverent about the material and to try constantly to improve it in order to create something magical. There is no such thing as a perfect script; the producer who believes he has one is in trouble. When a director is hired, he has his own vision. Sometimes there is a schism between director and writer, or writer and actor, or director, writer, and actor, and this must be controlled by the producer. I want to emphasize the importance of the development stage because any weakness in the script haunts the project in subsequent stages. No matter how talented the director or actors are, a poor script will overshadow their gifts and cause the picture to suffer

15

on the screen. To me, the biggest star of any picture is the writer. I'd rather have the next five films of Robert Towne than Robert Redford because extraordinary writing is a filmmaker's greatest magnet.

Pre-production begins when a start date is set for the picture. The financier-distributor gives the approvals then to go beyond the director and writer and start hiring actors, the heads of departments, and other below-the-line personnel. The hiring of department heads usually requires negotiations between lawyers and Paramount's business affairs executives. (There's probably more legal work per dollar spent in the motion picture industry than in any other industry in the world.) Pre-production is defined by the spending of money on such hiring and on the securing of equipment and locations.

Meanwhile, as producer, I have been working with the director and production manager on the budget, figuring the number of days and the shooting sequence, and consulting on the visual identity of the picture before a frame of film is shot. The cinematographer, director, and I discuss the look, texture, and visual style of the picture. I'm involved in many decisions during pre-production, from the collar an actor wears in a scene to the way his hair is cut.

A start date is usually set six months in advance. This can be a problem. On *Players,* I had a start date pegged to Wimbledon that could not be changed. The script was being rewritten, but I had to start shooting. The result was that the picture failed. The most expensive mistake on a picture is to be unprepared. It's better to push back a start date and spend more time in preparation. Each day in production is very expensive; each day spent preparing before most of the workers are hired is cheap. Being prepared is the most economical discipline a producer can learn.

Before turning to production, let me cover some issues involving the high cost of pictures. Inflation is a burden on all sectors of the country. In the making of pictures, everyone is paid too much—directors, actors, and producers—including me. Below-the-line costs have more than tripled since 1967. The difference is that most people above-the-line (producers, writers, actors, and directors) can afford to cut, but most personnel below-the-line (everyone else) cannot. One solution would be if actors, directors, writers, and producers got a fair accounting from their financier-distributors with regard to profit or gross participations; then high-priced creators might work for less salary or for free just to see more pictures made. If a given company has, say, $90-million a year to spend on pictures, it can make either nine pictures for $10-million each or fifteen pictures for $6-million each, which would put more people to work. This is a simplification, but it does point to the dissatisfaction most net profit participants feel regarding the report-

ing of their shares. There is fairness in accounting when one participates on a gross basis, or on some form of adjusted gross basis. Otherwise, because of growing interest rates, there's a long wait before
anyone sees net profit shares. This is why, if a creator is not a gross
participant, his lawyers and agents are looking for a large cash salary
for him up front.

It's impossible to make a small picture today on a union basis.
That doesn't hurt me because I'm established and have access to financing. It hurts the young filmmaker who is struggling to fund a picture. The United States is the most important filmmaking country in the
world, but there is no tax incentive for investors in movies. Investors in
oil and gas enjoy certain tax incentives that give them the opportunity
to gamble. The same should be true for investors in pictures. The
American film (next to Coca-Cola) is our country's greatest ambassador.
Today, American-made motion pictures are the number one films in
every country in terms of interest and box-office success. The government should be very proud of this, but they pay little attention to it.

In production, one early crisis occurs when the picture is running over budget and the cutting of scenes is required. Sometimes
there are early cast changes if things aren't working during rehearsal;
sometimes locations must be changed. When cutting scenes, the collaborative relationship of producer, director, and writer emerges again.
Perhaps the shooting schedule has to be restructured or reduced to
save money. This is achieved in a joint effort, sometimes punctuated by
angry fights. But through tactful negotiation, discussion, and recognition of economic realities, the parties (who usually hold a financial
stake in delivering the picture on schedule and on budget) can work it
out.

In my style of producing, I stay very close to the shooting, but
I don't go on the set. I have nothing to contribute there besides making
people nervous. I view every foot of film that is shot, make notes of
takes I prefer, and keep them to myself. The director is the captain of
the ship during principal photography. Usually there are hostilities or
tensions between actors or between director and actors, and the producer must be involved in keeping peace. I've had artists who wanted
to walk off pictures. At various times, Roman Polanski, Robert Towne,
and Faye Dunaway wanted to walk off *Chinatown*. Again, diplomacy
and reason must be applied to such problems. At all costs, I try to keep
the front office away from anyone involved in making my picture. I
want to be the only conduit between the picture and the studio.

During the production stage, certain marketing decisions are
being made. The trailer is being cut while the picture is shooting. This
vital selling device, which I personally work on, will be shown directly

17

to moviegoers as a captive audience inside theatres. A 90-second teaser trailer should play in theatres six months before the picture's release to plant an image in the audience's memory. As for the print campaign, there are usually various agencies working on ideas for campaigns while the picture is shooting because it can take a year to perfect an effective campaign. I don't believe in production publicity at all; it's forgotten by the time the picture comes out and distracts the actors from making the film. Publicity counts most in the month before the picture opens.

I often fight with Paramount about overselling and overpublicizing films. The best example of this danger is *The Great Gatsby*. Months before the film opened, the country was Gatsbyized; the effect snowballed with Gatsby hats, shoes, suits, and so on. By the time the picture came out, most people thought they had already seen it. Excitement about the film peaked well before it opened, rather than just at its release. There was no mystery about it. Part of the attraction of any film is the mystery that makes an audience want to see it. There was no pre-opening exposure to *Star Wars;* when it opened, the lines were around the block.

In post-production, I work most closely on the editing. It's taken me many years to build respect with directors and editors, and this, too, is very much a collaborative effort. The director has the prerogative to mold and shape the film in his cut. Then, I work with him and the editor to fine tune the editing process, which is critical to the form and impact of the final picture. I've pushed back release dates because the editing process needed more time. This happened on *The Godfather* and *Chinatown. Marathon Man* was supposed to open in June, 1976, but in April I told management the picture wasn't ready. They said, "It's impossible, we have 800 theatres booked for June, it's the best time of the year." I said, "I'll give you a picture, but you won't want it." We set a new opening date in October and continued working on the problems of structure in the film until ten days before release. Each picture is different, but post-production must be given enough time. Miracles in editing and scoring can cover a myriad of production flaws.

During post-production, I get further involved in the marketing and release strategy. The teaser has played in theatres; the theatrical and television trailers are prepared; print campaigns are locked in. I fight for play dates, terms, and specific theatres. I'd rather take less in the form of guarantees and have the proper theatres, but the sales staff doesn't often agree. If I've spent two and a half years of my life on a picture, I don't want it to play in a theatre where the arcs are bad or the screen is small or the sound is poor. For some reason, most of the theatres in America are ill or cheaply equipped. I don't have a solution to this problem, but exhibitors who spend more money on equipment and furnishings will find filmmakers insisting on booking their theatres.

Once the picture is locked in, attention must be paid to the European versions. An American picture is dubbed in four languages: Spanish, Italian, French, and German. Dubbing is as much a creative process as making the picture itself is. The work is generally done in each country, and distributors spend extra money on dubbing only if they have confidence in it overseas. Usually, dubbing actors are hired locally, and a new script is hastily written. The local actors try to recreate the performances on the screen by synchronizing their language to the lip movements on the screen. I insisted that Louis Malle take over the French version of *The Godfather*. He hired the writer of the French dialogue, selected all the actors, and directed the dubbing meticulously. Eventually, this cost Paramount $100,000, but it was worth it. On *Players*, however, they didn't spend much money dubbing the overseas versions because they didn't expect to recoup it. American distributors should spend more time and money on dubbing because there's a valid and discerning market overseas that could account for half of a picture's worldwide revenue.

Once the picture is cut and scored, previews are scheduled. This is similar to taking a theatrical play on the road. For a true audience reaction, pictures should be previewed in cities like Seattle, St. Louis, Dallas, or New Orleans, rather than Los Angeles, San Francisco, or San Diego, where there are professional preview-goers. A preview can be very instructive. John Schlesinger and I made many changes in *Marathon Man* after the preview, even though we both thought we wouldn't have to touch it. One becomes so subjectively involved in four months of editing that it's hard to see mistakes. At a preview, one learns about audience reactions, timing, laughs, tensions, and the general pulse of the picture. If reactions are not as expected, proper changes can be made before the picture is tested at a second preview. I preview pictures from two to four times. When the director and studio are satisfied, the picture goes through the final mix and is locked in; prints are struck, checked, and made ready for release.

When a picture opens in 500 theatres, the first three days can often determine whether it's a success or not. Sometimes, it's deceptive. The exhibitors thought *Black Sunday* was going to be bigger than *Jaws*. It opened in 500 theatres on a Friday, and I visited the Loew's State and Loew's Tower East in New York opening night and saw lines around the block. I went to bed thinking I had a hit and woke up to learn that those were the only good engagements in the entire country. On Monday we revised the entire ad campaign, quoting from the best reviews one could want and spending lots of money. Nothing helped. When a picture opens wide to weak business, it's almost impossible to revitalize it. If it opens strongly, the second weekend will determine whether it has "legs," or staying power. Aside from the summer and Christmas seasons, ours is a weekend business. Finally, all the money, work, and passion are tested when the picture is released. Then, it's in the hands of the people.

The Director

by **Sydney Pollack,** who has earned distinction as a director in motion pictures and television. Among his theatrical feature credits are *Tootsie, Absence of Malice, The Electric Horseman, Bobby Deerfield, Three Days of the Condor, The Yakuza, The Way We Were, Jeremiah Johnson,* and *They Shoot Horses, Don't They?,* which won him a nomination for Outstanding Directorial Achievement from the Academy of Motion Picture Arts and Sciences and the Directors Guild. Mr. Pollack has also directed numerous television series episodes and is the recipient of an Emmy Award from the Television Academy.

director can find his next movie through a variety of sources: pre-publication galleys of a novel, a completed screenplay, a treatment (a long synopsis of the events of a story), first-hand discussions with writers or a producer, or magazine or newspaper articles. Whatever the form, the first critical stage in creating a movie is developing this material.

Development is simply bringing the project from a nonproduceable state to a produceable state; that's a strict definition. What it means to me is tailoring a project to my own personal vision. A screenplay of *Doctor Zhivago* developed by David Lean, Fred Zinnemann, John Frankenheimer, or Arthur Penn would result in four different visions of the novel. Each would satisfy the strict definition, since each would make the novel into a screenplay ready to be shot. The variety would stem from the process of tailoring a screenplay to express a particular director's view. This is accomplished through plain hard work with the screenwriter.

Some writers like to have lots of meetings, get the director's input, and then go off alone to complete an entire first draft screenplay that is then turned in. This is a gamble that sometimes leads to success and sometimes doesn't. If the writer is off on an unwanted story tangent, the problem will be compounded throughout the screenplay. There are other writers who are willing to give a director 4–5 pages at a time, discuss them, and rewrite them as necessary. A middle ground finds the director and writer meeting several times before the writer goes off and completes half the screenplay, perhaps 50 to 60 pages. Then they meet again and discuss any disagreements growing out of those pages. Another method can find the writer and director writing together in the same room, arguing about the characters and dialogue. This is the closest form of collaboration and depends on a strong relationship between the two creators. Naturally, whatever choice is made stems from the personalities and work habits of those involved.

The development process on *The Electric Horseman* was dictated by economic realities. We had two major stars, Robert Redford and Jane Fonda, committed for a specific time period. We had a start date from the studio, which wanted to release the picture in a certain season. For these business reasons, the project reversed the usual process. The screenplay was being developed *after* the studio had committed all monies necessary to make the picture.

It's a seller's market. The studios desperately need product, which puts filmmakers in a stronger position than they have ever known. When pictures hit, they hit for higher revenues than ever before. There are many huge hits and many terrible flops, but very few moderately successful pictures. If a picture costs $8-million to make, another $4–6-million is often spent on advertising and print costs to open it. Interest charges are applied in addition to these figures. If the picture grosses over $20-million, theoretically it should be into profits, and those owning a percentage in the form of a profit participation should be paid.

It is only in rare instances, however, that one realizes money from a profit participation. When a picture has grossed $20-million without paying any profit money and people ask why, they are shown an array of figures, probably all accurate, having to do with costs of distribution, advertising, prints, overhead, executive entertainment, and so on. These figures are all added into the negative cost. On a big-grossing picture, it *is* possible to make money on a percentage deal, but it takes months and sometimes years. Most of the time, however, there is no percentage return.

Economics is the most inhibiting factor for a director making a film. Most creative people, with the exception of actors and directors, create alone and in silence. With actors and directors it's a little like taking your clothes off in front of a mob of people. There are hundreds of technicians; if we are on a street, there are horns honking and the clock is ticking away. Every time the director says, "Let's *try* it this way," and not, "Let's *do* it this way," he is spending money at enormous rates. The average Hollywood studio company out on location spends anywhere between $30,000 and $50,000 a day. Breaking that down into eight-hour segments, it averages $5,000 an hour. If the director wants to take an hour to play with a scene and try it two or three ways, $5,000 is added to the cost of production.

The economic pressures funnel down to the unit manager and the first assistant director. The unit manager is being leaned on by a production manager; the production manager is being leaned on by a producer; the producer is being leaned on by a studio. A director does not *want* to have a reputation for being wasteful because that is harmful to a career. When you shoot a scene ten or twelve times looking for some special expression from an actor, you are always vulnerable to production office criticism. Is Take Ten *really* better than Take One? How much better is better? $1,000 better? $2,000 better? No one can decide that except the director. He must try ultimately to be intransigent, while hoping that everything he is doing contributes to making a better picture and is, therefore, not wasteful.

The first thing usually asked a director when he is signed is "How much do you think it will cost?" Sometimes it is difficult to know in the beginning, but I usually make a guess. Then I work with an assistant director and a production manager to make what is called a *breakdown*,* a scene-by-scene itemizing of what will be required: How many extras? Should a set be rented or built? Will we be on location or in a studio? How much will living expenses be? How many days will it take? How large a crew? Will we need multiple cameras? How much action will there be? How many sequences involve large numbers of people? What will the weather be like? With sequences involving large numbers of people, will we be more than 300 miles from Hollywood so that we can get unemployed local personnel for extras, or do we have to pay Hollywood rates to the extras? If we have 100 people getting the Hollywood rate of $65 per day, that is a considerable sum of money. In *They Shoot Horses, Don't They?* we had between 700 and 1,000 extras a day.

Finally, we see that we have a 60-day shooting schedule and that the picture is going to cost, say, $6-million below-the-line. This price does not include above-the-line costs, which cover all the creative people—the salaries of the writer, the producer, the director, and the actors. The studio then says, "We can't spend that much money; we must cut it down to $5-million." So we start to cut.

Instead of building a detailed log cabin for a certain scene, we erect only a frame and perhaps cover it with canvas. That savings is knocked off the budget. We forget the 300 extras in Scene 42 and do it with 100 well-spaced extras. Instead of carrying a crane and the two additional men required to operate it for ten weeks, which would cost some $50,000 (including transportation, room and board, and fringe benefits for these men), I might agree to group all the crane shots into a two-week period. This change would save us some $40,000. But nothing saves money on a film as much as cutting days off the schedule. Other changes become relatively minor. When we have finally worked out the shooting schedule, the production department makes a budget. It is usually higher than the studio wants to go and more cutting or discussion takes place until finally we have a schedule and budget that is approved by everyone.

The choice of crew is next and obviously is extremely important. Not only do their various creative and mechanical abilities contribute to the final effect of the film, but every moment they save you

---

* For a specimen of a breakdown sheet, see the example from *China Syndrome*, p. 231.

is an extra moment you can spend creatively. Every director researches the background of a tentative crew member religiously. What pictures have they done? How fast are they? Do they get on well with other crew members?

The early stages of production depend upon the nature of the individual picture. If it requires an enormous amount of set construction, for example, then the art director is one of the first people hired. He has a practical problem: he has to build a town that will take two and a half months to construct, and we are three months from shooting. I start thinking about a cinematographer from the first day I come on the picture. But we usually do not hire one until a couple of weeks before shooting starts. I sometimes sit down with a cinematographer two months before shooting, just to talk to him. He may be finishing another picture, but we get together for a couple of evenings, run two or three pictures together, talk about an effect, a concept, or a way of working.

I try to be as involved as possible with the photographic techniques of the film. I like to choose the lens, discuss the f-stop, the light level, the color level, what the focus will be like. These aspects of photography are all part of the vocabulary of the director. It's possible to shoot a scene twice, doing the same thing with the same actors; yet, if they are photographed in two different ways, they will be entirely different in mood and emotional effect. A good example occurs in *Sweet Smell of Success*, in which they reversed the normal shooting concept. They shot almost every master shot with long-focus lenses, from very far away, in order to pack the buildings and the street in tightly behind the people. Then they shot their close-ups with wide-angle lenses to keep the background in focus and, again, to maintain an awareness of the buildings. This technique creates an overall effect in which the lay moviegoer feels oppressed by the city, by the sense of the city's closing in, without necessarily understanding why.

One of the first problems I had with *They Shoot Horses* is a common problem in films shot in color: how to make it look unglamorous. Color film tends to glamorize and enrich. Phil Lathrop, the cinematographer, and I finally did two things. Since we were shooting the entire picture on one set, I needed the freedom to shoot 360 degrees for purposes of variety. That meant no standing lights; otherwise, they would be photographed. Lighting people from above, from over their heads, is usually ugly, casting harsh shadows. That happened to be perfect for the story. The second thing we did was to force-develop the film. In other words, we underexposed the film and kept it in the developer a few minutes longer, making it grainier, milkier and taking some of the glamorous texture off it. In the picture *This Property Is Condemned*, which I did with James Wong Howe, we made tests to try to desaturate the color for the same reason—it was a 1930s picture, a poverty picture. We took a gray shirtboard and set it up in front of the camera. We photographed the gray cardboard, filling the frame, but with perhaps one-tenth of the proper amount of exposure. Then, we wound the film back and shot the scene with nine-tenths of the exposure, so that it was pre-fogged a bit. This process took some of the color out of it. One cannot underestimate the technical end—it's a technical medium, like architecture.

I do not usually rehearse much; rehearsal is a concept that comes from the theatre. In a film, because we do not have the luxury of time, I try to catch a performance before it starts to become aware of itself. Just before each new scene, I do some rehearsing, but very little. Some of the scenes in *Horses* between Jane Fonda and Michael Sarrazin were three and four pages long, and I rehearsed them for maybe 20 minutes. There were many critical shots in that picture in which people had perhaps a tenth of an inch of movement possible, because I was shooting through 40 people out of focus. Instead of cutting to a close-up, we tried to make the focus work like a close-up, so that we would not lose a sense of the environment. The frame covered perhaps 20 couples, but there was only one pair of heads sharply visible in the center of it.

During principal photography, I view the dailies each day with the editor, pointing out which take I like best. We might, for instance, use the first part of take one and the third part of take two. The editor makes a note each time. After shooting, I see a first assembly and then begin work on a first cut. An *assembly* means that the editor has simply organized all the film chosen from the rushes. Seeing it is usually a disastrous moment for me. But then we start from the beginning to trim, rearrange, accent, and find the rhythms and moods.

Somewhere along the way we bring in a sound-effects man. Probably by this time we already have a composer. I have a few meetings with him and then show him the final cut. Then we have a *spotting session* where we sit together with a footage counter. I might say, "Start the music when she turns her head there, and go to the point where he walks out the door." Now he knows that he has 130 feet that he has to fill with music.

Next, there is optical work to do. We figure out where the dissolves are going to be. Then a title man comes in, and we space the titles out, figuring how many feet they are going to run.

If the sound quality is poor, or if it does not match from scene to scene, *looping* must be done. For instance, if an airplane goes overhead during a master shot, but when the close-up is shot there is no airplane, the two cannot be intercut; it is necessary to loop the whole master. This process involves lip-syncing, bringing actors into the studio to repeat their dialogue and match it to the screen. It is boring, difficult work that usually has an artificial sound. It is worth great pains to get good original sound tracks.

With the final cut made, the film is ready for music *scoring*, which has been anticipated in the budget. After scoring, we take the film into a dubbing room, where three or four people control audio-mixing channels. There may be as many as 32 channels: one has all the men's dialogue; another has all the women's dialogue; another the looped, post-sync lines, because they have to be treated. (Since they have been recorded in a soundproof room, they have to be made to sound as if they originated outside.) The director spends days in the dubbing room, supervising the delicate mixing of all the available sound with the picture and into the final sound track.

Post-production radically affects a film; in certain films, it's as important as the shooting. The less dependent a film is on a linear story line, the more important the post-production period is. *Three Days of the Condor* was on the market eight weeks after we finished shooting because post-production was simplified by a strict narrative story line. *Jeremiah Johnson* took many months in post-production because there was hardly a narrative line at all; it's a picture made of rhythms, mood, pace, and a sense that is between the cuts. Many of these values are created in post-production. It's possible to radically alter what an audience feels when watching a picture by tiny variations from literal reality incorporated in the sound track: where a sound starts and where it fades; whether it cuts off or overlaps slightly into the next scene; whether it previews the coming scene by beginning just a touch before the cut occurs. Quite often, I'll make straight cuts in the visual, softened by cross-fading the sound behind it, rather than cutting from one sound to another.

There are certain moments in films that are very musical moments, and these must be handled sensitively in the mix. In a scene containing music and live sound effects, there is a tendency to use both. Sometimes this can become a cacophony that is distracting. I usually try to select one above the other. In one scene, I'll forget the reality of the street traffic and other sounds and let the music carry the scene. For example, in a nonverbal sequence in *Bobby Deerfield*, Al Pacino and Marthe Keller are in Florence having a contest over how soon he will be recognized if he removes his sunglasses. I could never get the scene to feel right the realistic way, hearing all the street sounds with the music underneath. So we faded the realistic sound a few seconds before the music began. This gave the audience the sense that something was about to happen, but then the audio void was filled by the music. At that point, we brought the realistic sound back, but very low. In this way, something is created for the audience, though

27

they may not know how. The sound track guides the audience as to how they should feel, often more so than the visual.

The next step is to look at what is called a *mute answer print.* It has no sound because until now we have been working with magnetic sound on a strip of film separate from the picture. The merger of sound and picture will happen in the printing process. This is a dead silent print that we look at for the colors. Invariably, it is not right the first try, and the lab makes corrections. When the picture is approved, we are ready to add the sound, which has been transferred to an optical negative. A bunch of squiggly black lines will become squiggly white lines on the positive, which an exciter lamp will pick up on a projector and translate into sound. This sound negative, which is made in the studio, is then sent to the laboratory. The laboratory takes all of the technical data from the viewing of the mute answer print, joins the sound negative with it, and strikes the first final-viewing *answer print.* From there, all the other prints are made.

Two technical advances have greatly affected picture making recently. One is faster film and lenses, and the other is the increased portability of the equipment. The two have a related effect. Faster film and smaller equipment allow more flexibility in production. We can shoot in available light and let an actor go into a live situation without attracting attention. Lenses are so fast today that it's possible to overexpose film shooting at night with no lights. The normal film used indoors, which has an ASA of 100, can be pushed two full f-stops (to the equivalent of ASA 400) and give a result that is quite usable. The Panaflex camera is much lighter and easier to use than older equipment, and the *Steadicam* and *Panaglide* systems, which allow for smooth handheld work, can eliminate the use of bulky dollies or building tracks.

Probably the most radically changed function over the past 20 years is that of the producer. At one time, it was very much a producer's medium. Gentlemen like Sam Spiegel and Hal Wallis were filmmakers in that they conceived a project, developed the screenplay, assembled the creative personnel, and were involved in the choice of locations, cameraman, director, and crew. Today, a producer is often anyone who buys an option on a literary property and interests a director or star in it. Often, they are not men who are experienced in realizing a screenplay; rather, they are entrepreneurs trained in business who have learned how to put deals together. As a result, many directors function as their own producers, though they are not credited as such.

My Movies: The Collision of Art and Money

by **Mel Brooks,** who was born in Brooklyn and first gained notoriety as one of the writers on Sid Caesar's classic television program *Your Show of Shows*. This led to an association with another Caesar alumnus, Carl Reiner, in the creation of "The 2,000-Year-Old Man" record albums, which became hugely successful. Brooks collaborated with Buck Henry on the television series *Get Smart* before turning to movies, where he won an Oscar for writing and directing a short subject, *The Critic*. He won another Oscar for writing *The Producers*, also the first feature he directed, and went on to co-write and direct *The Twelve Chairs*, *Blazing Saddles*, and *Young Frankenstein*. Brooks managed to add more hyphens to his credits for subsequent pictures *Silent Movie* (actor–director–co-writer), *High Anxiety*, and *History of the World, Part I* (producer-actor-director-writer). His production company, Brooksfilms, has produced such pictures as *The Elephant Man* and *My Favorite Year*.

What's the toughest thing about making film? Putting in the little holes.

'm primarily an observer of life who formalizes his observations by writing them down. Some of us have no need to tell anybody else about those observations. I happen to have a need to pronounce myself. I started my career as a drummer; I'm sorry I stopped because it still is the best and the loudest way of calling attention to myself.

I began as a writer and I'm still basically a writer. I directed a summer stock company when I was a little boy in Red Bank, New Jersey; I also directed some theatre in the borscht belt and was a drummer-comic there. I'd been writing *Your Show of Shows* and then *Caesar's Hour* on television for years when I decided that it was time for me to leave and do something else with my life. Maybe become a housewife.

When I moved away from Sid Caesar and went into the real world of writing television specials, it was very difficult when the director or producer would say "Thank you" and that was it; I had no control over the material. When I wrote my first movie, *The Producers*, I decided that I would also direct it to protect my vision.

The Producers was first written as a novel. It talked too much, so I made it into a play, which ended up with too many locations, so I turned it into a film. It was right out of my own life experience; I once worked with a man who did make serious love to very old ladies late at night on an old leather office couch. They would give him blank checks, and he would produce phony plays. I can't mention his name because he would go to jail. Just for the old ladies alone, he would go to jail. I wrote my heart out, and the movie, I think, is one of my best, though it was not very commercial.

I directed *The Producers* because I didn't want anybody interfering with my words. It was a very difficult course for me to chart because I didn't realize that movies are so expensive. If you make a record, the record sells for $7.00. It may cost anywhere from $500, $15,000 or, if it's a big record, $150,000 to produce. The smallest movie shot on a union basis would cost $1,000,000 and the average film today costs somewhere around ten million dollars.

30

I spent roughly eleven months editing *The Producers.* With each succeeding film, I've put more time into pre-production and less time into post-production. I edited for ten months on *The Twelve Chairs;* nine months on *Blazing Saddles;* five months on *Young Frankenstein,* about four months on *Silent Movie;* and three and a half months on *High Anxiety.*

The story of *The Producers* is a very interesting one. I wrote the script together with help from Alfa-Betty Olsen, and every studio said, "Please no. Try not to come back here." An agent, Barry Levinson, knew producer Sidney Glazier. Barry set a meeting (in those days, you didn't "take" a meeting) with me and Sidney, who read it, shook my hand, and said, "It's the funniest thing I've ever heard. We're going to make a movie out of this." He went to Joseph E. Levine (Embassy Pictures at that time) and said to Joe, "I will raise half a million dollars if you put up half a million dollars. You distribute the film; it will cost a million dollars to make." Joe Levine said yes but "Brooks can't direct." I said no.

Levine wanted a real director. At a luncheon meeting, I ate very nicely; I didn't want to make any mistakes, nothing dropped out of my mouth. I didn't eat bread and butter because I didn't know whether you should cut the bread or break it. Meanwhile, Joe ate everything; I had nothing to worry about. At the end of the meal, Levine turned to me casually and said, "Hey, kid, you think you can direct a picture?" I said, "Sure." He said, "Swear to God?" I said, "Yes." He said, "O.K. Go ahead," and shook my hand. He was impressed with me; he thought I was nice and cute and funny. He hadn't read the script, but he liked the idea. Like the old Hollywood producers who never read anything, he liked to hear things. "Tell it to me," they'd say. "He goes to this place called Shangri-La." "Yeah?" "And there are these people, they look young, but they're really old." "Sounds good, sounds good."

Sidney Glazier raised half a million dollars from a company called Universal Marion Corporation and Joe Levine and Embassy put up half a million. I cast the picture with Zero Mostel and Gene Wilder, and we shot it in eight weeks; the budget was $946,000.

When we finished the picture, we took it to the Lane Theatre in Philadelphia for a sneak preview around Christmas, 1967. Nobody came. Twelve hundred seats. Eleven people showed up. The movie was over, and I got on a slow train back to New York. Then, since we had shown the picture to some critics earlier in Philadelphia, the reviews came out. They were horrible. Joe Levine was going to shelve it, but Sidney Glazier prevailed upon him to wait and to start a little campaign of sneak previews in New York. We opened at the Fine Arts Theatre in Manhattan. Word of mouth had spread; there was a line around the block; you couldn't get in. Levine opened the picture slowly elsewhere, handling it carefully. Eventually it became a moneymaker, though it took four years to get its money back. Levine had risked almost a million dollars. He put up $500,000 for the negative and about $400,000 for prints, advertising, and openings. It took a lot of perseverance and work to make that picture become profitable.

I learned a little about movie financing from *The Producers* because I had a participation in the movie, and it was important for me to learn why I wasn't getting any money for my participation. It's impossible for a profit participant outside the studio to make any money on a movie unless it's a gigantic hit because overhead and interest are always being charged to the film.

My second picture was *The Twelve Chairs*. For it I actually went to Yugoslavia and learned there are two basic costs in a movie: *below-the-line*, which refers to materials and the technical aspects of the film, such as personnel, set construction, wires, lights, cameras, and transportation; and *above-the-line*, the more creative aspects of the film, such as the property itself, writers, producer, director, stars, and principals. Extras are (no offense) below-the-line.

When I finished my next picture, *Blazing Saddles*, I screened it for the Warner Brothers executives. It was quiet. Not even the world-famous bean scene got a laugh. I turned very pale. Thank God it was dark. John Calley, who was in charge of production at the time, and Ted Ashley, who was running Warner Brothers, were very nice to me and said, "It's crazy. We like it. Forgive the fact that there was no laughter. These people are studying their various jobs in connection with the picture, and they don't know what to make of it." I said to myself, "It's a failure."

Mike Hertzberg, the producer, was alone with me after they had all cleared out of that screening room, and suddenly he's on the telephone saying, "Yes, yes, screening room 12, 8 o'clock. Be there; invite people." I said, "What are you doing?" He said, "We're having a screening of the same movie. Tonight. All the secretaries at Warner Brothers. I'm getting 200 people to see it." 8 o'clock comes, 200 plain humans are packed into this room. They're very quiet and polite. Frankie Laine sings the title song. The whip cracks start; laughter begins. We go to the railroad segment. Lyle, the cruel overseer, says to Cleavon Little, "How about a little good old nigger work song?" The audience gets a little chilled. Cleavon Little and the other guys working on the railroad begin to sing, "I Get No Kick From Champagne." People leave their chairs in ecstasy, float upside down, and the laughter never stops from that moment on.

32

We next had a sneak preview in Westwood, and that too was successful. It was then that the studio executives screened *Blazing Saddles* again and changed their minds. The picture opened to mixed reviews. My films have never gotten unanimously good reviews; I hope they never will. "Everything Mel Brooks has learned about films," said *The New York Times*, "seems to have been forgotten in this mess called *Blazing Saddles*." When my next picture, *Young Frankenstein*, was released, one critic said, "Where was the great anarchic beauty of *Blazing Saddles*?" It takes them a while to like my films.

When *Blazing Saddles* opened, it got fairly bad reviews and was an instant hit in New York. But Warner Brothers opened it in about 3,500 theatres in one day across the country. It did well only in fifteen big cities. In every other place, like Lubbock, Amarillo, Pittsfield, and Des Moines, it died. The picture didn't get the word of mouth it needed, so it closed. The Warners advertising executive, Dick Lederer, was my guardian angel. He said, "I think we should spend $3-million to advertise it. Pull it out of all these little cities, open it in the summer when it's gained a reputation, and spend $3-million to support it." There was a mixed vote in the room; the deciding votes belonged to Ted Ashley and John Calley. They said, "O.K., we go with you. Let's spend $3-million, and we'll try and see what we can do." To their credit, *Blazing Saddles* opened wide in June to tremendous business around the country. It's done over $40-million in rentals worldwide.

In my experience directing comedies, I've found that timing for laughs is critical. How much space should you leave on screen for laughter before you go on to the next sound on the sound track? Once you've shown the picture to an audience, you and the editor decide. You say, "Look, they're laughing pretty heavily here. Can I have some more frames before we cut away from that shot?" That helps. There are ways to find the proper rhythm of jokes and laughter. The Marx Brothers actually went on the road with some of the comedy sequences from their films to test the timing on live audiences.

After a while, I can judge within a few seconds either way just how much laughter we can get. Sometimes, I'm dead wrong. In *Silent Movie*, there was a sequence that no one will ever see; it's on the cutting room floor. The sequence is called "Lobsters in New York." It starts with a shot of a neon sign that reads "Chez Lobster." The camera drops down to restaurant doors and pulls back. The doors open, the camera goes inside, and we see greeting us a huge well-dressed lobster with claws and tails; around the camera come two other very well-dressed lobsters in evening clothes. The maitre d' lobster leads them to a waiter lobster in a white jacket, who leads them to a table. They order, then follow the waiter lobster to a huge tank. In the tank, little people are swimming around. We thought this was hysterical. The lobsters choose some people, pick them up squirming around, and the sequence ends. Every time we saw this sequence, we were on the floor laughing. When we showed it to an audience of secretaries—the first audience to see any of my films—they did not laugh at all at "Lobsters in New York." They stared at each other. Not one snicker. Finally we got some embarrassed sounds and yawns. We threw out the entire sequence as a result. That was one of the surprises that comedy screenwriters get from time to time.

When I did *Silent Movie*, I used a Sony videotape camera that showed us exactly what we'd just shot when we played it back. I also consulted on the set with the three writers who had written the picture with me. The same team later wrote *High Anxiety* with me, and I wanted them around to be harsh critics. Film is such a collaborative process that unless you're writing a very personal story, it's helpful to write with another person. You become a mini-audience right there and then; multiple judgments enter into what you're doing, and that's important early on.

Writers! Do not discuss embryonic ideas. Incipient ideas are your own and nobody else's. When you have coffee, don't talk to other people in the business about your ideas until they are fully written and registered with the Writers Guild. You will not get help; you'll get envy and you'll get stealing. Your ideas are private. Not only will an idea get stolen, but you will let the vapor of creation escape when you tell it. Talk to yourself through the paper; write it down. It's a good exercise, and sometimes it makes money for you.

Comedy is a rough form to sell to studios and independent producers. It's the most mercurial cinematic item. Every once in a while a good comedy comes along. *Smile*, Michael Ritchie's film, is a terrific comedy, but nobody saw it because the studio didn't support it. Studios rarely take a chance on comedy. When I made my studio deal at Twentieth Century–Fox, I didn't know *Blazing Saddles* was going to go through the roof. I just wanted security, a place to work, and an assurance that I would make at least three movies. I still respect Fox for taking a chance on me when I was relatively unknown and for giving me the opportunity to make my three movies for them. I don't need studio front money now; all I really need is a studio's distribution expertise and muscle.

When I presented the idea of *Silent Movie* to Fox, their mouths dropped open. They were very shocked, but they didn't want to turn me down because of my track record. That's "The Green Awning Syndrome." After Mike Nichols made *The Graduate*, I said, "If Mike Nichols went to Joe Levine and said, 'I want to do *The Green Awning*,' the answer would be, 'The what?' '*The Green Awning*.' 'What is it?'

'It's a movie about a green awning.' 'Does any famous star walk under the green awning?' 'No, all unknowns.' 'Are there any naked women near the green awning?' 'No, no naked women.' 'Are people talking and eating sandwiches and scrambled eggs on outdoor tables under the green awning?' 'No, it's just a green awning.' 'Panavision?' 'Just a green awning. It doesn't move.' 'How long would it be?' 'Two hours, nothing but a green awning on the screen. No talking, no dialogue, nothing.' 'Alright, we'll do it.' " That's the Green Awning Syndrome. When I said "Silent Movie" in 1976, they said, "Sounds interesting." I knew in their hearts they were saying, "Oh, God! How can we say no without hurting his feelings, without losing him?" I explained later that there might be some great movie stars in it.

As it happened, I worked with five stars in *Silent Movie:* Liza Minnelli, Paul Newman, Anne Bancroft, Jimmy Caan, and Burt Reynolds. I chose them because I knew they were pleasures to work with. Fox was more amenable to the idea of *Silent Movie* when I told them there would be stars in it. "No dialogue in 1976? That's a toughie." They were very brave to make that picture. I wasn't frightened at all until the first dailies. I said, "What the hell are we doing? I can't hear anybody! This is crazy. You've done it, Brooks, this is it. Sanity has finally caught up with you." But it all worked out, and the picture was a huge success.

I wanted to keep the writing team on *Silent Movie* together, but they were ready to go off in different directions when the picture was over. Casually at lunch one day I said, "What about a movie called *High Anxiety*?" "What's that?" "It's Hitchcock." "Oh, yeah?" We discussed it and then wrote it in sixteen weeks. We knew that we had to have the Psychoneurotic Institute for the Very, Very Nervous, and I knew that I would be Professor Richard Harpo Thorndyke. Six years I was in analysis, and I wanted to get even with them. *High Anxiety* is a tribute to Alfred Hitchcock; there were many scenes from his films in it and stylistically it's very much like him. Through that picture, I could talk about psychoanalysis and psychiatry, which I care about a lot. I can't make fun of anything I don't care about. The budget of *High Anxiety* was $4,300,000; I brought it in for $3,400,000.

In order to direct comedy, the first step is to thoroughly understand the script: how it translates into sound and action, and how the characters relate to each other. Once it is understood, you get a picture in your mind that is always altered by the specific gifts of the actors and actresses. My secret is very simple. Early on, I have three or four casual readings of the entire movie script around a big table with all the principal players. Questions come up. I will say things like, "Gee, that's a strange approach to that line; I heard it differently. But I like it." An actor will invariably say, "What do you mean? How did you hear it?"

35

I'll say, "Well, forget it." He'll say, "No, no, please." In that way, he thinks he discovered it himself.

I try to keep the atmosphere on the set buoyant and relaxed because there's a lot of tension in making a movie. The cinematographer is always worried about the lights. If he's outdoors, he's a maniac because a cloud might go by. The actors are always worried about getting the scene right, and often when they've done it perfectly, they will ask for one more take because they're not sure. First, there is the artistic pressure of capturing life itself through that one-eyed monster; second, there is the budget, in which every dollar is a second that is ticking away. The pressure is especially great when you're doing a big scene with a lot of extras.

For the writer-director, there is often a conflict when you'd like to do something lavish in a scene, but you're not sure whether it's worth the cost. For example, at the same time that I'm writing a big grand salon scene in *History of the World, Part I* for the French Revolution sequence, I think of the budget and how much it will cost to reconstruct the Palace of Versailles. How am I going to get those verisimilitudinous qualities . . . which is very difficult to say and to get. In this case, I spoke to my friend Albert Whitlock, who paints the greatest mattes in the world. He can paint on glass and take a few live characters and paint Versailles around them. If I were to try to construct Versailles, the picture would cost $100-million.

I direct a film to protect the writing. I produce a film to have total business control as well as creative control over the film's future. Little by little, in defense of the initial vision, I've learned to put on other hats. In the movie business, it's important to understand the nature of money and how to sail through those terrible waters with reefs and sharks, where art and money meet.

Generally, in production, I take as much time as each film needs. Now, I take even more time in the distribution of the picture. What does the one-sheet look like? Where is the picture opening? Is there a good sound system? Is the theatre equipped with Dolby? Newspaper advertising is archaic and very costly; I would rather spend money on a good television campaign. Three or four months after the first opening, I would turn to television advertising to sell the picture. I wouldn't make a network buy unless I could amortize that cost over 800 to 1,000 theatres. Television helped boost the grosses of *High Anxiety* tremendously.

Since I'm very proud of my image abroad as a filmmaker, I'll travel to help sell my films. It's possible to get a lot of coverage in European newspapers simply by going there and doing interviews. I won't do that in the States because I don't want the same high level of exposure here. My pictures do very well in Sweden, Germany, Italy, and France; in England, they do pretty well, but not as well as I'd like (I'm greedy). China is an exciting market. They're going to love *Silent Movie;* they'll understand that we don't want conglomerates like Engulf & Devour chewing up our art. They may make me a Vice Premier; everybody knows I love Chinese food.

My advice as to the best way to break into the business is to write. Or be a big movie star. If Paul Newman wants to direct a picture, they'll let him. Very few of us are going to become big movie stars, but we can write if we apply ourselves. To me, the vapor of human existence is best captured in film; it's a great molding of all the primary creative arts. If a writer is talented, his talent can open the door to directing. The director, in the end, is the real author of a movie.

It's very important for a creative personality—writer, director, or actor—to have good advisors. I have a lawyer who has been a friend for 25 years. I also have a good business manager-accountant who protects me. Studio accounting should be a Busby Berkeley musical. When do they stop taking money? They take overhead on overhead and interest. If a picture costs a million dollars to make, it's a third more just because of studio accounting procedures. If it's $15-million to honestly and actually produce, it will cost $22-million for the same picture to be done at a major studio. For their part, they're risking a lot of money, which is how they justify it.

As for the future of the business, I see bigger profits on fewer pictures. It's a thrilling business, but it's sad to think that we're making a third of the movies we made 20 years ago. The new home entertainment technology scares me more than anything because I want an audience to laugh at my movies. I want people to sit in a dark theatre, let the silver screen bathe them with images, and have them laugh as a group. It's thrilling to hear a lot of people laughing together. But with the direction of current technology, it seems we'll have tiny little groups at home, or sometimes even one skinny person watching a big fat Mel Brooks movie. You can't get a lot of laughs that way. I wasn't born to make one thin person laugh; I was born to make a lot of fat and skinny people sit in the dark together and laugh.

What is the toughest thing about making film? Putting in the little holes. The sprocket holes are the hardest thing to make. Everything else is easy, but all night you have to sit with that little puncher and make the holes on the side of the film. You could faint from that work. The rest is easy: the script is easy, the acting is easy, the directing is a breeze . . . but the sprockets will tear your heart out.

The Writer-Director

by **Joan Micklin Silver,** who wrote and directed *Hester Street* in 1973 after gaining experience writing and directing educational films. The picture went on to become one of the most widely praised independently financed features; it was produced and distributed by Ms. Silver's husband, Raphael D. Silver. In 1976, she directed her second feature, *Between The Lines,* which was also distributed by their independent distribution company, Midwest Films. In 1977, Joan Silver served as producer for her husband's directing debut, *On The Yard,* distributed by Midwest. In 1979, she directed *Head Over Heels,* which was distributed by United Artists, from her own adaptation of Ann Beattie's novel.

The advice I have for women in film is to toughen up and leave your sensitivities at the back door. . . .

I began my career as a screenwriter. After writing several screenplays, I finally sold one to a studio, which put on a second screenwriter with whom I shared screen credit. That screenwriter worked very closely with the director on his particular vision of the material. The result was that the finished film didn't represent my conception of the picture. I learned quickly that the only way I would have half a chance to get what I wanted up on the screen was to direct it myself.

I approached the educational film company for whom I'd already written some scenarios and asked if they would let me *direct* a short film for them as well as write it, and they did. It was a scripted educational film with actors that described the immigrant experience to high school students. The story dealt with a Polish Catholic family that comes to America in 1907; the main character was a 12-year-old boy. After directing two more short films for that company, I very much wanted to direct something longer. I remember meeting a television producer who was extremely fond of one of my short films. He was doing an hour show, 46 minutes of material (minus the commercials), and told me he could not in good conscience hire me because, although I had done 30-minute projects, I hadn't demonstrated the ability to do 46-minute ones. Well, I remember running out on Sixth Avenue, screaming, and realizing that opportunities were going to be extremely rare for me as a woman who wanted to direct.

My husband Ray was aware of my troubles, and he said if I could write a low-budget film I wanted to direct, he would try to raise the money for it. That became *Hester Street*. The technical expertise necessary to direct a feature was learned right there on the job. One advantage on that first picture was the support of a terrific crew, such as the cameraman, Ken Van Sickle, who was unusually sympathetic, patient, and willing to take me through the ropes. There were also two friends working for the same educational film company who recommended crew and provided equipment rental lists and other guidance.

In the screenwriting, *Hester Street* was deliberately designed as a low-budget film. There was a small cast, a limited number of exterior production sequences, and a minimum number of locations. The screenplay was based on a novella written in the 1890s by Abraham Cahan.

During production, I was faced with a number of handicaps that stemmed from the limited budget of $350,000 and a 35-day shooting schedule. For example, there's a scene where the husband goes to meet his wife and child on Ellis Island. We didn't have the money to re-create it as it was done in *Godfather II*, but we could create a part and make it seem like the whole. The dramatic high point of that sequence was the separation between those coming to meet people and the new arrivals waiting to be recognized. By limiting the action to an area around a wire fence separating the two groups, we captured the drama that suggested what was going on beyond camera range. Another example of this technique can be found in a television film I directed, *Bernice Bobs Her Hair*. The story begins with a dance at a country club, but we could not afford enough extras to really mount a dance. My solution was to have the action take place everywhere but the dance floor: in the ladies' dressing room, on the veranda outside, and so on. We hear the music and have a sense of the dance going on, but never actually see it; still we lose none of the drama.

When the time came to re-create the *Hester Street* exterior, we had scheduled only four and a half days. By some miracle, it didn't rain. This was the big physical production sequence; a lot of money went into dressing that large exterior location, which was actually a section of Morton Street in Greenwich Village. With the help of an excellent production designer, Stuart Wurtzel, we redressed that street, removing signs and street lights and adding pushcarts and other props. The people who lived on Morton Street were extraordinarily helpful. For example, for the last scene of the picture, the camera had to be placed on a fire escape for an overhead shot of the wife, boarder, and child walking down the street, talking. The fire escape we wanted for our camera placement was outside the apartment of a student, and we had to leave the windows open because of the cables. He sat inside with his overcoat on all that time, studying.

One thing that afflicts low-budget filmmakers is a nagging worry about money. During shooting, time literally *is* money. On *Hester Street*, the location of a particular scene hadn't been properly secured, and it took two hours for us to gain access. Even while we were shooting the scene, I was thinking of the loss of those two hours and how to make up for it.

Another problem of low-budget filming is the level of technical expertise in the crew. A less-experienced crew requires more rehearsal time, particularly if there is a complicated camera move. The problem is not only the time passing, but also the need for extra crew rehearsals that can tire the actors unnecessarily. (Stand-ins are a luxury not available on low-budget films.)

Although I'm a writer, I'm not so fiercely attached to my dialogue. Some directors who don't write feel a little more in awe of the screenplay, a greater responsibility to it. But since I'm also the writer, I don't feel any compunction about cutting or changing the script—and I always cut it. Being a writer-director is a happy combination on the set, because there are times when something unforeseen happens dramatically, and I'm able to do a new scene on the spot.

Hester Street was my first directed feature. As one goes along in directing, more confidence is developed. I remember once we did a master of an important scene that included a lot of camera moves; it was the scene in which the wife makes a marriage proposal to the boarder. I thought the master was glorious, but since it was such an important scene, I covered it with two-shots, singles, etc. Of course, when I looked at the rushes, the master was great and I used it. If I had been more experienced, I'd have known that I didn't need further coverage. I felt the master was beautiful; I was just afraid to trust that first reaction.

Hester Street enjoyed wonderful critical acclaim and had the advantage of being distributed in 1975, when movie production by the studios was lower than usual, so securing theatres wasn't terribly difficult. All of the distribution and advertising was Ray's job. He nurtured the release and publicity of the picture very carefully and handcrafted the distribution pattern into a strong commercial success. (See article by Raphael Silver, p. 293.)

After *Hester Street*, some of the studios wanted me to bring them my next project, "anything you want to do." So I brought them *Between the Lines*, and they said, "Well, not that one." But that was the picture I wanted to make. Ray said we could either continue trying to raise studio financing or take our share of the profits from *Hester Street* and make the movie ourselves. We might have spent years trying to raise all the financing, which would have further delayed the project; so, we decided to finance it internally.

Between the Lines was screenwriter Fred Barron's original project. Although I supervised his rewrites, it was basically his script. We had an extremely spirited cast, and there was a lot of improvisational work done during the 44-day schedule. The picture was budgeted at a little under $800,000 in 1976. Although there was more money than on *Hester Street*, budget limitations were still a problem. It was a New York–based union production, though the action of the story takes place in Boston. I would have preferred shooting the whole picture in Boston, but on location everybody's hotel bills and *per diems* must be added to the budget. Therefore, we shot only two weeks in Boston and built the interior of the newspaper set in a New York studio. Shooting went faster in the studio, though, since there were not a lot of distractions such as noise problems.

In 1978, I read that three young actors had purchased Ann Beattie's book *Chilly Scenes of Winter*, which I'd known and loved and actually looked into acquiring at one time. I said to Ray, "Somebody bought my book. Do you think I ought to get in touch with them?" He said, "Yes." I contracted them; they were looking for a writer-director, and we got together. We submitted the project to Twentieth Century–Fox, which put up the development money for the screenplay. Then, United Artists bought the project from Fox and it was made as a UA picture with a new title, *Head Over Heels*.

On *Head Over Heels*, the budget was $2.2-million—small by Hollywood standards in 1979—on a 42-day shooting schedule. Our actors cost more than on the prior picture, and we were paying for a big Hollywood crew, but we benefited from their expertise. For example, the first assistant cameraman did a remarkable job following focus, just by eyeballing it. There was one scene in which the main character is at a candy stand going back and forth in front of the camera. In each take the actor did it differently, yet each take was in sharp focus. The assistant cameraman was maintaining focus, and he wasn't even looking through the camera eyepiece; the camera operator does that. That level of expertise is *de rigueur* in Hollywood.

As a writer-director, my role changes through the course of a picture. At first the screenwriter dominates, since it's from the screenplay that one budgets and finds locations; the screenplay is the blueprint of the film. Sometimes I write things into the screenplay that are not strictly necessary but are helpful to readers. For example, I am usually quite deliberate about descriptions or specifying how an actor says a line. Also, sometimes a scene contains more dialogue than I intend to use when I direct, because dialogue makes the scene more comprehensible to the reader. As I write, I'm very careful to include the information that the production manager, assistant directors, cameraman, prop man, set designer, and others need to plan their jobs. Through the screenplay, I'm leading these creative people, giving them guidance for their respective planning from the printed page. Once we're rehearsing, I pare away at the script and work with the actors, who find new ideas and make suggestions. Then the screenplay begins to shift and take on the life that the actors bring to it. This may require dialogue changes.

Once I'm directing, I think about the movie in a different way. I'm always considering the editing, how one scene ends and another begins, for example. During shooting, I'm cutting in my head and thinking about getting in and out of scenes. Also, on the set, I'm always conferring with the cameraman, not only on camera placement and lighting but on cutting as well.

As an actor's director, I'd rather use a slightly less beautiful shot if it contains a better performance. In one shot in *Head Over Heels,* the main character and his stepfather walk out of a hospital, stop at a certain point, and talk. The actors kept rehearsing and missing their marks, moving to where they were not lit. I wanted to tell them, but I didn't want to break the dramatic momentum they were building. The cameraman, Bobby Byrne, offered to relight the situation so that the actors were still well lit even if they missed their marks. Because of the cameraman's understanding, the actors did not have to be interrupted.

There are always business decisions that are part of the creative process in filmmaking. For example, good actors want to try scenes over. But the director must decide whether new ideas or extra takes are worth it, and whether there is time and money to try them. The luxury that a higher budget brings to a shoot is the luxury of time. Time can be badly used; directors can become self-indulgent. But, for the most part, those directors who have more money and therefore more time have a chance to make a better film.

The editing process is fascinating, and the relationship between the editor and the director is usually a close one. I'm delighted with and eager to try editors' suggestions in the cutting room. Films have so many components, and the shifting and layering of these components during editing and sound mixing is a really interesting process.

As a woman, I've had to overcome certain obstacles in order to direct features. Happily, I'm married to somebody who wanted to help me overcome them, who thought I was being unjustly denied opportunities and that what I needed to do was simply to make a feature. When I started working, I looked to people like Barbara Loden, who made *Wanda,* and Shirley Clarke (*Jason, The Cool World*). Today, I see the industry easing up; a number of women now have projects in development at different studios, though the attitude of that television producer is still around. There is a higher consciousness generally; there are more female production executives, more women on production crews. The only place where there seems to be a lack of women is in the camera department. Not too many camerawomen have opportunities to work on feature films, particularly union films.

The advice I have for women in film is to toughen up and leave your sensitivities at the back door. There will be a lot of rejection, which goes with the territory. Writing and making short films is a good way to break into the industry; those who persist will probably prevail. That's the advice I'd probably give to a young man who wants to be a filmmaker, too.

The Low-Budget Producer

by **Russ Meyer,** who began his career as a combat camera-man in World War II, followed by a post-war career in magazine photography and industrial film. A success in quality low-budget filming, Mr. Meyer is a forerunner among independent filmmakers for handling the production, promotion, and distri-bution elements of his films, which include *Vixen, Lorna, Cherry, Harry & Raquel, Beyond the Valley of the Dolls, The Seven Minutes, Super Vixens,* and *Beneath the Valley of the Ul-tra Vixens.* He has produced 23 films, none of which has lost money.

have had considerable success in making and distributing what are tagged *exploitation movies,* ranging from the pioneering film *The Immoral Mr. Teas* in 1958, *Beyond the Valley of the Dolls* for Twentieth Century–Fox in 1970, to *Beneath the Valley of the Ultra Vixens* in 1979. My success can be attributed to a background in combat photography during World War II, magazine photojournalism, and vast experience as an industrial filmmaker. I developed my particular genre of "sex-ploitation" film realistically and inexpensively. *Lorna,* for example, a takeoff on the Italian sex pictures, was made for $37,000 in 1962. I distributed it myself, with the aid of Eve Meyer, and made a substantial profit.

The market was largely mine and Radley Metzger's for several years until the introduction of hard-core films that initially came from Denmark. As a result, I was hard pressed to compete in the area that I had been playing—the outrageous spoofing of sex. Nevertheless, my name plus my heroines continued to sell my pictures.

The budget formula I applied to my earlier films was simple. I would hit upon an idea and then impose strict limitations upon myself before even considering budget. I knew we had to have a villain, a hero, a heroine, perhaps two fallen women, and another rather "klutzy" villain, a victim of circumstance. With just a thin outline in mind, I would find a location; then and there, I would proceed to develop my story line. It is like putting the cart before the horse; yet, instead of getting hung up requiring locations in Yuma, Kansas City, and Portland, I would work with what we had at a given place, with a four- or five-man crew operating without outside interference. *Vixen*—a film that has grossed over $17-million—was shot on a six-acre mountain ranch. My modest cast and crew lived in the cabin, and I shot the footage on a creek that rambled through the property. Except for some airport scenes, which we filmed in four days, and some pickup scenes in Canada, the entire film was completed within the six-acre location. This is an example of finding a location and successfully making your story fit that location.

45

I was the producer, director, cameraman, camera operator, and gaffer on *Vixen*. I also cooked, as if we were camping out. I had an assistant cameraman who was responsible for loading the magazine, following focus, and hustling the camera around. I handled the exposures, operated the camera, and gaffed the lights. A lone grip handled the reflectors and assisted the sound man, who rounded out the crew. There were no problems with unions, simply because I was not a signatory to any union agreements. I hired good, journeymen actors and paid them at least scale. Once you sign with one union, it begets another. I am not opposed to unions, but if you have only $72,000 to make a film, there is no point in signing with even one local; what was once $72,000 can become $750,000.

On *Beneath the Valley of the Ultra Vixens*, made in 1979, I found a house with high ceilings and built all the sets within this house. On an eight-week shooting schedule, the entire film was shot there, except for three days' location on the Colorado River. That film was completed for $233,000, plus $150,000 for prints and advertising. That doesn't include the cost of the equipment, which I own, nor of my services as director-producer. It also does not include the cost of nine months of post-production. All of the financing for that picture came out of my own pocket, and I expect a strong return on that investment. For example, *Super Vixens* was made for $219,000 in 1975 and has enjoyed a box-office gross in excess of $16,000,000 one of the top one-hundred grossers of all time as reported in *Variety*.

My budgets are kept low through direct economies during production and post-production. For instance, I am always conscious of the fact that film costs so much per foot and for processing. Also, I try to schedule the cast carefully. My budgets cannot afford the luxury of an actor working the first day and not working again until the third week. He still has to be paid every day/week. In post-production, I do all the cutting, with my soundman, Dick Brummer—who also acts as my sound-effects cutter—working alongside me. Formerly, I employed film cutters to cut sequences but was never completely satisfied with anyone. In *Beyond the Valley of the Dolls*, I recut the entire picture, even though I had two picture editors. This took three months. Editing, in my opinion, is the most important creative contribution one can make to a film.

Although it is possible to effect savings in nearly every area, laboratory costs must remain a fixed item. Of the total $72,000 budget for *Vixen*, laboratory costs (including the answer print, interpositive, titles, opticals, and dubbing) came to over $42,000—more than half of the total budget. The picture was made in six weeks, and the acting budget was not over $5,000, with the crew approximately the same. The balance went for logistics—food, gasoline, and car and airplane rental. Because most of the crew members were also friends and prior associates, some were paid their overtime in partial shares of the picture. They received a flat $500 a week and, in effect, invested their overtime pay in the production. A film such as *Vixen*, made in 1968 at a cost of $72,000, would cost over $225,000 today. This is partially due to the steadily increasing production cost in three areas: film stock, processing, and post-production services or facilities. Frankly, because of rising costs, I fear for the future of independent production.

Importantly, I took the time to establish my own distribution representatives around the country—21 local distributors (called *sub-distributors*) who also represent other independently owned pictures. I try to know each and every one of them personally. When I make a picture, I know that—through the efforts of these salesmen—when it plays in a theatre, I'll eventually get a check. I don't wait six months for one, and that's an advantage that few independent filmmakers have.

My distribution network is broken down into exchange areas. For distribution, I believe you have to get people who are real shirt-sleeve salesmen, not order-takers. They go out and sell, whether it's in the breadbasket of the country or in densely populated areas. As a matter of contrast, they can go into Marietta, Ohio and come out after a weekend with a $3,700 film rental; over another weekend, the picture can play a theatre in Chicago for only a $300 net because of an exaggerated house nut (overhead) and costly newspaper advertising.

Thanks to the independents, the majors are now becoming more aware of the "sticks" and of their grossing potential. They used to send a film out to a small community and get only $100 back, with the theatre owner banking a bundle on Monday morning. Independent producer-distributors, aided by sub-distributor salesmen, have shown the majors the real value of small communities by going in with percentage deals. An independent will seldom sell his picture on flat terms, but will ask for and receive a percentage contract with shared advertising and a 50% floor. For example, when *Beneath the Valley of the Ultra Vixens* plays a major market, about $38,000 is required for advertising and publicity in order to adequately launch the picture. If the exhibitor comes up with only $3,200, I have to bear the balance of $34,800. But our first-run deal in Chicago, say, is 90/10, so we retain 90% of the theatre's revenue after the exhibitor covers his house expenses along with his profit. That 90% is split 75/25 between me and my sub-distributor; 25% is the sub's distribution fee; the majors usually charge as much as 30%.

To me, it is always reassuring to know there are 21 people out there waiting to push a can of my film. Any independent can have his can of film, but if he lacks a good distribution setup, he most likely will not be able to do much with it. Perhaps his last quarter is in the picture, and he has post-production bills and lab charges due. He may then be forced to go to a "scruffy" sub-distributor who will offer him a measly $5,000 advance (or more often nothing at all), with an unjust 50/50 split of rental, or even less—a bad deal created by an "ace" who is taking advantage of someone who worked hard to make a picture. In the 40s and 50s, many independent producers accepted this, ending up with a lot of accounting forms and perhaps little or no money, while the real take went to the exhibitor and to the distributor. The independent may have heard excuses like, "Well, we didn't do too well because it rained" or "A lot of major opposition" or "Walt Disney was here." All mumbo jumbo—everything but decent film rental. Having a completed film of good commercial value is hardly enough—an independent filmmaker requires a reliable distribution facility.

One of the satisfying things about my pictures is their longevity. *Lorna,* made in 1960, is still playing, as are many others. They unspool constantly, and for percentage, not flat deals. Further, I don't allow them to play with a major's film as a second feature. Of my pictures made after 1969, the terms are generally 50% to 60% of the box-office gross, with a 35% floor on the second week. I'm beginning to be recognized more and more in foreign territories. For years, almost all my films had been banned overseas, but now they are being shown widely.

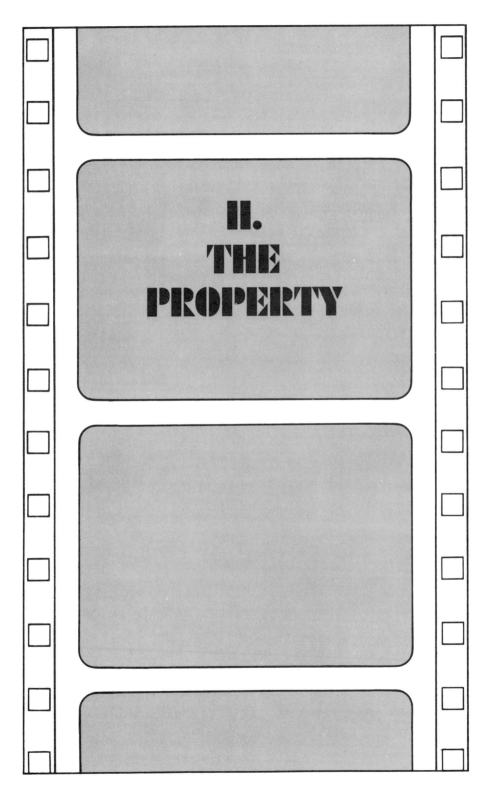

II.
THE
PROPERTY

The Screenwriter

by **William Goldman,** a distinguished novelist and also a screenwriter who has won Academy Awards for his original screenplay *Butch Cassidy and the Sundance Kid,* and for his adaptation of *All The President's Men.* He has adapted his novels *Marathon Man* and *Magic* for the screen and has written the screenplays for *Harper, The Hot Rock,* and *A Bridge Too Far.* Among his other novels are *The Temple of Gold, Soldier in the Rain, Boys and Girls Together, The Princess Bride, Tinsel,* and *Control.*

Writers have always been secondary in Hollywood. But ask *any* director and he will tell you he is only as good as his screenplay. There is no picture without a script. When you read that a producer announces a new $15-million picture from a novel he has bought, that's nonsense. No one knows what a film will cost until there is a screenplay. There is no film; there is no anything at all in this world until there is a screenplay. A screenplay is gold. And right now, with movie companies fragmented and dying and with money coming from all kinds of strange new sources, it is a golden time to write screenplays. It's a whole new and unpredictable ballgame. Now one can write anything. Since no one knows any more what will or won't go, almost anything has a chance of getting made. Now it seems possible for a writer to say what he wants through film and make a living at it.

One of the things that no one tells an eager author in college is that if he writes a novel, the chances are that he won't get it published. And if he does get it published, he might make a thousand dollars or maybe even two. It takes years and years to become an established fiction writer, and one can hardly support a family that way. No one buys hard-cover books anymore. There aren't more than a handful of writers who can actually make a living out of hard-cover fiction writing. Film writing, on the other hand, not only pays, it overpays. And it is a way for one to exercise his craft and still feed his children—both critical aspects of a writer's life.

There is more interest in screenwriters today than ever before because of money. People are beginning to wonder why screenwriters get so much money since the star makes up his part and the director has all the visual concepts. The answer is that it all starts with the word: the screenplay. The reason that the director gets all the publicity is because he's the most visible person during shooting, which is the only time the press is allowed around a picture. They are not present during pre-shooting, when the writer, producer, and director are working on the script or are assembling the cast with the help of the casting director. No one is present post-shooting, when the editors and composer are working their magic. And though the press may be on the set

52

during a day's shooting, they're not around the night before, when that day's schedule is mapped out. At this critical session, the production designer will say, "We must have the door here," and the cinematographer will say, "Well, if you move the door here, I can give you this shot coming in which will scare everybody," and the director will agree or disagree, or he won't know. He's just one of many people going down the river on this boat, hoping they get past the rapids.

Movies are a group endeavor. There is a group of six or eight technicians who are essential to the collaborative process: the writer, director, cinematographer, cutter, production designer, producer, production manager, and sometimes the composer. As for writers, we are more essential than the public gives us credit for, but no more essential than the other technicians. But our visibility is low because few of us go out on publicity junkets. Basically, we are very dull people.

Some authors start out, no doubt, knowing they want to write screenplays. I am basically a novelist, and I fell into screenplay writing rather by misinterpretation. It happened at a time when I was in the middle of a monstrous novel called *Boys and Girls Together*. I was hung up in the thing, and to try to unstick myself I wrote a ten-day book called *No Way to Treat a Lady*, which was published under another name. It is a short book with 50 or 60 chapters. Cliff Robertson got hold of it and thought it was a screen treatment rather than a novel. At the time he had a short story called *Flowers for Algernon*, which eventually became *Charly*. He asked me to do the screenplay, but when he saw the results, he promptly fired me, hired a new writer, and went on to win the Oscar for Best Actor.

The whole sequence of events did prompt me to learn more about screenwriting. I bought the only book available—called *How to Write a Screenplay*, or some such title—and discovered that screenplays are unreadable. The style is impossible and must be dispensed with. It always has those big capital letter things that say, "305 EXT. JOHN'S HOUSE. DAY." I realized that I cannot write this way. Instead, I use run-on sentences. I use the phrase *cut to* the way I use *said* in a novel—strictly for rhythm. And I am perfectly willing to let one sentence fill a whole page. Here's an example from the ending of *Butch Cassidy and the Sundance Kid:*

```
                                              CUT TO:


BUTCH

   streaking, diving again, then up, and the bullets
   landing around him aren't even close as --
```

CUT TO:

SUNDANCE

whirling and spinning, continuing to fire and --

CUT TO:

SEVERAL POLICEMEN

dropping for safety behind the wall and --

CUT TO:

BUTCH

really moving now, dodging, diving, up again and --

CUT TO:

SUNDANCE

flinging away one gun, grabbing another from his holster,
continuing to turn and fire and --

CUT TO:

TWO POLICEMEN

falling wounded to the ground and --

CUT TO:

BUTCH

letting out a notch, then launching into another dive
forward and --

CUT TO:

SUNDANCE

whirling, but you never know which way he's going to
spin and --

CUT TO:

THE HEAD POLICEMAN

cursing, forced to drop for safety behind the wall and --

CUT TO:

BUTCH

racing to the mules, and then he is there, grabbing at the near mule for ammunition and --

CUT TO:

SUNDANCE

throwing the second gun away, reaching into his holster for another, continuing to spin and fire and --

CUT TO:

BUTCH

He has the ammunition now and --

CUT TO:

ANOTHER POLICEMAN

screaming as he falls and --

CUT TO:

BUTCH

his arms loaded, tearing away from the mules and they're still not even coming close to him as they fire and the mules are behind him now as he runs and cuts and cuts again, going full out and --

CUT TO:

THE HEAD POLICEMAN

cursing incoherently at what is happening and --

CUT TO:

SUNDANCE

whirling faster than ever and --

CUT TO:

BUTCH

dodging and cutting and as a pattern of bullets rips
into his body he somersaults and lies there, pouring
blood and --

CUT TO:

SUNDANCE

running toward him and --

CUT TO:

ALL THE POLICEMEN

rising up behind the wall now, firing, and --

CUT TO:

SUNDANCE

as he falls.

In this sequence, I've used the proper form, but I never want to let the reader's eye go—it's all one sentence.

A writer needs to find his own style, something he is comfortable with. For example, I use tons of camera directions, all for rhythm. It often upsets the directors, who shoot the scenes the way they want them anyway. But it *looks* like a screenplay, and yet it is *readable*. The standard form cannot be read by man or beast.

Anyone wanting to be a screenwriter should write a screenplay—not an outline or a screen treatment or a novel that then has to be adapted. One of the reasons that Hollywood is dying is that there is such incredible waste. A studio can have a million dollars tied up in a property between the time it is purchased as a novel and the time a script is ready. And this is aside from subsequent production costs. If an author writes a screenplay, it is already there to be seen and judged. The company can say right off, "Yeah, we'll shoot it," or "No, we won't." If it sells, it pays the bills. And, besides this essential aspect, it is a legitimate and honorable kind of piece to write.

Background reading and research can be important for a writer. For one thing, sometimes he just stumbles upon something that really grabs him and that he knows he wants to do something with. It was way back in 1958 or '59 that I first came across the material about Butch Cassidy and was moved by it and knew I wanted some day to write a movie about it. I continued researching the subject off and on for ten years, finding things to read that added background and depth. There is a lot available on Cassidy but almost nothing on Longbaugh (Sundance). Larry Turman, a good friend who produced *The Graduate,* was very important in helping me to structure it.

Since I am basically a novelist, it never occurred to me to ask for advance money on "spec" based on an outline that I might sell to someone. I just wrote as if I were writing a novel. This is an unusual occurrence, at least for a Class A picture. The professional screenwriter doesn't usually just write an original screenplay and then look for a market. If he makes his living as a screenwriter, what he probably does is "buckshot" it. That is, he writes ten outlines and circulates them, hoping that one of the ten clicks and someone gives him money for it. He then writes the full screenplay with financial backing.

I wrote the first draft of *Butch Cassidy and the Sundance Kid* in 1965 and showed it to a few people, none of whom was interested. I rewrote it, really changing very little, and suddenly, for whatever reason, everyone went mad for it. Five out of the seven sources in Hollywood who could buy a screenplay were after it. It was this unexpected competition—not my particular skill with the rewrite—that sent the price so high.

Authors who write in various other forms of fiction and nonfiction besides screenplays often have two agents, one on each coast. The one on the west coast handles the film material, while the New York agent handles all of the other manuscripts. It was my Hollywood agent, Evarts Ziegler, who handled all the negotiations for *Butch Cassidy.* My only contact with the deal was that he called me in New York every day to keep me posted on the bidding and warned me to stand by the phone to get his call when the bidding was over. It was up to me to give the final okay. The screenplay was finally bought by Fox.

No doubt many authors write a film imagining a certain actor in a specific role. Right from the beginning I had Paul Newman in mind. Actually, as I wrote the picture originally, I saw Paul Newman and Jack Lemmon in the main roles. Jack Lemmon had just done a movie called *Cowboy,* and I thought he would do a fine Butch Cassidy. Paul Newman had done a movie about Billy the Kid, and I saw him as the Sundance Kid. As the years went on, Lemmon disappeared from my mind, but Newman agreed that he would play the Sundance Kid. Then, when George Hill (who was eventually signed as director) read the script, he mistakenly assumed that Newman was going to play Butch. When that happened, Newman, who wasn't really eager to play Sundance, was delighted to change roles. Then the long search began for the actor who would play the Sundance Kid. Every star in Hollywood was up for it. There were arguments about certain choices. Under such circumstances an author doesn't have very much power. Long ago, Hollywood decided that the way to keep people quiet is to overpay them. An author paid all that money should go home and count it and be content. I was in there arguing, and so were others who had more influence, notably Newman and Hill. We finally won the battle, and Robert Redford, who in those days was not nearly so well-known as some of the other candidates, got the part.

I was really fortunate. Overall, I happen to be delighted with *Butch Cassidy*. In many ways it is better than what I wrote; in many ways it isn't; and in many ways it's different. My script was much darker and, I think, would not have been so successful. And most of the credit for its coming off so well I give to George Roy Hill, the director.

Butch Cassidy is an example of an original screenplay. I've also adapted my own novels *(Marathon Man, Magic)* and books written by others *(All The President's Men, A Bridge Too Far)*. The hardest thing to write is an original because it's creative; the easiest thing is an adaptation of somebody else's. On a straight adaptation, I don't have to deal with the anguish of the original writer. But when I'm adapting my own work, I think, "That was so hard to write, I'd like to keep it." I'm not as ruthless as I should be. The Faulkner phrase "You must kill all your darlings" is basically true.

For example, one scene in *Marathon Man* that I cared about was the run. The hero runs along and fantasizes that legendary runners come alongside him and get him out of a scrape. In the first draft screenplay, I wrote it as a fantasy, as in the book. John Schlesinger, the director, said, "I can't shoot this; it's a literary conceit and it won't play." When a director says, "I don't know how to make that play," it's best to change it, rather than risking that his uncertainty will show through in the film.

The assignment on *A Bridge Too Far* was unique because it was financed not by a studio, but by one man, Joseph E. Levine. In order for the story to be told properly and for it to be faithful to Cornelius Ryan's book, one had to have a lot of stars. The use of stars would help the audience organize the several parallel stories to be told. This affected the writing of the screenplay since, in a scene of two characters talking, if the scene legitimately belonged to character A but character B was cast with a star, I would flip the scene so that it would favor character B.

Films that become successful tend to reinforce our expectations; films that are not as successful, but are equally competent, tell audiences things they don't want to know. For example, everyone in this country thinks of *A Bridge Too Far* as being a commercial failure.

In fact, it was a giant success in Japan and Great Britain and did very well all over the world, except for the United States. It told Americans something they didn't want to know: battles and wars can be lost. All over the world people have lost wars and know that kind of suffering and agony firsthand; we don't.

On *All The President's Men*, if there was a contribution in the screenplay that was valid, it was deciding to end the film in the middle of the book, on a less-than-triumphant note for Woodward and Bernstein. Instead of having them get saved by the cavalry at the end, the idea was to have the audience apply what they knew and fill in the ultimate victory. No one knew at the time that *President's Men* would become a very successful film. People were saying, "Haven't we had enough of Watergate?" Nobody knows what's going to work. Hollywood is based on a search for past magic. "Redford and Newman worked twice *(Butch Cassidy* and *The Sting); if we could only get Redford and Newman in a picture, we'd all be rich." The reality is that nobody knows. One can guess that a movie about some robots in the future will work, and that George Lucas will handle it well, but Universal didn't think so. They passed on *Star Wars* when they had *American Graffiti.*

How close is a writer allowed to the actual production? To a degree the answer lies in how big a writer he is. The bigger the name, the more likely he is to have a say about the details of production. Generally, the answer is that the writer gets as close to the production as his director allows. The production is really the director's baby. If he has faith in the author's judgment, the director will be more willing to tolerate his presence during filming. If the director doesn't want him, there is nothing the writer can do about it.

An author is blessed if he has a director who is interested in working closely with him as he prepares for production. The time when the author is most essential is in the story conferences with the director prior to filming. It is during these very crucial days that he tells the director over and over again exactly what he meant. And sometimes an author really hasn't written what he meant. Talking it all out in minute detail with the director can clarify the content and insure the director's chance of a clean and accurate interpretation. It is during these conferences that scenes are cut, added, or otherwise modified. In *Butch Cassidy,* for example, the screenplay was changed, but never basically. Certain scenes were cut; the musical numbers were added, but the thing that makes the movie work—the basic relationship established between the two men—was left essentially unchanged.

In one specific instance, I had written an atrocious scene, the opening scene of Robert Redford and the card game. Everyone said, "Get rid of it! It stinks!" And I kept saying, "I know it stinks, but it's the best I can do." And all the time that I was going through that pressure, George Hill kept saying, "You're not going to change it!" George knew how to make it play. He took the scene and put it in sepia, which gave it an old look. And he had what is probably the longest close-up in modern film history on Bob Redford. It's about 90 seconds of solid Redford, and the scene really plays. He gets a tremendous tension out of it. This is a striking example of how a good director can take even a rotten scene and make it work.

I went out to Hollywood in June of 1968. George Hill was already there. For about 90 days, he and I met every day, spending most of each day talking about every aspect of the script and coming up with ideas for it. These meetings lasted until mid-September and included a two-week rehearsal period prior to actual filming. Until the filming began, I was involved in many decisions that were made, but the final work necessarily was that of the director. I returned in the middle of production for one week of shooting at the studio between location work in Utah and Colorado and in Mexico. On this visit, I saw four or five hours of rushes that George had shot in Utah and Colorado and gave him my reactions. That basically was my contact with the production of the film.

My own feeling is that I don't want to be around on a film I have written. There are times when an author can be helpful. In *Butch Cassidy,* for example, there were a couple of scenes misdone. Had I been around, I could have said, "Oh, no, no, no, no—I meant this." You see, they were actually miswritten, and I didn't realize it until I saw them on film. They are not, incidentally, in the final film. Had I been around, I could have said, "I miswrote that. Don't play what I wrote; play it this way."

Generally, however, I don't like to be around for two reasons. First of all, because I am the screenwriter, nobody really wants me around. If a line is misspoken with the proper emotion or spoken properly without the proper emotion, there can be problems. The writer thinks the actors are ruining his lines and the actors resent the author's presence. And similar tensions can arise between director and author over interpretation. Second, although there is nothing more exciting than your first day on a movie-star-laden set seeing all your dreams come true, by the second day you are bored with it. By the third day, everything is so technical that you are ready to scream, "Let me out of here!" The idea of standing around for 72 days of shooting, bothering people, and saying such insignificant things as, "The line is 'There's the fireplace,' not 'Where's the fireplace,'" is madness. Since the author just doesn't know when he might be really helpful, he might as well stay away and avoid the agony for himself and everyone else.

What movies get made reflect the executive mentality; what movies are successful reflect the audience. I have no idea what they will like; I try to write a screenplay that I will like, and I pray. If I want to continue working in pictures, it's essential first that my screenplay gets made and second that it gets made properly. After all, the business pays attention only to writers who write movies that are commercially viable. But, beyond it all, nobody really knows which films will be big. There are no sure-fire commercial ideas anymore. And there are no unbreakable rules. Classically, westerns have villains. *Butch Cassidy*, however, the most successful western ever made, has no tangible villain, no confrontation in the usual sense. Perhaps the success of the movie with kids is in the concept of the "super posse," a force that follows them and makes them do terrible things that they cannot control.

I love movies and I enjoy writing screenplays enormously. In addition, it's how I support my family. If it were the only kind of writing I did, however, I think I would find it desperately frustrating. When I write a novel, I take it to my editor. He says, "This stinks and I want you to change it." If I agree with him, I say, "Okay," and I change it. If I don't agree with him, I can say, "Goodbye." It is my baby and I can fight to the death. I can either not get it published at all or get it published as I want elsewhere. At least it is *my* fight to make if I choose. In films, an author doesn't have that right. In films, he must assume the director or producer will be ultimately responsible for what the finished product is and whether it works or not. And, of course, there is no guarantee that he will get a director or producer who will listen to him.

One thing that really pleases me about movies today is that advertising and publicity and critical reviews don't mean anything any more. *Butch Cassidy* opened in New York to pretty bad notices but tremendous business. If *Bonnie and Clyde* had been a play, it would have closed on Saturday because before it opened it got terrible notices from *The New York Times* critic who had seen it at a film festival. Happily, the reviews are totally unimportant on a film. No one except maybe the critic's mother is going to go to a film or stay away from a film because the critic says it's good or bad. Movie audiences will not be lectured to. It is a golden time.

The Literary Agent

by **Lee G. Rosenberg,** a partner in Adams, Ray & Rosenberg, Inc., a talent agency in Los Angeles. Educated at the Choate School and Harvard (B.A. 1956), Mr. Rosenberg held various production positions in films and television before cofounding the agency in 1963. Adams, Ray & Rosenberg currently represents writers, directors, and producers in both the motion picture and television industries and also engages in packaging for television.

Agencies serving literary clients can be divided into two categories, compound and independent. The compound agencies, such as William Morris and International Creative Management, represent a vast array of talent, including writers, directors, producers, actors, actresses, Olympic stars, and former Presidents, for the disposition of rights as well as services. The independent, smaller agency will more often represent a more homogeneous list of clients. Larger agencies are compartmentalized, and crossover between departments becomes a complicated and time-consuming administrative task.

Compound agencies represent their people well but are less likely to be interested in or actively solicit representation of "unknowns." The independent agent's concentration on a specific genre of client inevitably produces better work and more time available for the client, as opposed to the agent who must divide himself between the varying needs and demands of a variegated list of clients. The independent is in a far better position to offer this concentrated activity and to serve the needs of the newcomer as well as the established client. It's also characteristic of the independent agency that it must solicit new and untried talent, since any thoughtful agent must be aware that this is the fuel of a successful and ongoing agency. Accordingly, new talent becomes the lifeblood of the agency.

In our case, the early concentration of the agency was on writers in television. That emphasis changed as those clients became more established, so that there is now an equal emphasis on television and motion pictures. Some writer clients have become producers and directors in features as well as television, and the agency has therefore expanded its purview to include these creative areas as well. We have enlarged our staff in order to serve all of these clients. We operate as a collective, in contrast to many other agencies that assign clients to individual agents. The only division of responsibility internally is made with respect to the marketplace, where each agent is assigned an area of concentration that might include studios, independent producers, production companies, and networks. Each agent is accessible to all of the clients, and conversely all of the agents represent all of the clients without any specific client assignments. However, if a client enjoys an easier rapport with a particular agent, he can emphasize his relationship with that agent.

Each of our agents gathers information from that segment of the marketplace for which he or she is responsible, information that is pooled in two weekly staff meetings and other informal sessions. An agent might be responsible for coverage of MGM/UA, Disney, NBC, a handful of independent producers and buyers, and a group of publishers in New York. Coverage is maintained by personal visits with these buyers and by daily contact by phone, as well as through correspondence and periodic visits to New York, so that each agent is constantly gathering information and selling at the same time.

Our office includes six agents serving a client list that ranges between 200 and 250 clients. A large number of these clients are usually employed, rendering them unavailable for long periods of time; on any day, a small number of clients are available and are actively soliciting employment. Many clients don't look for assignments; rather, they perform their services in the speculative writing of books (which takes months if not years) or original screenplays.

Novelists are generally handled by agencies in New York. With the west coast's emphasis upon film, agencies here become outlets to New York agencies for the published works of their authors. Occasionally we work with a writer from the genesis of a novel through its screen version. In such an instance, we might assign responsibility for publication of the novel manuscript to an agency in New York, making certain commission arrangements to accommodate the circumstances. Often, we handle publication rights without a New York co-agent.

Playwrights, too, come within the scope of the agency. We might, for example, represent them in the licensing of their plays here in Los Angeles through such local theatres as The Mark Taper Forum. In fact, this is an area in which we hope to expand activity in the near future. Playwrights based primarily in New York who wish to translate their works to film, as well as European writers who wish to work in American films, are also potential clients. At the moment, this organization does not handle performing talent. We feel the time and energy required for handling performers are such that we would not be able to maintain a desired level of effectiveness on behalf of the clients we now handle.

To begin a study of the agent–client symbiosis, let us examine a writer's initial problem: finding and engaging an agent.

Securing an agent is a critical and often difficult accomplishment for the unknown writer. First, just saying that one is a writer doesn't make it so. Second, once one has written something, the product must be read by others who might be impressed with its potential. Reading takes time. Once a writer has something to offer—novel, play-script, screenplay—he can, through a number of devices, attempt to interest an agent. Consider the direct phone call, for example. The impression of personality and intellect the writer might make on an agent willing to take the call is possibly more important than coming to the office and saying, "Here's my script." Getting the agent to take the call may depend upon whether the agent has received a prior contact about the writer from someone he trusts, or whether he has received a letter from the writer that sounds reasonable, intelligent, and perhaps reflects the writer's ability to communicate and the originality of his point of view. Basically, the inventive applicant is likely to attract the interest of even a busy agent, who might then agree to listen to him.

However the writer manages it, after the initial connection, he then must put a manuscript on the agent's desk. Sitting and conversing accomplishes little; the agent must read the script. And this necessity points out the greatest problem of all: finding time for reading. With all the other demands upon his time, an agent is fortunate to find an hour a day to devote to reading. Following the submission of a manuscript, the writer must be patient.

If the agent is impressed with the manuscript, he calls the writer and tells him he likes the work—perhaps with a few reservations—and arranges a meeting to talk things over. Considering this meeting a first date that may lead to marriage, the agent inevitably projects his own personal chemistry while at the same time seeking to get acquainted with the author as a person. As in a marriage, a couple never knows whether they have made the right move until they have lived together for a few years. At this first encounter, the parties begin to assess each other. The agent will react to the material as a sample of the author's work and an index of his ability to handle the visual medium: how he dramatizes and how he writes dialogue and action. The agent will also include his judgment on the salability of the script.

This initial procedure is nearly the same in all agencies, whatever their size. There is, however, one significant way in which an agency such as ours modifies the process. The agent explains to the writer that the script is going to be recommended for reading by other agents in the firm. A larger agency usually doesn't have time for this extra consideration. In an enterprise involving so subjective a judgment on the part of the reader, there is likely to be added insurance of success if the agents comprising the firm—and ultimately responsible for shouldering the work of representation—are all enthusiastic about the property. If just one of the group has a positive reaction, it would be inappropriate to sign the writer to an agreement. For the alliance to succeed, there must be mutual trust and genuine enthusiasm between agency and client, and the broader the exposure between the two the more confidently they can work together.

In contrast to the west coast film-oriented agencies, the publication agents in New York rarely have a contract with a client. A novelist who takes three years to write a novel is not likely to shift loyalties very often. In the faster-paced world of film and television, however, the agent must have constant fluid contact with the market and with the client. In this world, general and specific problems and the loneliness of the writer are daily rather than annual or even triennial issues. It is not good business sense to ignore these needs.

The initial contract between agency and author is generally a document that provides an "out" for the writer if he is not employed for a certain period of time. He can say, "I'm canceling the contract," and, unless he has earned a certain fixed sum within the stipulated time, he is free to separate himself from the agency. Again, a client might come in and say, "Look, I'm not happy with you. You're not functioning well. I'm not getting anywhere." There might be adequate reason for the agency to allow him to break the contract, even though legally he has no right to leave. The agency must be realistic. If forced to stay under what he considers intolerable conditions, a client may give the firm the worst kind of public relations.

There may be, however, poor conditions in the relationship that can be improved. Perhaps there has been such insufficient or inadequate communication between the writer and his agent that the writer feels his interests are being neglected. His complaint may clarify the situation and initiate satisfactory correction. In this case, the contract binds agent and client together for a cooling-off period. It also allows the agency to legally hold the client while the parties have an opportunity to reassess their position and attitudes. If the parties still can't resolve their differences, the agency may then allow the writer to go with another agency under an agreement to split commission with the other agency. Or, if real hostilities prevail, the agency may release the client completely.

The Writers Guild limits the duration of an agency contract to two years. An agency may, of course, contract for a shorter period, such as one year, if it chooses. However, since the initial investment in attempting to introduce and sell new talent is substantial, one year is generally not long enough for agents to realize any material return for their efforts. By building on what an agent has done that first year, a client who moves on to another agent might subsequently find work in a deal for which groundwork had been laid by the first agent. A two-year bond, therefore, is usually desirable for both parties.

Once the contract has been signed, the agent begins the process of submitting material to potentially interested parties. He will decide who among his list of studios, producers, story editors, directors, actors, distributors, and the like might be interested in this client and/or specific property. In some instances, just two or three people may seem particularly good prospects. For example, a property might appear to be a "director's script" particularly suited to the talents of directors X, Y, and Z. The agent submits the script to these three, perhaps simultaneously to save time and to stir up a little competition for the property. Another property might be submitted to as many as 20 separate buyers within as short a time as 48 hours. The aim, of course, is to stimulate maximum response. An agent with more than one positive response to a property is obviously an agent in clover.

While there may be occasions when a very limited submission is made, in today's highly horizontal, fragmented market, institutions such as studios and distributors rarely buy just a manuscript. An agent must be inventive in putting together a salable package. He may need to coordinate several interests, combining writer with director and/or star. The ultimate source of money is usually the studio or the independent production company. Individuals with sufficient funds to make such a deal on their own are rarities. No matter how many parties are involved, the agent remains with the negotiations through the general licensing and establishing of rights. Thereafter, the property is in the hands of the party who buys it.

As the agent moves in to close the deal, he tries to nail down as many specific details as possible. If he is dealing with people he knows, people who are resourceful and knowledgeable and who have studio bureaucracies backing them, he is usually safe in making verbal commitments. With anyone who isn't with a studio, however, he will be wise, before proceeding, to insist that a memorandum agreement be drawn up and, in extreme cases, that funds be put in escrow. Proving damages in a renege on a verbal agreement is excessively difficult and costly. Our agency frequently executes a seven-page *deal letter* outlining substantive points including price, general rights acquired, and certain exotic stipulations that may be implicit in a given case. Details are set down so a lawyer can actually draft a contract from our letter. Once the deal letter has been initialed by the parties concerned, for our own agency records we put it into a *deal memo* including the client's name, commission, the buyer's corporate designation, the starting date of services, and many other items distilled from the deal letter. After the deal has been made, there is an administrative period while contracts are drawn up and payments are made. The agent can help to keep lines of communication open between writer and producer and to work out problems that might arise from misunderstandings or differences of opinion. It is the agent's obligation to continue to serve the best interests of the client. This is not to suggest that most producers are exploiters. Most deals go very smoothly in a happy alliance. But it is the agent's primary job to help each client develop to the fullest extent of his talents.

When writers were called upon to write material years ago, on occasion they weren't paid if the producer didn't like the result. Further, there was no machinery to guarantee the writer credit on the screen for what he had written. The Guild has now established that no writer may speculate his writing for an employer or potential employer; he must be paid for what he writes. In addition, every writer must receive credit for what he has written. Occasionally, because it's a highly subjective business, one writer's work may be combined with that of another in the course of a rewrite or an adaptation of a story. In such a case the Writers Guild, not the studio or the employer, is the final arbiter as to who receives credit.

If arbitration seems necessary, the Guild will submit proposed credits to selected member writers who will read the material and make recommendations that will determine who gets what credit. In this arbitration procedure, the writer is given an opportunity to examine the list of potential arbitrators and eliminate a reasonable number of those he thinks might have some bias.

It might be helpful at this point to explain the issue of "separation of rights" as it affects the writer client. The Writers Guild, through negotiation with management, has established among other minimums that certain rights are the property of the writer or writers who receive story credit in motion pictures and television. The precise definition of these rights and the conditions that surround them are available in the Writers Guild Basic Agreement.* The rights separated out for such a writer include publishing, dramatic stage, and merchandising.

There are limitations on the writer's use of these separated rights, such as the "holdback" theory. A writer might have reserved dramatic stage rights for himself, then exercised them so a play could run coincident with the release of a motion picture on which the purchaser of the writer's services (for the screen material or story) may have spent millions of dollars. Since this would cause a substantial conflict, a *holdback* is enforced that allows for time to elapse between screen and stage presentations. Finally, regarding separated rights,

---

* Editor's Note: Inquiries as to the content of the current Writers Guild of America Theatrical and Television Basic Agreement should be addressed to the Writers Guild of America West, 8955 Beverly Boulevard, Los Angeles, CA 90048 (phone number 213-550-1000) or Writers Guild of America East, 555 West 57 Street, New York, NY 10019 (phone number 212-245-6180).

there are certain minimum sums of money that can be paid to enable the employer or purchaser of the screen rights (as long as such rights are covered by the WGA Agreement) to acquire the separated rights on certain preestablished conditions.

Publishing rights carry with them further complications, since publishing tie-ins for motion pictures and television have become a very valuable source of income not only to writers, but also to producers. (See article by Roberta Kent, p. 86.) Hard-cover publication rights are generally reserved for the author, but he may not use them for a substantial holdback period. It's often unlikely that a writer would be able to use them at all in a published tie-in to the theatrical or television film since in order to publish a hard-cover book and aim it at a date current with the release of the film, he'd need a minimum of nine months lead time. Another problem is the securing of rights to use the film title and "artwork" (including stills, title logo, etc.) that are critical to a publisher's interest in the book tie-in. Since the studio or financier-distributor controls these elements, the writer must deal with the studio or financier to acquire them. There is a routine set forth in the Guild agreement that provides certain minimums for these elements, but we usually negotiate higher terms for those rights.

The paperback or novelization rights are determined first on the basis of what the Guild calls *designated writer* procedures. If more than one writer shares story credit, the Guild designates the writer or writers entitled to the advantages of paperback publication rights. The designated writer or writers then must deal on a specified basis with the studio to acquire the artwork elements needed to publish the book.

In 1973, the enormous success of David Seltzer's novelization of his screenplay *The Omen* caused the industry to recognize that paperback publication was a highly lucrative ancillary right. Other books, such as *Love Story* and *The Godfather*, helped prove there is a synergy between books and movies. Today, agents and publishers are very much aware of the value of these tie-ins. When making development arrangements for a television mini-series, a two-hour television movie, or a theatrical feature, the publishing rights are treated as a valuable and negotiable point. Naturally, the agent wants to make a deal as early as possible to have the necessary lead time to get the book published.

The studio may invest thousands of dollars in the development of a screenplay and millions in the production of a film. Since they're contributing heavily to the existence and desirability of the literary property from a publication standpoint, they insist upon a sizable chunk of publication revenue. The agent resolves this in many instances by giving the studio 20% of net publication revenue after agency commissions have been deducted. In a typical transaction, our client recently retained 80% of net publication revenue and the studio retained 20%. We were fortunate that the studio allowed our commission off the top rather than simply off the client's share. (Occasionally, commissions can go as high as 25% in foreign publication deals, since the base agent has to share with the agent abroad; to motivate that overseas agent, 5%—half of our usual commission—is not enough. Sometimes, the overseas agent receives as much as 12½% while our agency receives a like amount, for a total of 25% worth of commissions.)

Publication revenue includes advances as well as royalties earned after recoupment of advances. An advance is simply a royalty paid in advance. If a client has received a $300,000 advance for writing a book, the studio gets 20% and the client 80%; the payments generally will be $100,000 upon signing the contract, $100,000 when the manuscript is delivered, and $100,000 when the film is released. From the $300,000, the agent takes his 10% commission, and the balance is divided between the author and the studio in the 80/20 relationship. If the book earns the advance, and there are subsequent additional royalties paid, the treatment is the same: agency commission off the top, then an 80/20 split to the writer and the studio. A studio might justifiably insist on a larger share of the book if the studio contributes towards advertising the book, thereby making not only their share more valuable, but our share as well, since the book would enjoy more exposure.

Recently a book was published based on an original screenplay written by a client who had also been hired to write the book. However, he did not succeed in the prose form. Another writer was hired by the publisher for a flat cash payment. The studio put up hundreds of thousands of dollars towards exploitation and advertising of the book, matched almost dollar for dollar by the publisher. This created a huge advertising and publicity campaign and made the book an instant best seller; unfortunately, the film's release was delayed and as a result some of the initial advertising impact was lost.

For an independently financed picture, an agent faces basically the same issues. The writer wants to get a book published, and the producer wants as much of the action as possible. There are all kinds of compromises. However, when a picture deal is made very quickly, and timing makes book publication impractical, we ignore the issue entirely.

For the writer who has not yet determined whether he or she wishes to write exclusively for motion pictures or for publication, it's useful to be aware of the economics of both industries and some of the attendant selling problems. In the case of a first novelist, less money is available for a book than for a screenplay written for hire and based upon an original idea. If the novel is enormously successful, the economics even out. Also, writing a book produces certain collateral economic problems that relate to the producer–buyer's attitude towards the risk involved in acquiring the book rights and then investing even more risk capital in the development of a screenplay. When a development deal is made exclusively for a screenplay, there is only one investment and one assessable risk. As an example, if a book seems desirable for film purposes, it must either be optioned or acquired outright, depending on conditions imposed by the author. The producer knows that in addition to the money spent for the option or outright purchase, he still has to arrange a substantial additional investment for development of the screenplay The same story might have been developed for somewhat less money as a screenplay. Obviously, it's not unwise to write a book; it simply adds a dimension of time and risk to the entire process, which might diminish marketability of the property.

Establishing a Literary Agency

by **Lew Weitzman,** who founded Lew Weitzman and Associates, Inc., an agency specializing in literary clients, in 1973, after working as a literary agent at the William Morris Agency in Beverly Hills for several years. Before joining William Morris, he had served as a literary agent with MCA Artists, Ltd., and as an associate agent with other firms.

> *In the agency business, what one is selling is ideas, so there's no need for a warehouse. ... What I needed during the first few months of existence was a table and a phone. ...*

In the fall of 1972, as a literary agent at William Morris, I became concerned that specific clients in whom I had great faith were not being given the best opportunities to have themselves and their product presented to the marketplace. I felt frustrated over the fact that clients whom I personally worked with and was responsible for were not being regarded with special care by the other agents, who had their own preferred-client lists. I began thinking that if I could work in a smaller operation, I'd have a greater opportunity to promote the specific talents of those people I felt close to.

From the writer client's point of view, if he's on a list with many other writers, his particular talents may go a little less noticed when compared with those people who are the biggest money earners for an agency. If a writer can earn hundreds of thousands of dollars and thereby higher commissions, he will be presented to the marketplace in a stronger position than someone who perhaps could do the job as well, but who at this career point cannot guarantee such sums. The result has been a branching out from the larger agencies of a number of experienced agents who have joined to form their own agencies for the express purpose of being more responsive to the needs of their clients. This trend has been characterized by the desire on the part of these agents to establish their own identities and to be able to personally and independently guide the careers of those clients who the agents believe are entitled to greater opportunities.

I wanted to know if I could be more effective on my own in representing those people I felt strongly about, so in January, 1973, I left the Morris office and asked thirteen clients to join me. In the agency business, what one is selling is ideas, so there's no need for a warehouse to store cartons of merchandise. What I needed during the first months of existence was a table and a phone. The filing cabinets were contained in my briefcase and the client list was on one side of a small piece of paper.

All theatrical agencies in Los Angeles are licensed by the Labor Commission of the State of California. In addition, literary agents are franchised by the Writers Guild of America, and we adhere to the provisions outlined by the Guild in its franchise agreement. (The Labor Commissioner has now designated all agencies, literary and otherwise, as talent agencies.)

Our agency represents writers in theatrical motion pictures and television, with an emphasis on television, where the material is written for an American audience, has a budgetary restriction, and usually should be based on a contemporary theme. A writer who is not widely known in TV sometimes finds it more difficult to get a project launched because there is a reluctance on the part of certain network executives to allow writers to cross over from one-hour episodes into a longer form. There is less crossover resistance from theatrical feature buyers. In motion pictures, there is a greater variety of salaries, depending upon the writer's stature in the industry, and on whether the work is a treatment with options for a screenplay or a full screenplay ready to be purchased. For two-hour television movies, fees are much more structured. The average currently is between $25,000 and $30,000, with maximums around double that.

When an agent looks at material, he's looking for a number of assets, some of them quite intangible. He considers professionalism, of course. Many aspiring writers unwisely submit manuscripts in all shapes and forms, probably not really knowing what a screenplay is and how the mechanics of it are set up. An agent is much more likely to consider a script if it is in proper form. Beyond this criterion, he looks for the kind of content that he thinks makes sense commercially in the marketplace. Can it be cast? Can it be made for a reasonable cost? Is it entertaining?

At best, the agency business depends on personal judgment and educated guesses. There is no guarantee that anything that comes across a desk will appeal to any buyer at a particular time. Appeal is a matter of mood—specific mood of the individual evaluator and general mood of the times—a matter of attitude and feeling about what producers or other buyers are looking for. It does appear at present, for example, that there is a great deal more interest in the original screenplay than there used to be.

Once an author client has a salable manuscript to show, the agent goes through his list of potential buyers and lets them know what he has and how he feels about it. This contact can be by a phone call, by personal visit, or, in cases where speed is essential, can mean sending material immediately to the prospective buyer by messenger, with a letter. The agent must act with speed if there are other projects of a similar nature in the marketplace. Naturally, the "firstest with the mostest" is the one who sells.

While some agencies use a "scattergun" technique when submitting a manuscript, making it generally available to all of their buyer contacts, our agency tends to be selective in our submissions in an effort to reach the one or two buyers we believe would have the best chance of getting the project launched. To be successful in these judgments, an agent must know the market extremely well.

Although the order of events varies to suit the agent or a given need of the day, a typical day in the life of an agent can be fairly easily predicted. An agent is likely to spend the morning in his office either making calls or attending meetings. He might have lunch with an author client or a prospective buyer to talk about material. The afternoon he may spend visiting the studios and talking to producers and to clients who are on assignments, learning how things are proceeding and what new needs may have developed. By late afternoon, he will return to the office to complete calls that came in regarding projects and services for various clients. There is no set situation, of course; rather, each agent develops the kind of operation with which he feels most comfortable.

The purpose of making regular daily rounds is to be in close contact with buyers in order to keep them informed about new material and to learn firsthand what their specific needs are. Beyond the strictly business aspect of it, however, is the importance of a good personal rapport with buyers. An agent is, after all, a sales representative. If a producer trusts him personally, he will have more faith in the agent's opinions and the product he has to sell.

In the past, an author would normally leave the matter of negotiations in the hands of his agent alone. Today's business sophistication calls for the agent to coordinate strategy with the writer's support team: his accountant/business manager for purposes of tax and financial planning and his lawyer for immediate and long-term legal results of the deal.

When the agent receives a positive response on a script, he gets in touch with the author and provides him with background on the buyer's position in the industry: what he has made, what he is working on currently, and what sort of arrangement he may have with a financing entity. Then they discuss price.

One way the agent and author can control who might buy the material is through the price they place on it. If an important, high-priced writer is approached by someone who has little reputation in the industry, the agent must take extra measures to insure that this new buyer is not only financially solvent, but also that he has the background and contacts necessary to insure that the picture has a good chance of being produced. In the final analysis, however, authors and their agents are as much interested in getting the material off the ground as they are in making high-priced, high-class deals. The aim, after all, is to get the picture made.

Whatever the circumstances, all negotiations are delicate and need careful handling. If a writer in the marketplace has received a certain price for past performance, this can help shape a deal. On the other hand, if the writer is not established, there may be a good deal more jockeying about price. The agent tries to establish a price level that is compatible with the market and that protects his client's interests. With the approval of the client, he then approaches the buyer with the terms outlined. When the agent puts a price on the material, the buyer may claim that the price is out of line and counter with a lower offer. Then the agent returns to his client, perhaps suggesting, "He is saying this; I think we can get that." It's a matter of give and take, of what the agent thinks the market will bear, how eagerly the producer wants the material, and how keenly the client thinks he has to have the deal. "Get all you can, but don't blow the deal," is often the client's instruction. There's nothing like a good haggle!

Deals are blown, and sometimes rightly, because client and agent refuse an offer they feel is too low for a good property. If there is a timelessness about the piece and money is tight, it might not be wise to sell just for the sake of the deal. As the market improves, the agent should be able to get a fairer price. Conversely, there are certain screenplays that are quite contemporary. An agent will try to move them as soon as possible, because their worth will drop or even disappear within a short period of time.

Today, agents negotiate not only for cash compensation for the writer and material, but in addition for "a piece of the action," or a percentage of the profits of the venture. If he can't get a percentage, the agent might attempt to have certain other monies taken out of first profits of a picture as a deferment that would be shared by the producer, the writer, and anyone else who is written into the deal. Often, a writer's deal will call for cash to be paid up front and in addition certain monies to be paid once the producer launches the project. That is, further monies would perhaps be paid at the start of principal photography, with more monies paid at the close of photography or upon the first general release of the picture, plus possible participation in the profits. Writers are not likely, however, to share in gross receipts. Nevertheless, anticipating the revenue impact that the growing home entertainment market will have on theatrical film, agencies are now including a proviso in contracts that entitles the writer to share in the proceeds from future markets.

It would be remiss not to discuss another very important characteristic of the business today. A real sign of the times is the tendency for the literary agent to be concerned with more than just selling the writer's work. Often he finds himself attempting to include the manuscript into a "package deal." In the motion picture vernacular, a *pack-*

age is a salable coalition of two or more elements of a potential motion picture. There can, of course, be disadvantages to packaging. Any time a literary agent suggests a deal between his writer and a director, star, producer, or combination thereof, he may place the material in a slower market. No matter how hard he tries to get the right combination, part of the package may not be held in high regard at one studio or another. For example, an agent will try to avoid jeopardizing a writer's project by involving a director who has a lesser reputation. Nor would it be practical to package a project that has been seen all over town unless a new element (star, director, partial financier, etc.) would move the project forward where it had previously been rejected.

There is another side to the question of the value of packaging. The chief source of money for production is still the studio, although there are new funding sources providing venture capital for movies. The motion picture studios have changed from all-out production units into financing and distributing bodies—virtually banks of a sort—interested in backing ready-made packages rather than developing the various elements from within. An agent finds, then, that more and more he is not submitting a manuscript to a studio directly. Rather, he approaches a producer, director, or star who might be interested in joining a package deal with the manuscript that in turn would spark interest in a studio with the money to finance it. An agent derives great satisfaction from arranging the production of a creative and profitable motion picture.

The Story Editor

by **Eleanor Breese,** executive story editor for Lorimar Productions. She has served in the same capacity at Brut Productions and for producer Joe Wizan at Twentieth Century–Fox. Prior to that, she worked as assistant story editor in the features division of ABC and at Metromedia, David Wolper, Inc., and for the Rand Corporation. Ms. Breese has written three novels and several screenplays in addition to short stories.

New or unproduced writers are encouraged to write complete screenplays . . . even if this must be done on speculation. . . .

The title *story editor* is gradually becoming a misnomer in large production companies because the person holding the title doesn't really edit or develop stories, screenplays, or other literary material; that is the function of the production executive and the producer working on a specific project. But the story editor does perform an essential service involving all literary material circulating within a company by acting as a sort of creative traffic director for all submissions and coverage, consulting with producers, writers, directors, and production executives, and overseeing a staff of readers.

A basic requirement of the job is the recognition and appreciation of good dramatic writing and a thorough familiarity with writers working in movies and theatre, including credits. Most creative executives in the movie business carry with them a mental storehouse of writers' and directors' credits, based on hours of movie-going and television viewing. This familiarity with talent and credits becomes part of their lexicon. It's not unusual for a story editor, production executive, or agent to come home with a pile of scripts to read at night or over a weekend. To place the story editor in perspective, let me "widen to a long shot."

Lorimar first emerged as a force in entertainment through the production of such successful television series as *The Waltons*. It has since widened its perimeters to include television movies and theatrical motion pictures, which are independently financed by Lorimar and distributed in the United States and Canada through major distributors and in the rest of world markets by Lorimar. Lorimar has been variously described as a mini-major or a high-rolling independent. In a business requiring investments of millions of dollars for the product merely to be made available to the consumer, Lorimar is equipped to furnish financing, facilities, business services, and personnel to movie makers with credentials.

The company is governed by an executive committee consisting of the board chairman, president, executive vice-president, executive vice-president of administration, and executive vice-president of feature films, all of whom apply their knowledge and experience to make gambling judgments as to which specific projects to take on. Next in line in the creative area are the vice-presidents of features and television (and their staffs), who are actively involved in development. Studios and major independents such as Lorimar also sign exclusive contracts with production entities (often a producer or producing partners and their support staff) to supply the company with theatrical or television projects in exchange for the security of a financing base and a link to distribution. In features, an agreement may be made with one producer offering only one project in the form of a joint venture with Lorimar. In television, salaried staff producers are free to find material that interests them for two-hour movies, multi-hour mini-series, or episodic series. The story editor serves all of these creative executives by handling, in the language of the business, "submissions of material." After all, literary material is the coin of the realm.

Once the executive committee approves a project as a theatrical feature, Lorimar will finance the development of the screenplay to its final form, organize the financing of the picture, organize and control all of the mechanics involved in physical production, and make the finished picture part of the release schedule. After executive committee approval of a television movie project, the producer attached will endeavor to interest a network buyer, and the network will reimburse Lorimar's development costs on the screenplay. Then, the project journeys up through a chain of approvals at the network before a commitment to film is made. When production is set, Lorimar initially puts up the production money, and at stipulated steps of completion the network reimburses the agreed-upon costs up to a limit, called the *network license fee*. Any overages are borne solely by Lorimar. In exchange for the license fee, the network has the right to televise the picture for two network runs. All subsequent exhibition rights, such as domestic or foreign theatrical, domestic or foreign television syndication, pay cable, or other home format, are all retained by Lorimar.

There is a normal daily flow of submissions to the company from writers and agents. Submissions come in a variety of forms. The one technically closest to production is the screenplay, averaging about 120 pages of dialogue and description. Over the years, the industry has developed an accepted screenplay form, which is a departure from the dialogue and description form used by dramatists for stage plays. (See excerpts from screenplays of *Butch Cassidy and the Sundance Kid*, p. 53, and from *The China Syndrome*, p. 224.) The novice screenwriter is advised to follow this form in order to be competitive. A screenplay is rewritten in a sequence of drafts, so one may bear the reference *first draft, second draft, revised second draft*, or no such reference at all on the title page. A *revision* is generally a reworking of a prior draft that is not as much work as a full draft; a *polish* is even less work, usually the making of minor corrections in and additions to a prior draft. These terms are often used in a business sense to define the point at which a writer is to be paid. In a *step deal* with a writer, for example, he or she may be paid for a first draft, one set of revisions and a polish, or any variation thereof, and the agreement may stipulate payments to be made upon delivery of each step. If a screenplay is being developed in-house, such title page references are instructive; if one is submitted from the outside bearing the legend *first draft,* it cannot be verified as such. An agent or producer might submit a fifth rewrite as a first draft to create the impression of freshness.

Projects may be submitted variously in the form of a *treatment, story outline,* or *format,* which are like short stories of varying lengths. What distinguishes them is that they are not in screenplay form. They convey the writer's story in prose style, perhaps with some examples of dialogue, concentrating on story points, sequence of events, and characters. This form of presentation is often used by established writers as a shortcut method in selling their stories to a financier-distributor who would then finance the writing of the screenplay by the same writer. New or unproduced writers are encouraged to write complete screenplays, however, even if this must be done on speculation, that is, without advance compensation. This way, the new writer communicates writing ability as well as story sense. If a new writer were to submit a treatment only, there would be no evidence of screenwriting ability, especially in the handling of dialogue. This also makes sense from a business standpoint, for the new writer's bargaining power is enhanced with the buyer if a screenplay, rather than a treatment, is to be acquired.

Books are submitted from agents or producers in various stages of pre-publication. The latest stage would obviously be the hardback or paperback edition, prior to release to bookstores. Working backwards, an earlier step would be a bound copy of the *uncorrected page proofs,* available several months before publication and possibly including errors, used to gather early reviews or for selling subsidiary rights such as motion picture rights. A typewritten *manuscript* is the earliest form in which a full book would be available. There is rivalry among some story editors, especially in New York where most publishers are based, to have access to desirable manuscripts at the earliest possible time, so that a producer or financier may have an advantage over the competition.

Other types of submissions are as varied as any source material for movies can be. *Urban Cowboy* and *Saturday Night Fever* were based on magazine articles; *Superman* was from the comic book; *Ode to Billy Joe* was from the song.

The story editor receives literary material from either outside the company (from agents and other creative personnel) or inside the company (from production executives or creators under contract) and oversees coverage of the material by a reader. *Coverage* refers to a reader's synopsis that is the objective retelling of a story in condensed form. Rendering a synopsis, which may fill from two to a dozen pages including a reader's comment, is the main function of a story department.

Many writers deplore the system of readers writing a synopsis of their work that is placed in a story file, available for possible destructive reference forever, but this is the only way yet devised to cope with the mass of material submitted to any single company for consideration. It is simply a matter of saving an executive's time, a shortcut method to sift through the material; an aid, rather than a decision maker. A synopsis is useful to an executive in deciding whether to read a project and is seldom a substitute for firsthand reading of something under serious consideration. Writers suspect that an unfair evaluation may be made by a reader who happens to be in a bad mood, or who may be predisposed against a certain kind of story.

Just as experts in art or cooking develop taste in their fields by exposure and experience, a good reader develops judgment by reading hundreds of screenplays, viewing movies regularly, and discussing aspects of evaluating and reporting projects with the story editor and other readers. As he reads, there is a movie going on in the reader's head; scenes are visualized and dialogue is heard. The reader hears and sees a work as a possible theatrical film (different, attractive, commanding, big), as a television movie (an effective personal story that would be intriguing on the small screen), or as a pilot for an episodic series.

Following years when readers were paid only a few dollars for reading, synopsizing, and evaluating material, there is now a Story Analysts Guild within the IATSE, the motion picture multi-union, with a graduated pay scale determined periodically by contract negotiation between management and the union. If the workload in a story department exceeds the amount the staff readers can cover quickly, the editor may hire free-lance readers from the industry experience roster for a minimum of one week's work.

The daily routine of a story editor can best be described by reviewing the mail that arrives, which can be broken down as follows:

1. Material from Lorimar executives. This includes submissions to them from agents representing a writer or a whole production package, from producers who hope to engage Lorimar in a project, and from acquaintances and friends of executives.

2. Scripts or books from individual producers working within the Lorimar framework. Sometimes a fast synopsis is required, and overnight service is given on such priority requests. Usually, no more than

a week passes before coverage is returned to the executive or producer along with the material.

3.   Books from Lorimar's New York office, which are submissions from east coast agents as potential films. Some books are covered by readers in New York and the synopses are sent to the west coast, but most of the books are transported by overnight pouch to Los Angeles for evaluation. (Writers live all over the country, and while life experience elsewhere can be enriching for a writer, I believe writing for the motion picture market usually requires the writer's presence within a reasonable distance of the marketplace. A writer cannot judge current film interests by released films playing in theatres or on the television screen, for these represent buying decisions made eight months to two years earlier.)

4.   Scripts or books submitted directly to the story editor by agents or friends. These may be accompanied by personal letters with information about a new writer or something of the history of the project. Agents who are selective in sending material to a likely buyer are appreciated, while the few agents known for their scattergun approach of submitting projects indiscriminately receive low priority for coverage. Projects from the editor's friends may receive personal attention, but recommendation to management is made on the same basis as other material.

5.   Projects that come in "off the street" or unsolicited; that is, not represented by agents. These must be accompanied by a release signed by the writer. If an unknown writer who does not have an agent wants his work to be read by a production company, it is advisable to request and sign a legal release to protect the company from a lawsuit in case they pass and later produce a film on a similar theme. Many companies will not read unsolicited projects. Material submitted by a licensed agent is protected by agreement between agents and film companies, so a release is unnecessary.

With all submissions, the appearance of the material is a factor; with the work of a writer who is not established, appearance is often the deciding factor between initial attention and indifference. A screenplay submitted to a potential buyer should be clean and fresh, not dirty or rumpled; readably typed in the established screenplay form, from 100 to 130 pages in length; and as free as possible from distracting typos and errors of spelling. Samples of screenplay form may be found in textbooks or mass-market paperback versions of certain movies.

After sorting the submitted material according to priorities and by the speed of coverage requested, the editor decides which reader reads what project. The never-settled debate among writers over whether it is better to have a prominent agent and risk getting lost in the shuffle of volume or a less prestigious agent who will provide more personal representation intrudes on the issue of priorities of material to be covered. The story editor is inclined to give precedence to the "important" agent, even though the other agent may be more careful in selecting the target buyer and generally works more closely with the writer client. So the debate continues.

The reader's coverage is returned with the material to the producer or executive to whom it was first submitted. (An internal system of identifying cards attached to the property prevents mix-ups.) After reading the synopsis, the producer may want to read the material thoroughly or merely skim it. Or the synopsis may simply aid him in returning the project to the agent or author with an appropriate letter. Copies of all coverage are distributed internally to all Lorimar executives and producers and to the New York office, unless someone stops such a distribution to protect a confidential submission. It's possible that another producer in the company may read a certain synopsis, spark to it, and ask to read the material itself.

Sometimes an executive or a producer may ask for a *selling synopsis* for presentation to a director, star, or network. A reader writing a selling synopsis would not make creative changes in the story, but would emphasize, without comment, its exploitable aspects. Normally, the language of a synopsis should not reflect editorial comment by the reader, as in "a silly chase ensues," but should objectively convey the style and substance of the material. The reader's separate comment following the synopsis can be more personal but should be an evaluation of the material specifically for the market.

When material submitted to the story editor is turned down, it is returned to the agent or writer, usually with a note. A story editor's helpful comments in a rejection letter will sometimes result in an appreciative response from the writer. A noncommittal rejection leaves a writer baffled, wondering if there is anything to be done to improve the salability of his work.

There are other services the story department performs. An executive or a producer may ask for a copy of a certain book from a bookstore or publisher. As many as 100 copies of a book have been requested at one time by a producer of an ongoing project. There may be a query about the availability of film rights in a literary property, in which case the name of the book's agent can be obtained from the publisher's subsidiary rights department and the answer learned from the agent. Further, a producer may ask the story editor to do research on a subject being considered or ask for a list of suitable writers for a specific project. There are also daily calls from executives requesting old coverage from the story files.

For early scouting of potential movie projects, publications containing capsule synopses of forthcoming books are read in the story department, such as *Publishers Weekly* magazine and *Kirkus Reviews,* a private reviewing service. The industry trade papers, weekly *Variety* from New York and *Daily Variety* and *The Hollywood Reporter* from Los Angeles, are read to keep up with the activity of people in the business and to follow film grosses; the Nielsen ratings are studied as an index of television audience response. The story editor's rounds include being aware of plays produced locally, lunching with agents, writers, and other story editors, and attending special screenings and parties. The annual budget for the story department is projected through meetings between the story editor and company budget officers, and it is the responsibility of the story editor to see that the operation of the department stays within these budget guidelines.

It used to be that all story editors were heavily involved in the development of projects, meeting often with writers and executives, helping to evolve a screenplay through draft after draft. This is still done by a story editor in a small production company, where only one or two projects may be in work at one time. But today in the major studios or a large independent such as Lorimar, the individual producer chooses his writers and works with them to develop a final script. The designation *story editor* more aptly describes the story editor on a television series who works with the producer of the series in determining the format, choosing material from episodes submitted by agents, and rewriting purchased material for the series with or without the collaboration of the original author. The movie business could do with a better term to distinguish between the TV series story editor, who really does edit scripts, and the studio story editor, but so far none has evolved.

Exploiting Book-Publishing Rights

by **Roberta Kent,** who has been active in the publishing and motion picture industries for over ten years. She has worked with Creative Management Associates (now International Creative Management), Curtis Brown, Ltd., and the W. B. Agency in New York, and at the Paul Kohner–Michael Levy Agency in Los Angeles. She is currently an agent with the Ufland Agency in Beverly Hills.

What every soft-cover publisher dreams of is paying $7,500 for the novelization rights to a motion picture that . . . sells 5,000,000 copies of the paperback book. Then, everybody makes money.

The value of book-publishing rights in connection with motion pictures has spawned a new and important addition to the publishing industry, the movie tie-in or novelization. There have been movie tie-ins for years, but when David Seltzer's 1973 book version of *The Omen* (written after his original screenplay) sold over 3,000,000 copies, yielding royalties in six figures, the book-publishing world and movie makers recognized the increasing value of coordinating book sales with movie sales to their mutual benefit.

After the huge success of *The Omen* novelization (a made-up word that offends many novel writers), there followed years of escalating sales to paperback houses that wanted to publish book versions of screenplays projected to be successful films. Movie tie-ins that once brought in $3,500 as a total advance from a publisher began attracting prices of $100,000 and more. The market became as cutthroat as the paperback competition for a hardback best seller. Agents held auction sales, and every few months new price records were set. If *The Omen* heralded the market boom in 1973, *FIST* was the turning point in 1978. The $400,000 sales for Joe Eszterhas's powerful novelization of his original screenplay was associated with an unsuccessful film in the marketplace. Just as the movie company was shocked when it did not do well on the film, the book company was appalled when book sales were low. This taught the publishing industry that the only reliable value of a movie tie-in was as an adjunct to the picture. The result has been that guaranteed advances have leveled off to an average of $50,000 to $60,000 for novelization rights.

An important lesson is that the prices usually quoted as sales to paperback houses for movie tie-in rights are guaranteed advances against royalties to be earned by sales. High advances anticipate high sales. The paperback house pays this amount, which is nonrefundable, to the holder of the novelization rights. But whether the advance is $7,500 or $75,000, the money earned on a book (the royalty) will be the same if it sells 2,000,000 copies. The only difference is the spread of the initial advances spent. On a strong sale of 2,000,000 copies, the advance will, whether large or small, be earned back, and the extra earnings will be converted to royalties. Today, publishers have decided to rely more on the strength of the movie tie-in to attract sales (and therefore royalties) on its own, with decreased advances paid, rather than hoping that royalties from high sales will equal a strong advance.

One other factor that bottomed out the movie tie-in market was that publishers were buying novelization rights to television movies, but people were not buying these books. The success of the *Brian's Song* novelization followed its initial and subsequent television runs, and this led to increased bidding on other TV movie tie-ins. However, it was found that people who watched a high-rated, one-time TV movie did not necessarily buy the book, and publishers were stuck with unrecouped advances and unsold copies. The only television program that can usually succeed in selling tie-in books is the long form miniseries.

Although advances have leveled off for movie tie-ins, the market is still quite valuable and should be properly exploited by the studio and producer. It will be useful to follow the process with two types of source material: the original screenplay and the existing novel.

If an original screenplay is commissioned by a producer or written on spec by a writer and then purchased by a producer, there may be an effort to make a book deal before a financier-distributor gets involved. In this case, the screenplay will be submitted to publishers (hard-cover or soft-cover) for evaluation. If the publishers feel that the property will not succeed on its own as a book, they may want to review it when a movie deal is set (involving commitment of financing, a director, and stars). This is most common. But if the producer must wait, the issue of lead time becomes a factor.

It's appropriate to review the mechanics of publishing at this point because as a movie project gets further along, time pressure becomes more acute. A novel can take anywhere from three to eighteen months to write. The manuscript is turned in to the publisher, who starts the editing and then the printing process. It takes anywhere from six to nine months to get that hard-cover book into print and another month to distribute it to bookstores. A paperback generally comes out a year following the publication of the hardcover edition. Usually, timing calls for a hard-cover novel to be in bookstores at the time the picture is shooting, while the paperback tie-in will be published just about the time the motion picture is released. A paperback original requires about as much lead time for publication as does a hardcover, to allow for design, typesetting, and printing.

To return to the hypothetical example, assume the producer is having no success in preselling hard-cover or soft-cover publication rights to the original screenplay. When he makes a deal with a financier-distributor, however, it's a new ball game. Now the mass-market paperback houses (Bantam, Dell, Fawcett, Avon, Jove, New American Library, Warner Books, etc.) become interested because the screenplay will be a movie and therefore has new value. The financier-distributor usually takes over from here and makes a novelization deal with a paperback house that involves the screenwriter and producer. Essential to the movie tie-in deal is the acquisition of the movie logo (called *artwork*) and stills, which must be obtained from the distributor.

Before the elements of such a deal between financier-distributor and paperback publisher are described, the issue of who writes the movie tie-in for an original screenplay must be covered. Under the Writers Guild of America Basic Agreement, the Guild can tentatively name who will receive "story by" or "written by" credit prior to formal designation of screen credit, and that writer benefits from separated rights (including publication rights) and thereby has first chance to make the novelization deal. This would require his dealing with the producer for permission to use the artwork and stills from the movie as well as with an interested publisher. If the Guild-named writer does not make a novelization deal within a stipulated period of time, it falls to the producer to do so with another writer and then pay the Guild-named writer a percentage of the adjusted gross receipts from such a novelization deal. For example, a paperback publisher could pay a $100,000 advance to a studio for the novelization of an original screenplay that the screenwriter declines to novelize. (The Guild requires the studio to pay $2,500 separately to the Guild-named screenwriter in that event.) Then, the studio may pay a novelization specialist a flat fee of, say, $15,000 to do the job. The Guild permits a deduction of $5,000 from the studio's share covering a use fee for the artwork, which the studio pays to itself before reaching "adjusted gross receipts" of $80,000 (subtracting novelizer's fee and the fee for the artwork from $100,000 publisher's nonrefundable advance). Under the Guild rules, the Guild-named writer will receive 35% of the adjusted gross receipts, minus the $2,500 advance, or $25,500 in this example, a sum higher than the novelizer receives.

The elements to be negotiated in a novelization deal with a soft-cover house include the *advance*, which averages $50,000–$60,000 but can be as high as six figures or as low as $5,000. Usually, everyone involved in the project receives a slice of the advance: producer, financing entity, screenwriter, and writer of the novelization. Next, there is a *royalty*, which is generally 6% of the cover price for the first 150,000 copies sold, 8% thereafter. The royalty is also divided between the entities, but only a novelizer with strong bargaining power will share in this amount. The *territory* usually covers the United States and Canada only, but sometimes worldwide rights are sold, and the advance reflects that. *Timing* ideally is planned so that one month before the picture's release, the book is on the stands and the public can become familiar with it. Other negotiated points include completion of the manuscript and coordination of the artwork. Obviously, as soon as there is a logo design and production stills, the distributor should send them to the publisher in an effort to reduce the necessary lead time. If a publisher has paid a substantial sum to a financing entity for novelization rights, the contract will usually state that the financing entity will supply artwork at no extra charge.

The original screenplay is one type of source material that can be exploited in book publishing. A second type is the existing novel, which can be issued in paperback as a tie-in, timed with the release of the motion picture.

A publisher generally makes comparatively little money publishing and selling a hard-cover book. The primary source of income for a hard-cover house is the sale of subsidiary rights, such as book-club and paperback rights. Revenues from these sources are usually divided by giving 50% to the author and 50% to the hard-cover publisher. Movie rights are generally held by the author. Paperback rights are sold by competitive auction, which accounts for the huge sums often involved. Each year, several sales are made in the million-dollar area. However, a book must earn back that advance in sales before a dime of royalty is collected. There was an estimate that for Bantam Books to earn back the $3.2-million advance to Judith Krantz on *Princess Daisy*, 9-million copies must be sold. Usually, a best seller in hard-cover is one that has sold between 25,000 and 50,000 copies; a moderate-sized first printing in paperback is 80,000; if a paperback has sold a million copies, it is selling phenomenally.

On a prestige book, subsidiary rights deals are generally made when the book is in galley form, any time from two months to two weeks before publication. The paperback house, movie producer, and studio will work very closely on the timing of the book. If the film will be a long time in the making, the paperback house will publish one edition and then reissue it at the time of the movie's release. The difference is that the reissue would contain the artwork and stills that coincide with the marketing of the film.

There is a symbiosis that can take place among the sales of the various subsidiary rights. A book that is a book-club selection with large paperback sales will certainly be offered as an attractive and expensive movie sale. Conversely, if a book has been sold as a movie, the amount paid for the book by a book club or paperback house increases; the pressure goes both ways. The publisher pressures the agent to sell the movie rights to enhance the subsidiary value of the book, and the movie buyer pressures the agent or publisher to sell the rights to enhance the value of his screen property.

One issue that arises involves advertising costs. If a hardback publisher has benefited from a large paperback sale made on the heels of a major movie sale, the producer can ask the hardback publisher to share those benefits with the movie by committing sufficient money to successfully promote the book, "creating a best seller." The hard-cover publisher can argue that the big movie sale was made on the strength of the literary material alone and can suggest that the producer contribute to the book's advertising budget to boost sales potential. This issue is unresolved.

To review: If a movie's source material is an original screenplay, it can be sold as a hard-cover or soft-cover book before the movie becomes a reality. If the source material is an existing novel, a subsequent paperback edition can become a movie tie-in timed with the release of the picture. If a project originates as a magazine article, either the author of the article will expand it into a book, or a book will be derived from the eventual screenplay. *Saturday Night Fever,* which originated as a *New York* magazine article, became a novelization based on the screenplay. *King of the Gypsies* is an interesting case because it began as a *New York* magazine series by Peter Maas, who made a book and movie deal simultaneously. Bantam bought the soft-cover rights and sold hard-cover rights to Viking in a reverse of the usual procedure. Coinciding with the placement of the book rights, the motion picture rights were sold to Dino DeLaurentiis.

A new way a studio can exploit book-publishing rights is to finance the writing of a novel. Twentieth Century–Fox advanced money to author William Kinsolving to write *Born with the Century,* a deal that evolved from a meeting with Fox producer Michael Gruskoff. G. P. Putnam's Sons bought the hard-cover rights, and paperback rights went to Fawcett for $1.1-million, divided half to the author and half to the producer and Fox. Metro-Goldwyn-Mayer paid author Charles Sailor a $20,000 advance to write *The Second Son,* which was sold as a paperback original to Avon, and also financed *The Glory Hand,* a novel written by Sharon and Paul Boorstin. This way, the studio is involved in the earliest development of the property, generally helps in obtaining publishing deals, gets a screen property for a relatively small investment, and participates in the revenue from all deals made. Studios avoid having to pay enormous prices to acquire these books and are able to tailor the books to their own market, while trying to attract the book-buying public as well. The writers receive the seed money necessary to write a book and the opportunity generally to write the screenplay, all packaged by a financier-distributor devoted to exploiting the project in all media.

Book-publishing rights can be further exploited in the form of photo novels, "The Making of . . ." books, large-sized art books, and calendars. *Star Wars, Close Encounters of the Third Kind, The Empire Strikes Back,* and *E.T.* offer examples of the possibilities.

The future of publishing will find more paperback originals being developed, either from original screenplays or from novelists. The publishing business is going to become more dependent on non-print avenues of promotion, such as radio and television. Our society is becoming less a printed-word society and more an image society, and publishers will be more dependent on those images to sell the word. As far as novelization sales go, the market will find its own level. The extravagant advances are a thing of the past. Advances against royalties will be moderate, in the hope that the royalties will bring publishers a substantial amount of money. What every soft-cover publisher dreams of is paying $7,500 for the novelization rights to a motion picture that ultimately sells 5,000,000 copies of the paperback book. Then, everybody makes money.

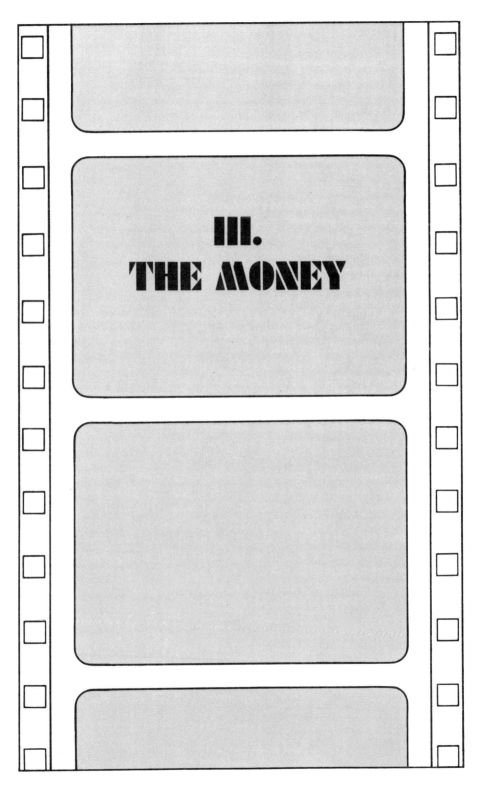

III.
THE MONEY

Elements
of Feature Financing

by **Norman H. Garey,** who was a partner in the law firm of Garey, Mason & Sloane, based in the west side of Los Angeles. He represented actors, directors, writers, producers, and production companies in the motion picture and television industries. Mr. Garey graduated from Stanford University and Stanford Law School, lectured at Stanford, at the USC Entertainment Law Institute, and at the UCLA Entertainment Law Symposium, and was a member of the Los Angeles Copyright Society and the California Bar. He died shortly before publication of this book.

An important lesson is to define at what point one's gross or net profit position is achieved. . . . another lesson is not to use phrases like net *or* gross, *but rather to define* net *of what* or *gross after what. . . .*

The matter of feature motion picture financing usually begins with the philosophy of the entrepreneurial producer. There are many established producers, for example, who are not particularly interested in buying or optioning a big, best-selling book or a finished original screenplay by a "star" screenwriter because these are very costly items, and many producers don't wish to spend a lot of money out of their own pockets. They would prefer to be original and either create ideas themselves and hire writers to develop them or induce financial sources to hire these writers. Or a producer may want to buy or option a screenplay that comes in from a relatively unknown source, perhaps a young writer who is a graduate student at UCLA or USC. It may be that the writer who is a bit better established, and who has an agent, in the normal professional course of events makes a submission of his material through the agent to the producer, who reads it and decides to buy it.

First, the producer's lawyer will commission the requisite title search to make sure that the material (and hopefully its title as well) can safely be used and that there aren't any conflicting claims, at least as disclosed by the copyright records in Washington. Next, the producer will decide how much to spend in option money and what kind of price to establish with the writer's agent. If it's a finished screenplay that the writer has written on speculation, he deserves some reward for it, which is generally reflected in the purchase price due on option exercise. The price would be constructed not only in terms of the cash payment due upon exercise of option and/or commencement of photography, but also (in many cases) in terms of contingent compensation as well.

As an example, suppose that the writer is an established one with at least one produced screen credit and that the producer is negotiating for an original screenplay. If the producer is putting up $5,000 for a year's option with the right of a renewal for a second year for another $5,000 (usually the first payment applies against the purchase price, and perhaps the second does as well), the purchase price may easily be $100,000 or more. That second option period for the second

$5,000 may be necessary because it takes that long to mount the production, to secure the elements necessary to put the financing in place, and to know that there will in fact be a movie which then warrants exercising the option and paying the $100,000.

On the "back end," this deal may provide that 5% of 100% of the picture's net profits will be payable to the writer. But both the cash payment due on option exercise and the 5% of 100% of net could be made to depend on that writer's having received sole screenplay credit. If another writer has to be brought in, then the first writer arguably hasn't completely delivered the value expected. The Writers Guild, in making its credit determination, may find that there was material in the shooting script that was created by the second writer, who naturally has also been paid. Some flexibility must be allowed in constructing the first writer's deal for the potential necessity of bringing in a second writer and for the economic consequences of that eventuality. Thus, both the cash and the contingent compensation of the first writer may be reducible in the event that he shares screenplay credit.

Suppose, as another example, that the writer is even more well established than the one just described. Perhaps he wants a lot more than $5,000 option money up front. Maybe he wants $25,000 or $30,000 up front in option money for a year, or even wants his work purchased outright rather than optioned at all. The producer doesn't want to spend that much out of his own pocket and doesn't want to go to a studio for it because that will mean giving too much away at the back end of his own deal. He may then establish a partnership with the writer, whereby the producer's profit points and the writer's profit points (and perhaps even their cash compensation) are pooled and divided in some way. Under such an arrangement, the writer takes a risk along with the producer, but he also stands to be rewarded along with the producer if they're successful. This doesn't mean that the pooling and division necessarily result in a 50/50 split. It could be 66/33, 75/25, 60/40, or some other percentage. But the pooling and division partnership has become a rather frequently used device to accomplish a deal between a producer and a writer or the owner of a piece of material when the producer doesn't want to lay out a lot of money and the writer doesn't want to accept short money up front without a commensurate back-end reward for doing so.

A more typical deal is the for-hire development deal, in which a producer creates the idea and will either hire a writer out of his own money or go to a studio for development money to hire a writer. In this deal, the writer will frequently ask for a large cash fee as well as for participation in the profits of the picture and the proceeds of the subsidiary or "separated" rights. These negotiations are frequently difficult ones. The writer may conceive that he is the originator of the material since he is creating certain of the characters and their inter-relationships, even though usually the story line and the plot premise at least have already been created by the producer. There is often some up-front ego conflict in these cases about who's contributing what. But these matters can be resolved by allowing the writer for hire to parti-cipate to some degree, beyond what the Writers Guild Minimum Basic Agreement requires, in the proceeds of the subsidiary or separated rights (such as theatrical and television sequel, print-publishing, and merchandising rights), or by rewarding the writer with a net profit par-ticipation, which the Guild agreement does not require at all. If a sig-nificant cash fee is being paid up front, then the writer generally doesn't deserve all that; he's performing an employee's function and taking no risk at all. If, on the other hand, he is taking less than his normal front money and is contributing a great deal, then perhaps he does deserve to participate in these back-end rights and/or in the movie's net profits.

Assuming that the screenplay is of very good quality, the pro-ducer will then want to go to the marketplace and seek production fi-nancing based on this material. He might approach either a financier-distributor (a major studio) or one of the major independent production financiers. There are five or six independent production companies that finance pictures but do not distribute their own product, and therein lies the distinction between them and the so-called majors. If the ma-terial is absolutely sensational, the producer may be fortunate enough to be able to sell the "mini package" consisting of script, rights, and producer's services. Knowing what the costs are, the producer should be in a position to construct a price, both in terms of guaranteed cash compensation (part of which may have to be earned out by producer services rendered over a future period) and contingent compensation, whether measured in terms of gross receipts, gross receipts from some future break-even point, or net profits.

On the other hand, it may be that the material, while very good, is only very good when allied with certain other creative elements. In that case, it may be necessary to do some prepackaging. This may in-volve negotiating for a certain director, either because his name will help attract financing and/or cast or because the material may need fur-ther development. In the latter case, it's wiser from a creative stand-point to involve the director who is actually going to make the movie in further developing the screenplay. It may also be desirable to attach some actors and thus complete a major package for delivery to the pro-duction financier; a complete package will improve the producer's deal vastly.

The philosophy that one must recognize and observe in making these decisions is that of the risk/reward ratio: The further a producer has moved the project—that is, the greater the investment he has made in terms of time, effort, and money and the more finished the product he is delivering—the more he's going to get for it both in cash and in back-end contingent interest. If he's in a position to bring in what is nearly a completed movie that just hasn't been shot yet, he's going to be able to make the best deal with the financier. However, there are some risks to this approach, both strategic and financial. That's what makes the game interesting. Perhaps the elements one involves may turn out to be liabilities. The director may be terrific for the material but turn out to be unacceptable to the financier. Or, although everybody may have thought that the actor's last picture did very well and therefore that he should provide a big advantage, a picture that he made a while ago may come out in the meantime and turn out to be a disaster, whereupon no financier wants him anymore. The producer may have to drop one or both of these gentlemen from the package politely and without creating any legal or economic liability in the process.

Sometimes it's necessary, in order to involve a director or an actor, to put up *holding money* or option money, just as one would do to secure rights to a literary property. An actor's time and a director's time are valuable, and they will not always pledge their availability to a certain project without knowing either that there is financing which guarantees their future compensation or that there's some money payable now for which they're willing to give the producer a temporary hold on their services. Naturally, the independent producer's lawyer must negotiate separately for the services of each of the creative people in the package before going into the final negotiation with the production financier.

Thus, if the producer is in a position to bring a finished script to a studio, and the studio has not taken the development risk (because the producer has done so), he can command a far better deal from the studio. If he's willing to take it a step further and put down some money to tie up a director and/or an actor, then he's entitled to even more from the studio. Perhaps that entrepreneurial producer can also independently raise production financing from private sources, either those who, as in the tax-shelter days, were seeking a write-off but also liked the movie business for its glamour, or genuine equity financiers. If he can take the project all the way to completed film and then merely seek distribution for it, the producer will make an even better deal.

There are other potential sources of production financing to consider. Assume the producer is beginning to assemble those creative and money elements necessary to physically produce the film. Those sources of money may be *territorial*; that is, he may sell off the theatrical distribution rights in certain territories of the world in order to raise money out of those territories with which to produce the movie. He may be able to raise money out of certain media of exploitation; for example, U.S. network television and/or pay (cable or over-the-air subscription) television will frequently pay fairly large advances or make guarantees for a certain number of runs of the picture after its initial theatrical release, particularly if the picture has some substantial stars in it. These guarantees received from television sources or from overseas territories can be taken to banks and discounted for cash, which is then used to finance the movie. The producer may wish to sell off or license in advance the right to receive income from certain ancillary rights sources, such as sound track album recording and publishing rights to the music used in the movie. It may be that the merchandising rights are extremely valuable; if it's a high-technology picture, there's a lot of gadgetry that can make good toys. The merchandising rights also may be presold for guarantees that can be turned into cash. Book publishing is another possible source. A publishing house may be willing to put up money in advance of the material being secured or written. This investment will come at the earliest possible time if the producer is going to presell the publishing rights.

One technique used to finance many low-budget films is raising money through *limited partnerships* formed by individual investors. Each investor is a "limited partner" (in that his liability for losses is limited to the amount he invests, and he incurs no personal liability beyond the amount) whose contribution, when aggregated with those of his partners, totals some proportion of the total production cost of the film. As a unit, these investors share a percentage of the "money's" share of the film's net profits (usually at least 50%) equal to the percentage that their total investment bears to the total production cost of the picture. The remaining net profit shares are retained by other "money" (who get the balance of that 50%) and by the producers and other creative elements who get the other 50% (or less) of the net profits. Broadway shows are traditionally financed in this manner. The individual investor can be attracted to films by means of the limited partnership, which finds doctors, accountants, farmers, realtors, and a whole cross section of society drawn to the glamour of movies.

If the producer is financing the picture privately, without going to a studio, it will be absolutely necessary that he secure a completion guarantee from one of the traditional sources (unless his own financial resources are so substantial that he can and will place at risk his own general assets). There are a handful of recognized, professional completion guarantors. (See article by Norman Rudman, p. 189.) A *completion guarantor* is a kind of cost insurer, or insurance company. He agrees (for a premium usually computed as a percentage of the picture's production cost) that out of his resources or financial contacts, he will guarantee the money necessary to complete the picture if the money that has been raised from other sources turns out to be inadequate; for example, if the picture runs well over the original budget. The producer must satisfy the completion guarantor that he has a good track record for cost responsibility going in and that the director also does, because the director is in a real sense the general contractor in the field. He's responsible for building the building, and if the costs are going to run over, it'll probably be because of him. The completion guarantor will want to put his own supervisor or production manager and location auditor on the picture to watch what's going on, in order to protect his risk. He may insist on the right to take over the picture, to take it out of the producer's and the director's control, if it's going substantially over budget. There may be penalty clauses in the completion guarantee stating that if the completion guarantor is required to come up with money, that is, if his guarantee is actually called upon, he has the right to invade the contingent compensation (or in some cases even the cash compensation) of the producer or director or both. The controls that the completion guarantor will insist upon may be at least as onerous as those which a major studio would impose upon a producer if the studio were putting up the money. The source that's ultimately answerable financially is the one considered entitled to impose those controls. The completion guarantee then has to be approved by the basic financing source(s) because they want to know that there's a real guarantee in place; they don't want to be confronted with the unwelcome choice of either accepting a three-fourths completed film after having put up all of the money or having to put up money beyond their original commitment in order to complete the picture.

Another way for a producer to finance a picture is through a *negative pickup*. It may be that he hasn't been able to raise all of the production money from nonstudio sources, but only a part of it. If there's a completion guarantor willing to back the ultimate cost of the project, the producer can then go to a studio (or other production financier) where the management believes in the picture enough to take a limited financial risk on it. They will agree to guarantee payment of part of the negative cost—for example, a million dollars—upon delivery of the negative. The studio is not taking a production risk because if the negative is not delivered, the studio has no obligation. On the other hand, if the negative is delivered, but the picture is not very good, the studio is still obligated to pay the "pickup" price. That negative pickup guarantee by the studio can be taken to a bank and turned into cash, which may give the producer the balance of his production cost.

One other way for a producer to proceed is to go directly to a bank and secure a production loan on the strength of all the other guarantees that he has assembled. The bank loan itself can be "taken out" (discharged or paid off) by a negative pickup guarantee from a studio. That's another little wrinkle in the financing package. Basically, the bank's loan is interim financing, and the negative pickup is permanent financing or the "takeout loan," as it would be called in real estate parlance. The financing devices used in the motion picture industry are strongly similar to those used in the real estate development and construction industry. Making a movie is analogous to building a building on a lot. The literary property is the lot, the piece of real property. The movie is analogous to the building. The screenwriter is the architect, the director is the contractor, and the producer is theoretically the owner. The major studio (if one is involved) can variously represent a lending institution, equity partner, and/or leasing agent for the finished building (in its capacity as distributor).

If the producer has completed the film entirely from nonstudio sources of financing and is now seeking distribution, he would screen it for a major studio distributor. If it was well received, the producer could possibly command a deal for the film in which the studio would advance all or more than all of the negative cost, thereby perhaps generating an immediate profit as a result of simply making the deal. He might further obtain a guarantee from the studio of a certain number of dollars toward print and advertising expenses. This guarantee is very important because the commitment of exploitation money frequently indicates the seriousness of the distributor's intent. Even the best film is not going to be successful if it's advertised poorly or inadequately promoted.

Next, the producer will probably be able to command some kind of gross receipts participation deal. This is structured so that once the studio has recouped its expenditures (its outlay for prints and advertising and the advance made to the producer to cover the negative cost outlay, enabling the producer in turn to pay off the various loans taken out along the way) the proceeds derived thereafter will be divided between the producer and the distributor on a gross basis, without any further deductions. The division could be 50/50 after recoupment by the studio, or it could be an alternating 60/40 deal. This might call for a 60% split in the studio's favor until the studio has recouped all of its outlay (prints and ads, its advance to the producer, etc.) with the percentage then shifting in the producer's favor up to a further point based on gross receipts before flattening out at 50/50 or some other split. There are varying combinations, depending on bargaining power.

If the producer does not require any advance whatsoever from the studio because money from foreign territorial sales and other sources has financed the picture as well as all print and advertising costs, he can hire the studio as pure distributor on a reduced distribution fee basis. There is conceded to be a variable profit factor in the standard 30% U.S. domestic distribution fee, so that it is possible, when the studio has taken no financial risk, for the producer to hire the studio as salesman only ("leasing agent" in the real estate analogy) and expect the studio to distribute the picture at a less-than-normal profit, for example at 22½% domestically instead of 30%, at 27½% in Canada instead of 35%, and at 32½% instead of 40% for any previously unsold foreign territories.

Producers raise production financing themselves to avoid having to go to the domestic distributor earlier than necessary because the further down the road one can go alone, the better the deal will be with that major studio distributor at the end of the line. The best position for a producer is to be able to walk into a distributor with a completed film under his arm and say, "Okay, we'd like to have you as distributor. What kind of a guarantee of prints and advertising are you willing to make, and what kind of reduced distribution fee are you willing to quote?" The more studio money the producer accepts and the earlier he accepts it, the greater the risk he asks the studio to take and the more the studio will expect to be rewarded for it. Again, the risk/reward ratio operates. If the financier-distributor is asked to take the entire production risk, the best the producer can expect—assuming he's assembled all the elements and has paid the entire development cost—is usually a 50/50 net profit deal. For that much risk, the financier-distributor is generally considered to be entitled to at least 50% of the net profits, and perhaps more, and to insist on the standard distribution fee of 30% for the U.S. and Canada.

The producer's profit percentage will be reducible by the profit participations he has had to give up along the way to raise the money or to obtain the creative elements. The writer will probably receive 5 to 10%, the director 10 to 15%. Immediately, the producer has given away perhaps 25% of 100% of the net profits, half his share, and that's with virtually no cast. If there is major casting, he may be giving away gross participations that, at best, come off the top and significantly reduce what constitutes net profits in the first place and, at worst, may also come to some extent from his end of the net profits. With studio financing, the producer may end up with somewhere between 10% and (if he is relatively fortunate or has been able to negotiate a net profit "floor" as a protection against further reductions) 20% of the net profits, with some gross participations off the top that reduce the net profit pie before it can be cut up.

To understand this in practical terms, one should track the money flow briefly. A ticket dollar comes in at the box office to the exhibitor during the first week of the picture's run in a major city. The distributor has been able to negotiate optimum terms from the exhibitor, a 90/10 split in favor of the distributor. First, we must deduct from that dollar the exhibitor's house nut (or expenses) of around 10%, so we're down to 90¢. If the 90/10 deal calls for the distributor to receive 90% of the remainder, that's about 80¢ out of the dollar that has come in at the box office; 80¢ of that dollar constitutes the distributor's rentals. In the U.S. and Canada, the distributor is entitled to a 30% distribution fee, which is 24¢, so now we're down to 56¢. The 30% distribution fee is to pay the distributor's own nut, or internal expenses, and is conceded to contain a profit factor the amount of which depends on how many pictures the distributor has in exploitation in a given year and thus how easily the fixed costs are covered that year. Advertising and publicity expenses are very high, especially television advertising; they generally run at 20 to 25% of rentals, and these expenses come next. If our rentals were 80¢, deduct 25% of that for advertising, or 20¢, bringing our 56¢ down to 36¢. We haven't even considered other distribution expenses, such as the cost of striking prints, taxes, dubbing, the MPAA seal, shipping, and transportation. With all these, the 36¢ will be reduced to less than 30¢. Now, the negative cost of the picture must be recovered. If it's supposed that the negative cost was roughly one-third of the total dollar that came in, we've got nothing left. Thus, if we're lucky, we've covered the negative cost of the picture, but we probably haven't. We're probably going to have to wait significantly far into the next dollars that come in to break even and to begin computing net profits, if any.

If we are barely into net profits, the studio is entitled to 50% for putting up the production money. They're the investing partner in this sense, not the salesman in the sense that they've received their distribution fee earlier. If there were 2¢ left out of that original dollar (let's be generous to ourselves), the studio gets 1¢. But wait—if there was a gross participation out to a major star, then that actor's participation would come off the original 80¢ that we took in at the box office. If he recieved a 10%-of-gross participation, there would have been another 8¢ gone before we even got this far. So instead of having 2¢ left, we'd be minus 6¢; we'd be unrecouped.

If you take that dollar and multiply it by many millions, it illustrates the difference between that actor's being a gross participant and that same actor's being a net profit participant. If he was a 10% net profit participant, that actor would wind up with nothing or with his minor share of 1¢. But because he is a popular actor and has a good enough agent, he commands a 10% gross participation from the first dollar and comes out of that sample dollar with 8¢ (which is far more than anyone else except the distributor) rather than (maybe) a fraction of 1¢.

There may be half a dozen directors in the world who command first dollar gross participations of a significant kind, and hardly any writers who can. However, there are many actors and directors, and even a few writers, who are given gross participations from break-even, that is, once break-even is achieved. So once we got down to that 1¢ and beyond, which is theoretically break-even, then and only then (on the next dollar) would this hypothetical actor or director or writer participant's gross participation be payable.

An important lesson is to define at what point one's gross or net profit position is achieved. If it's gross from first dollar, that's very different from gross after break-even or some other break point. In our hypothetical example, the gross-from-first-dollar participant would have gotten 8¢. The gross-from-break-even participant would have gotten nothing or nearly nothing because we barely reached break-even out of that last cent of the dollar. Another lesson is not to use phrases like *net* or *gross*, but rather to define net *of what* or gross *after what*.

The foregoing has used the producer with a track record as its focus. The new or impoverished producer is going to get stung when he goes to a studio because he has no leverage. In this case, there may be a small cash fee and an even smaller profit participation, certainly not 50% or anything very close to it.

Today, more than ever, difficulties exist in seeking independent financing for motion pictures. With tax-shelter financing having dried up in this country, at least at the individual-investor level, and costs on the increase across the board, the major studio financiers are at least for the moment back in a very powerful position. Several major independents have emerged that finance their own pictures, but they still turn to the studios for distribution. Exhibitors would like to become a source of financing in order to participate in film profits and to assure a constant flow of product into the theatres. But they can't presently join with the traditional distributors in joint ventures or in other combinations that might run afoul of the Paramount Consent Decree.* Producers and exhibitors have begun to join in financing arrangements, and the major distributors are generally very suspicious of these arrangements.

* Editor's Note: Before 1948, it was an industry standard for most studios to own major interests in theatre chains, thereby controlling production, distribution, and exhibition. The Justice Department deemed this triple involvement to be anticompetitive and began litigation against the companies. Following the landmark Supreme Court decision *U.S. v. Paramount, et al.* in 1948, Paramount, RKO, Warner Brothers, Twentieth Century–Fox, and Loew's-MGM entered into a "consent decree" in which they consented to divorce themselves of theatre ownership, while retaining production and distribution. In the following years, these companies slowly underwent reorganizations that complied with divorcement of theatre holdings. The result of the Consent Decree has been the emergence of many new theatre chains and small production entities that now compete with the majors. In October, 1981, the Justice Department announced the intention to review the Paramount and related decrees, which have governed the movie business for over 30 years.

It's an industry that, while shrinking economically in some ways, is not exploring its own potential in terms of financing. One reason is that the antitrust laws (as made manifest in the Consent Decree) prevent it from completely doing so. They will probably have to be modified in some fashion to permit greater participation by exhibitor-distributor combines in financing production because the exhibitors are the only major group that has the interest and wherewithal to do so. A recent decision points in that direction. In February, 1980, a Federal judge ruled that Loew's Corporation would be allowed to enter production and distribution, in a major alteration of the Consent Decree. Citing the lack of successful product, the judge reasoned that such an entry into the market would heighten competition. It's too early to assess the impact of this move, but other large theatre chains are expected to petition for similar permission.

Another problem is that ours is one of the few motion picture industries in the world that is in no way subsidized by the government. It was subsidized in an indirect fashion during the days of tax-shelter financing in that the investor, through favorable tax treatment, was in effect given a subsidy inducement to make the investment. There should be some other inducement created, though not a direct government subsidy, since that may lead to government control in some form. Another way of motivating new sources of financing to participate in the industry is to provide greater disclosure in the way distribution accounting is performed. If we were more able conscientiously to say to outside investors that we know we'll get a fair and honest count from distributors, we might be more successful in bringing more outside money into the business.

The Bank and Feature Financing

by **Peter W. Geiger,** a vice-president with the entertainment and media section of Bank of America's North American Division. Based in Los Angeles, the division manages wholesale banking activities for major corporate customers in the United States, Canada, and Mexico. Geiger has devoted his entire career to the motion picture industry. Before joining Bank of America in 1951, he was associated with RKO Radio Pictures and American-European Film Industries, Inc. Geiger was named head of the New York motion picture office of Bank of America in 1954 and was transferred to the bank's Los Angeles headquarters in 1958, where he was promoted to assistant vice-president in 1961 and to vice-president in 1968.

> *When a producer comes to a bank seeking financing, a secondary source of repayment is essential; we cannot look to the proceeds of the picture for the repayment of the loan. . . .*

Bank of America was a pioneer in the financing of pictures, which goes as far back as 1904, when the movie industry was in its infancy. In those days, banking was a person-to-person business. The founding family of the bank, the Gianninis, had a personal interest in the picture business and provided sums to pioneers such as Cecil B. DeMille, Sol Lesser, and Samuel Goldwyn. The first million-dollar loan was made to Mr. Goldwyn in the early 1930s, on the basis of his reputation and his consistent record of accomplishment. In the 1930s and 1940s, the bank lent up to 60–70% of a film's budget on a picture-by-picture basis. The producer-distributors controlled the theatres as well, and by block booking they would know how much money their picture would earn in their theatre circuit. This money was assured, and in those days pictures were generally completed within budget.

After the separation of distribution and production from exhibition in the late 1940s, proceeds were not so clearly determined. At the same time, television entered the scene, which caused the postwar era of the motion picture market to decline dramatically. The philosophy in the 1950s was to continue to finance on a picture-by-picture basis as long as there was some kind of backstop or guarantee.

In the late 1960s, a number of companies faced near extinction because they tried to top the success of *The Sound of Music*. Millions of dollars were lost in the financing of musicals and other extravaganzas that failed at the box office. This "Sound of Music Syndrome" resulted in an industry depression from 1969 to 1971. In the retrenching and refinancing that resulted, there emerged the long-term revolving bank loan formula, which most of the majors follow today.

The motion picture business today is the healthiest that it's ever been. Major companies have done extremely well; their cash flow is excellent, which is good for them and bad for the banks. Several companies don't even have to come to banks to borrow. They have a cash-rich balance sheet. To ensure this stability, movie companies are diversifying. For example, Twentieth Century–Fox has acquired Aspen Skiing Corporation in Colorado and Pebble Beach Golf Club on the Monterey Peninsula of California.

Most major financier-distributors borrow money on a commercial revolving loan basis, not picture by picture. Often the term of such a loan agreement runs over a number of years with figures of over a hundred million dollars. In some cases, two or more banks join in such a transaction because of the large amounts involved, making a consortium loan that is administered by a loan agreement typical of most commercial loan agreements, with certain financial ratio (such as debt to net worth), inventory, and other controls. This is done in such a way so that the financier-distributor itself determines how to allocate funds among its divisions and projects. The bank does not get involved in creative judgments. However, if a company is in deep financial trouble, we may put a ceiling on the cost of any one picture, but that is only in case of emergency.

A revolving loan commitment involving a consortium of banks would typically finance one major studio over, say, a period of seven years, with repayments primarily flowing from picture earnings. Principally, the bank looks at the strength, track record, and financial position of the company itself. These loans can continue on indefinitely as long as the company is a viable, ongoing business. The company involved would naturally have to live within the confines of certain financial ratios. If these are deemed not practical after a time, the company can amend the terms of or rewrite the whole agreement while it is still in force.

At the bank, we receive detailed periodic statements from the company, bringing us up to date on their projected picture budgets and on how they evaluate the results of certain of their pictures. For our part, we have made our own projections along with those of the company, and we both follow certain guidelines that realistically allow the company to operate and expand. For instance, if an acquisition is contemplated, some basic terms of the loan agreement would have to be renegotiated because the financial ratios will change accordingly. Sometimes, in a downturn of pictures or of business generally, if the bank feels that the company is not sufficiently covered, we may ask them to provide additional collateral, such as theatrical presales and television syndication contracts.

A bank provides interim funds. It doesn't share in a spectacularly profitable picture like *Star Wars* or *Raiders of the Lost Ark;* neither does it want to suffer from loss pictures. We look at a revolving loan as an interim advance, like a real estate construction loan, but there must be someone else responsible for the long-term risk. After all, the movie business is one of the riskiest businesses there is; we cannot foretell by any stretch of the imagination whether a given project is even going to be completed, much less if it will be acceptable in the marketplace. In addition, we cannot have realistic market studies done, such as those that define what types of cars or microwave ovens the public wants to buy next year. It's totally speculative. We must evaluate a motion picture company using the same guidelines we have for other industrial concerns seeking loans, by looking at the financial statement and making projections. The one distinct factor is the unusual risk involved.

At Bank of America, we structure our long-term revolving arrangements with major film companies in a manner consistent with their chief source of cash flow, which is from the distribution of pictures. The long-term aspect of such loans takes into account that in a given cycle, a picture will repay itself in 18 to 24 months. This covers the average lead time from the start of principal photography through its full exploitable life in the domestic and foreign theatrical markets. That's the primary income. During this period, the financier-distributor knows whether the particular picture will make a profit, break even, or lose money. Later on, it will gain the benefits of secondary income from such sources as television syndication and pay TV. These revolving long-term loans represent most of our involvement in the area of picture financing and relate to the major companies only.

With the small, independent producer, the bank looks at a number of contingencies that have to be covered before a bankable loan can be made. When a producer comes to a bank seeking financing, a secondary source of repayment is essential; we cannot look to the proceeds of the picture for the repayment of the loan. All kinds of things can jeopardize a picture in the course of production. It can be aborted during filming for causes not insurable. It can run way over budget, and, although a contingent amount should be secured to avoid that, this backstop doesn't always succeed. *Apocalypse Now* is a good example of a picture that had to be refinanced during production because it far exceeded the budget.

A producer will have to come up with some kind of financial strength other than the picture, because we do not ascribe any value to the picture itself. This secondary source of repayment for a loan may be in the form of some personal liquid assets, certain presales of theatrical exhibition, television exhibition, or book or music publishing or merchandising rights—something the bank can look upon with comfort; something that is collectable. Whether an independent producer makes a picture for $500,000 or $15-million, the ground rules are the same.

One popular financing technique involves presales to foreign countries. Let's assume a producer has a strong reputation and has assembled a talent package that is attractive to a certain distributor for the foreign market. For the privilege of distributing this picture overseas, that distributor may commit, say, $3-million in advance of production, payable one third now, one third when the picture is finished, and one third when it is delivered. The last two payments are contingent upon certain events happening. For the first payment, the producer may obtain an irrevocable letter of credit from the distributor, which the bank will discount for cash. The producer will then try to make a similar deal with a domestic distributor.

Overseas, a picture can also be sold territorially, as in the case of *A Bridge Too Far*. Joseph E. Levine presold that film in chunks of territories on a worldwide basis to the extent that the picture was assured a healthy profit before it was in production. In the case of territorial sales, a producer may obtain several letters of credit from several distributors that would guarantee a certain amount of dollars for certain territories in exchange for distribution rights in those territories. A bank can discount some of the amount guaranteed, as long as the letters of credit are written in such a way that they are not dependent on the delivery of the picture; otherwise, the producer would have to invoke the entrance of a completion guarantor.

A completion guarantor in this case would assure the bank that the overseas distributor will accept the picture offered to him. If anything happens to this picture on the way to completion, we want to be assured that completion and delivery are going to take place. Say, for example, that a producer makes a deal with Paramount for $2-million payable on delivery of the picture in exchange for domestic distribution rights. In the middle of production something unforeseen happens that is noninsurable, and the picture is aborted. Paramount is not on the hook because the picture has not been delivered to them. Rather, the completion guarantor has to pay the bank the production outlay plus interest in order for the bank to get its money back.

These examples have referred to established producers who have access to pools of money from industry or personal sources. New producers generally rely on studios for full financing (and thereby relinquish a portion of profits) or make low-budget pictures financed by independent sources.

A first-time producer has to have "angels" who provide him with the necessary support to make his picture. A classic example is *One Flew Over the Cuckoo's Nest*, which was independently financed by producers Saul Zaentz and Michael Douglas through private sources only after no studio would provide the necessary financing in advance of shooting. When the picture was completed, they shopped around for a distributor, and the picture went on to be a great commercial and artistic success and was awarded the Oscar for Best Picture of the Year. Certainly, if the head of a studio can't foretell such a success, a guy surrounded by a bank vault isn't going to try to determine which pictures will make money and which will not.

The entertainment division of Bank of America is an outgrowth of what was originally the motion picture loan department. Eight people are involved wholly in motion pictures, along with those handling broadcasting, theatres, cable television (a considerable new area where funds being sought offset the lack of demand of some of the studios), and other media, such as newspapers. The bulk of our financing is done in the feature film area. (Networks, for instance, function mostly on a cash basis and rely on their parent companies for funding.) We carefully track our major customers and follow their progress on a continuing basis, both in respect to their financial and operating results. There's never a dull moment; it's satisfying when a certain loan is accomplished or frustrating when a certain problem cannot be solved. We try to be prudent students of the industry but must view it objectively, in a strict business sense. The industry is artistic and creative, but nevertheless, as the name implies, it is show *business*.

Foreign Tax Incentives and Government Subsidies

by **Gary O. Concoff,** a partner in the law firm of Sidley & Austin in Los Angeles. He received his law degree from Harvard Law School after gaining a B.S. in business administration at UCLA. He is the author of various articles on legal questions relating to the motion picture business, with specific emphasis on finance aspects of motion pictures. Mr. Concoff is an Adjunct Professor of Law at UCLA Law School, teaching a course on motion picture transactions. In addition, he has spoken in many programs on both corporate and entertainment law sponsored by UCLA, USC, and the Practicing Law Institute, among others.

An American producer seeking financing from sources other than financier-distributors may find himself looking to tax incentives or subsidies available under the laws of foreign countries. Why would a producer turn to these sources of financing? One answer is that the producer may have shopped his project to all of the domestic majors and been turned down or may have been unable to get the kind of deal he wanted. A second, less cynical reason may be that the producer desires more autonomy and control over the product and therefore wants to finance the project outside the studio system. A middle category may find an American source of financing willing to put up part of the necessary money but not all, in which case the producer may try to qualify his picture for foreign tax incentive investors or subsidy for the balance.

To define terms, a tax incentive (or shelter) is generally established and overseen by a government taxing authority to encourage local investment (and therefore encourage the local industry) and to directly benefit the individual or corporate investor before a picture is made. A subsidy is also planned and regulated by a foreign government, but such subsidies usually benefit the owners of the completed picture once it qualifies under government rules.

From the point of view of the foreign country, there are some obvious antecedents leading to modern subsidies and tax incentives. The patrons of old in European countries were usually aristocrats who supported the arts. Films are generally considered in European countries to be an art form. There is, then, some logic in the government supplanting the patrons and supporting the arts and the development of young artists. A second reason is an attempt to compete with the American center of production and to encourage and enhance the local motion picture industry. That's true of the Canadian tax-incentive plan. A third reason is that a government decides to provide creative tax-incentive financial planning involving motion pictures in order to enhance domestic investments and the country's economy.

In the United States, the independent producer is at a disadvantage when compared with his foreign competitors because he does not have any government subsidy, or indirect subsidy through significant tax incentives, to aid him. I believe there should be some manner of tax incentive or subsidy supporting the low-budget picture to supplement the motion picture studios' ability to control financing. The response to this is that the United States government looks at our highly visible industry, sees people living in huge homes and driving expensive cars, and concludes that the industry doesn't need any subsidies. A tax-shelter plan for American movie investors flourished in the early 1970s but was ended by the government in 1976.

There is one relatively insignificant tax incentive that is of some substance domestically. the investment tax credit. The investment tax credit essentially treats a motion picture like any other kind of personal property or equipment. In an attempt to stoke the economy, the government gives a tax credit (about 7% of the production cost of the picture) as a credit against the income taxes of the entity that is at risk when the picture is first put into use (exhibited or broadcast). For example, a production company might undertake to produce a television motion picture, for, say, $1.5-million but may receive a license fee of only $1.3-million from a network; in the interim, it takes serious risks of completion. The government acknowledges that risk by providing the investment tax credit to the production company. In a theatrical feature, the credit would go to the financier-distributor who would likely be at risk. The question here is whether the producer or distributor is at risk financially at the time the property is put into use. For instance, if a picture is released domestically but was financed as a negative pickup wherein the distributor was at risk for $2-million and the producer was at risk for $400,000 (due to overbudget costs), the producer and distributor would share the investment tax credit (usually about 7%) proportionally. The Internal Revenue Service oversees and regulates these transactions from the standpoint of collecting tax and reviewing whether the investment tax credit is properly taken.

The following country-by-country review is current as of this writing, but because the entire area of tax incentives and government subsidies is changeable year to year, the reader is advised to seek counsel as to the updated policies of a specific country.

CANADA

In 1967, the Canadian Parliament established the Canadian Film Development Corporation, which invested seed money in the development of motion picture properties for Canadian producers. There were some low-budget Canadian pictures that the CFDC took substantial positions in without any tax incentive involved. Tax incentives were adopted by the government in 1978 with the clear purpose of enhancing and developing the Canadian film industry. In a short period of time, the expansion in Canadian production was very dramatic.

The American producer has to face the fact that the laws determining whether a picture is a certified Canadian production (thereby qualifying for the tax incentive) state that the picture must be owned, controlled, and produced by Canadian citizens or landed immigrants. Nonetheless, an American can develop a property, interest a Canadian producer, and take an executive producer or presentation credit. The non-Canadian cannot function as the producer or take a producer credit. Then, in an arrangement with the Canadian under which the Canadian has final say, the American can get his picture financed through Canadian sources.

Certification is the term used in Canada under which a picture can qualify for tax incentives. The system is quite technical and complicated. First and foremost, the producer must be a Canadian. There is a ten-point system used to determine whether a picture is primarily Canadian and therefore qualifies. The key creative personnel are assigned points or units. For example, the director is allocated two units; the screenwriter, two units; the actor or actress receiving the highest remuneration receives one unit; and the actor or actress whose pay is second highest, one unit. The list continues with one unit each for art director, director of photography, composer, and editor. There are no points for producer. The Canadian taxing authority, functioning with the advice and consultation of the Canadian Film Development Board, determines certification. Out of these ten units, six must be Canadian for a picture to qualify. For example, if a project involves an American screenwriter and two American leads, four points are gone. A Canadian director would then have to be used along with other Canadian personnel representing four more points. This puts great stress on the availability of first-class directors and writers in Canada.

After the point requirement of six out of ten is met, there is a second test. 75% of the aggregate remuneration paid to various persons other than those covered by the point system and 75% of the payments with respect to processing and final preparation of the film (laboratory work, etc.) must be paid to Canadian people or entities.

To summarize, first there must be a Canadian producer. Second, out of ten units, six must represent Canadian elements; third, 75% of the remaining production cost (substantially below-the-line) must be Canadian. It's possible, for example, in some cases to qualify a picture with an eight-week shooting schedule by shooting, say, five or six weeks in Canada and two or three weeks in the United States to achieve an American look so that the picture would attract the American audience and compete with product financed by the majors. Further, the remaining 25% of expenditure does allow for some latitude in including other American elements as well. However, this is a very tricky area requiring careful planning and good Canadian legal advice.

American investors cannot benefit from any tax incentive on a Canadian picture. This is a tax incentive device for Canadians only and is generated in the form of an offering. There are two types. One is the *private offering* made to a small group of wealthy Canadian investors who might finance a picture themselves and take the tax benefits. In this case, the investors would make a down payment of perhaps 20% of the budget and fund the remaining 80% over, say, a maximum of four years. This is accomplished by arranging for bank credit for the balance. The benefit for the investor is the right to write off or deduct 100% of the cost of the picture immediately. He gets a tax benefit for that year, but later when the income is returned, he must recognize it as income. The net effect is a deferral of taxes by reason of early deductibility of the 80% balance.

The same rule regarding tax benefits applies to a *public offering*. A public offering of $5-million to raise money to finance a picture can be divided into, say, $5,000 units, with the possibility of a thousand individual investors. In this situation, the producer would insist on letters of credit issued by banks for the balance or 80% that investors would write off. For example, if a Canadian dentist wants to invest in two units for $10,000, he puts $2,000 down and goes to the Toronto Dominion Bank to obtain a letter of credit for the $8,000 balance. The bank in effect is securing or guaranteeing his credit. In this way, there will be no question that when the producer needs the balance of the dentist's investment, he will have it from the bank. The producer has a call on the full $10,000, although the investor puts only 20% down and defers 80% over a period of years. The producer will then borrow against the various letters of credit on an interim basis to fund the production costs of the picture.

This is not a loan to the producer; it is an equity investment in the picture. The equity investor in Canada rides with the success or failure of the picture. If it's successful, he gets his investment back and perhaps makes a profit. If it's not successful, he may ultimately have a true loss, not a mere tax-benefit loss. The advantage for the investor is that regardless of eventual profit or loss, he has been allowed to write off four times his current investment in the investing year, which may be a real benefit depending on his tax bracket.

Care has to be taken that the tax incentive is not destroyed by guarantees or advances from distributors that could constitute income for the investors and thus remove their deductions. Advice from Canadian tax counsel must be sought by Canadian investors and producers to benefit properly from these procedures.

117

ENGLAND

The Eady Plan in England is a government-subsidy plan (as opposed to a tax-incentive plan) under which the British government sets aside a certain portion of box-office receipts from all pictures exhibited in the United Kingdom and refunds a certain portion of those proceeds as a subsidy to the producers of pictures made in the U.K. The subsidy is supplied from an admissions tax on all pictures exhibited in British theatres but is divided among Eady-qualifying pictures only. That tax money is placed into the British Film Fund and is then allocated to the qualifying pictures on a yearly basis. The British Film Fund Agency (under the Board of Trade) distributes to each eligible film an amount equal to that proportion of Eady money that the total proceeds of that picture bears to the total earnings of all eligible pictures.

In order to qualify as a subsidy picture, the producer of the picture must be a British resident or the production company must be registered in, and the control of business must be exercised in, the United Kingdom. The producer of an eligible picture must make his claim for payment under the plan in writing to the Film Fund within two months of the end of each eligible year, and payments are usually made a few months thereafter. Eady proceeds can be quite significant, and often the treatment of the Eady subsidy becomes a difficult part of a negotiation with a financier-distributor.

An American producer who wants to produce a picture in the U.K. and meet the standards of Eady could easily engage English counsel, form a British corporation, and make sure that the corporation owns the rights to the picture and engages the people employed on the picture. If that corporation, as the maker of the picture, spends some 75% of the cost of labor on British subjects or citizens of the Republic of Ireland, it will qualify under the Eady Plan for subsidy benefits. An actor and perhaps even an actor and director might be excluded in the calculation of that 75%. The financing of the picture does not have to be in British money, though it must be spent in England or the Republic of Ireland.

The Eady Plan was enacted by Parliament through the Cinematograph Film Act of 1957, which has been amended several times. It is a government subsidy, not a tax incentive. When making an agreement with a financier-distributor, one may encounter a demand that the picture qualify for Eady benefits and that warranties and representations be made to that effect. It would be necessary, therefore, to determine prior to commencement of production whether the picture will qualify, either through an opinion of counsel or unofficial soundings of the governmental regulatory body. After production, there is always the risk that the money was improperly spent or that through violation of some of the rules, one might lose the benefits. Further, if the picture is not distributed in the United Kingdom, it cannot receive the subsidy.

While the Eady Plan is an interesting incentive, in some ways similar to the investment tax credit, it is not usually sufficient in itself to cause an investor to invest in a multi-million dollar picture. Rather, it's a bonus for a picture shot in the U.K., available to the makers only after the fact. This is a distinction between a subsidy and the Canadian system of tax incentives, which can be helpful in attracting investors to cover 100% of a budget and thereby cause a picture to get made.

The English system is very much in flux. There may be dramatic changes, including the elimination of Eady, because the Conservative government is on record as being opposed to subsidies. As an eventual substitute for or supplement to the Eady Plan, tax-incentive devices are now being developed.

GERMANY

The German system of tax incentives has until recently been similar to the incentives that Americans enjoyed before the U.S. law was changed in 1976. Until October, 1979, Germany allowed American producers to receive substantial tax-incentive investments from West German taxpayers, the only investors who could benefit from the national system. The tax incentive took the form of an investment of perhaps 40–50% of the cost of a picture, the balance of which was financed by some third party, such as an American distributor or investor. The West German could deduct 100% of the picture cost, even though he invested only 40%, and then defer part of his tax obligation until the picture proceeds were realized.

In October, 1979, the tax-incentive rules (other than as relate to certain pictures financed out of Berlin) were substantially tightened. While many German advisors feel that the system of tax incentives remains viable, at this writing the matter is very much in doubt. Reliable German tax counsel must be consulted as part of any inquiry into a proposed German tax-shelter investment.

The practical applications of these tax-incentive rules vary within West Germany from taxing area to taxing area. One might get a slightly different opinion as to how to structure a transaction in Munich from how to do so in Frankfurt. Interestingly, the city of Berlin supplements the tax incentives through very desirable loans to encourage film production within Berlin.

The German arrangement has not required any particular expenditure of monies in Germany or use of German elements. However, there has been a tendency on the part of the groups that have financed

119

several pictures to shoot at least a portion of a group of pictures in Germany in order not to offend the German taxing authorities.

German tax-shelter financing has been organized through private or public offerings. The individual investor was, until October 1979, allowed to write off nearly twice his actual investment in a film. However, his liability was unclear. If a group of German investors put up half the budget of a film and a third-party distributor put up the balance, that remaining 50% was usually advanced by the distributor as a loan to the German production entity in advance of production. The question of whether this was a recourse loan or a nonrecourse loan has been unclear. There was some question as to whether the third-party distributor could look to those investors to repay the 50% the distributor had advanced if the picture did poorly.

Until recently, the American producer desiring to take advantage of German tax-incentive investments has not formed a German company. Rather, he would make an agreement with a German corporation that would act, in effect, as a general partner for the purposes of raising financing. Recently, formation of a German entity by non-German producers has become more prevalent. The German investors in this situation invest in a limited partnership-type vehicle and get the benefit of the deductions. The American would usually contract to grant ownership to, and the copyright would have to reside in, the German entity. Then, through a service agreement with that entity, the American producer would undertake certain production functions with the money all being spent through the German entity. In effect, the German limited partnership subcontracts to the American producer certain production functions. Naturally, competent German counsel must be involved from beginning to end in such a transaction. Again, all of the foregoing arrangements have been put in question by the changes in German tax law effective as of October 1979.

This covers the three major countries having tax incentives or subsidies for motion picture financing. For the American producer, proximity to Canada makes that country's incentives an intriguing prospect. One doesn't determine to make a picture in England because of its subsidy, but if that location suits the story, the producer might go to England rather than France because of the former's subsidy benefits.

France and Italy have subsidy systems, but their rules strictly limit qualification to national pictures. For instance, only a truly French producer can gain the benefit of the French subsidy, which then must be reinvested in the next French picture of that producing company. There are treaties among various countries, including Italy, Germany, England, and Canada, that allow co-productions to share certain subsidy benefits if specific elements from each country are employed. There is speculation that the European treaty countries may turn to some pan-European subsidy arrangement enabling projects to cross European boundaries easily and to benefit from a universal subsidy system. It should be emphasized that a producer planning to shoot a picture in Europe should consult a knowledgeable attorney in the country involved to learn what manner of subsidy might be available for a specific picture.

Another form of government dispensation to attract filmmaking finds below-the-line facilities available at particularly low costs, or at no cost. Morocco, Tunisia, and Australia provide breaks on equipment, personnel, and location facilities if a picture is shot there, in a general effort to attract production. This can result in substantial savings. A picture budgeted at $1.2-million if shot in the United States might be shot in Australia for perhaps $800,000. Latin American countries such as Mexico, Colombia, and Venezuela have also offered reductions in below-the-line facilities in order to attract movie production.

The prognosis for tax incentives and government subsidies varies. In Canada, one hears estimates of perhaps another four years of continued tax incentives. Ironically, if the industry succeeds overwhelmingly, that may shorten the duration of the incentives. My own feeling is that Canadians should continue their plan for as long as twenty years, because it takes that long to build a solid base for a financially sound motion picture industry. In the United Kingdom, one hears speculation that the Eady Plan might be abandoned by the Conservative government and, perhaps, replaced by a form of tax incentives. In Germany, there has been a refinement of the nature of tax-incentive investments that might make it more difficult to secure German tax-shelter money for American producers. Many of the underdeveloped countries, however, will continue to offer below-the-line benefits to attract production.

Financing and Foreign Distribution

by **Sylvie Schneble,** a journalist-screenwriter who resides in Pacific Palisades, California. Her work has appeared in *Crawdaddy* magazine, *Action, Fade-in,* and *Los Angeles Reader*. She wrote *Golden Needles* and *Invasion of the Bee Girls* for producers Paul Heller and Fred Weintraub, both released by American International Pictures. She won first prize for her play, *Heirs,* when it was produced at Jacksonville University in Florida.

and **Tristine Rainer,** a producer of television movies including *Games Mother Never Taught You* and *Having It All*. She has also served as development vice-president for George Englund Productions and director of development for Dan Curtis Productions. Ms. Rainer has been a professor of film and literature at the University of California at Los Angeles and has worked as a journalist for *Action* and *Emmy* magazines. This article originally appeared, in somewhat different form, in *Action* magazine, and is used here with permission of the authors and the Directors Guild of America.

. . . the independent producer may want to throw up his hands and simply turn his film over to a U.S. major for overseas distribution. At least they keep honest books, right? Don't you believe it. . . .

Foreign distribution is like the lady and the tiger. Send a film overseas through the wrong door, and it will be ravaged by crosscollateralization, overhead charges, distribution fees, improper marketing, and zero grosses. But choose the right door and a producer's dream materializes: a guaranteed global market and profits that are bankable *before* the film even enters production.

The game is played all year round, but most obviously at Cannes and the MIFED film-TV market in Milan.* Here, where American independent producers meet their foreign counterparts as well as salesmen, marketing representatives, and financiers, the talk is always the same: fewer pictures, bloated budgets, interest charges that escalate with the seasons, and a rumbling discontent with the distribution tactics of the U.S. majors. What they are *really* talking about, these independents with pictures to sell, is nothing less than their own survival.

Survival means expertise in foreign distribution. A producer must know how to negotiate the release of his or her film market by market beyond the United States and Canada. If you doubt this, consider the track records of Sandy Howard *(The Island of Dr. Moreau, Embryo, Sky Riders)*, George Barrie *(Fingers, Thieves, I Will, I Will . . . For Now)*, Michael Klinger *(Shout at the Devil, Gold)*, Lew Grade *(The Boys from Brazil, Raise the Titanic)*, Lee Rich and Merv Adelson *(The Choirboys, Twilight's Last Gleaming)*, and Elliott Kastner *(The Medusa Touch, A Little Night Music, The Missouri Breaks)*. Rarely do these men dent the domestic box office, yet each turns out "product" furiously. How? Because they find their revenue overseas.

It used to be that an American release grossed about 45% of its revenues abroad. Now, that figure can be as high as 90%, much of it recouped before production through territorial sales. For the smart independent, a film can flop dismally at home, yet profit handsomely abroad. Neither Lorimar's *The Next Man* nor *The Choirboys* made *Va-*

---

* Editor's Note: The American Film Market has since been established in Los Angeles as a third selling market by a group of domestic independent distributors, in an effort to bring international buyers for American pictures to the United States.

riety's list of top grossers ($4-million in domestic rentals required), but both eased comfortably into the black after release in Latin America, Europe, and Japan.

How do Howard, Barrie, Grade, Kastner, and others do it? First, they understand some basics. For half a chance at profitability, a producer needs the following:

— An international web of major distributors. *In all the foreign markets.*
— A sales and advertising staff experienced in first-run release outlets, ad budgets, and exhibition terms. *In all the foreign markets.*
— A service department to effect proper print utilization. *In all the foreign markets.*
— An accounting department for collections, ongoing distribution accounts, and first-run playoffs. *In all the foreign markets.*
— Proper representation at the major film festivals and markets.

That's an intimidating list of resources. Small wonder that, traditionally, most independent American producers let the majors handle their overseas distribution. There is a catch, though, for the majors have financial needs of their own. In each foreign market, a studio release must generate sufficient rentals to cover branch-office overheads *and* cross-collateralization bookkeeping, whereby profits from one market can be devoured to pay for losses in another market. And whereas a major's U.S.-Canadian distribution fee is normally 30% of incoming rentals, it can rise to 40% and higher abroad. The result? Too often, producers receive zero or minimal overseas revenue.

Consequently, independents are seeking new roads to Rome via (1) mini-majors like Orion and New World; (2) in-house distribution arms, such as those established by Dino De Laurentiis and CBS Theatrical; (3) brokerage services along the lines of Mark Damon's Producers Sales Organization; (4) personal attendance at Cannes and MIFED; and (5) working with knowledgeable attorneys and agents, as Francis Coppola has done with *Apocalypse Now*.

The majors, of course, still proclaim the superiority of *their* foreign distribution channels. Columbia, Warner Brothers, Twentieth Century–Fox, MGM/UA, Paramount, Universal, and Disney all see themselves as having the necessary "muscle" to get the best play dates and theatres. Certainly, they have a quasi monopoly abroad because they still make the biggest films. "When Warners comes along overseas, we say, 'Hey, fellas, you'd better treat us well with this picture, or you won't get the one coming up—*Superman II*,' " says Myron Karlin, vice-president in charge of international operations for Warners. "We sell groups of pictures overseas. That gives us leverage. If a foreign exhibitor wants *Superman II*, he may have to play four other Warners pictures."

In the U.S., that kind of block booking is illegal. When Fox block-booked *The Other Side of Midnight* with *Star Wars* in transactions in Boston-Minneapolis film exchanges, a Federal grand jury in New York indicted the company for criminal contempt of the Consent Decree. (For background on the Consent Decree, see footnote, p. 105.) Overseas, no such legal censure exists.

To enforce block booking and otherwise maintain their international muscle, Warners operates 104 branch offices in 53 countries outside the U.S. In Italy alone they have 13 offices. That creates a pretty hefty overhead, which someone has to pay for. In decades past, overhead charges were divided among 40–50 pictures a year; now, a major studio may release only 10 films a year. The question is, with soaring production and promotion costs, has that enormous foreign overhead, combined with the majors' 35–40% overseas distribution fee, turned into fat, dragging down the profitability of each film?

Myron Karlin denies it: "The allocation Warners makes to the various countries is so small, it's insignificant."

Yet Universal and Paramount were forced to streamline their overseas operations into one joint company, Cinema International Corporation (now the world's largest film distributor, netting about 35% of American global theatrical revenues; CIC also picked up MGM and Disney territories in 1973), while Fox is closing out foreign branches, preferring to use local distributors in major markets like Japan and France.*

More disconcerting to profit participants is the majors' policy of cross-collateralizing profits made in one country against losses in another. Myron Karlin modestly says, "We take the world as our oyster," but cross-collateralization means your pearl found in Australia will be spent to make up for your losses in Italy. Since the majors usually insist on rights "anywhere in the universe," a film can screen on the moon and they'd still own it and cross-collateralize it.

Independent producer Sandy Howard asserts, "Had I distributed *A Man Called Horse* through a major, I wouldn't have seen a penny." Howard's film performed well in every country in the world except Japan and Holland. Distributed in 1970 by the short-lived Cinema Center Films, a CBS subsidiary, *Horse* was not cross-collateralized, so Japanese and Dutch losses didn't affect overall rentals. Cinema Center also charged low overheads and distribution fees, and "we

---

* Editor's Note: In November 1981, CIC was broadened into a new organization, United International Pictures, handling overseas distribution of product from Universal, Paramount, and Metro-Goldwyn-Mayer/United Artists (MGM/UA).

made a great deal of money from foreign markets," recalls Howard. "I'm happy to say I participated for a change."

IN-HOUSE DISTRIBUTION

Let's say a film makes a million dollar profit in the United Kingdom. The producer pays 35% of that to the major distributing the film. That's $350,000. But go directly to a British distributor, such as EMI, Rank, or Brent Walker, and the fee may be 25%, or $250,000. There's an immediate savings of $100,000. Multiply that kind of savings worldwide, and the lesson is clear. If you can, deal directly with the territories.

If you can?

That's the catch. A producer needs the sound financial base of a Dino De Laurentiis or Sir Lew Grade before plunging ahead with an expensive, complex in-house distribution arm. The producer also needs the kind of international reputation and moxie built up by De Laurentiis and Grade over the decades.

De Laurentiis, like the mini-majors, has overcome the problems of cross-collateralization. The distributors with whom he negotiates must assume all territorial losses, forcing them to hustle harder than the secure manager of a major's branch office. Many foreign distributors are actually stronger than the branch offices of majors. In Japan, where revenues of imported films exceed those of locally made movies, distributors like Toho, Nikkatsu, Toei, Shochiku, and Nippon Herald frequently wrest greater rentals from American films in their market than do the U.S. branch offices.

Working with reliable foreign distributors, De Laurentiis is able to raise pre-production financial commitments that are readily bankable. In other words, he's making money before the camera even turns—money that allows for a long-range program of feature productions. Sandy Howard and Elliott Kastner are other old hands at this game. While there are exceptions, it's no accident that most presold films tend to be "safe," based on predictable material, most often a novel. Almost every one of Lew Grade's films, for example, had a literary antecedent. And the number of "all-star" casts has risen in direct proportion to the number of foreign presales. Ironically, this built-in safety factor, which works so well overseas, is perhaps the very quality that *prevents* most of these films from performing well in the U.S. Artistic considerations aside, the important point is that "foreign rights are now looked upon as a phenomenal source of income," according to Edmond Saran, president of Best International Films, veteran of handling foreign rights to U.S. pictures (*The Next Man, Search and Destroy*).

126

THE BROKER

Negotiating market by market may be the ideal for an independent producer, but few have the resources to pull it off. A more realistic alternative might be to hire an experienced service company to handle foreign sales, maybe Mark Damon's Producers Sales Organization.

Mark Damon was once consigned to the ranks of expatriate American actors in Rome (*Black Sabbath, Ringo And His Golden Gun*). Now, like De Laurentiis, Damon negotiates advance guarantees with independent distributors in the territories. He works for an up-front fee. "Producers are becoming aware of the tremendous advantages of doing business this way," he says. "Three pictures that I handled were in profit before release anywhere: *The Choirboys, Matilda,* and *The Wanderers.*" Damon was executive producer in charge of foreign sales on *The Choirboys,* co-produced by Lorimar and a European consortium and distributed by Universal in the U.S. and Canada. "Universal wanted to give it to CIC for foreign distribution," continues Damon, "but I knew that would be disastrous for profit potential. Peter Guber told me *The Deep,* which grossed $80-million worldwide through Columbia, has yet to pay any monies to the profit participants." Damon expects to realize $50-million gross rentals overseas on *The Choirboys,* whereas it grossed less than $4-million domestically.

Damon maintains ongoing relationships with distributors around the world—and hires accountants to check on them. Could an independent American producer do all that himself? Probably not. There are too many variables to confront, too much specialized knowledge of foreign law and procedures required. How can a producer understand the validity of a contract if he or she doesn't know the country itself?

For example, in some countries contracts say 25% of the advance guarantee is due the producer by a certain date. But the producer needs to know about licenses to export monies from those countries. Without such licenses, the contract becomes invalid. The producer may not know that there are certain withholding taxes on certain kinds of distribution deals amounting to as much as 60–70%. He or she may not know that for a letter of credit to be paid in Israel, the Censor Board must first give approval. "Almost every country has some different loophole in which the average individual can go out and get killed," says Damon with a smile.

ATTENDING THE MARKETS

Nevertheless, there are always independent producers hustling at Cannes and MIFED, trying to sell foreign territories on their own. They may even be *forced* to act independently if no one else wants to sell their films. As a glance through *Variety*'s market issues indicates, they are out in force every year. These people are at a clear disadvantage because foreign sales are often a matter of established relationships and procedures. The leverage that De Laurentiis and Damon's PSO have is simple: continuity. They've lasted for years. The films they promise *are* delivered. They don't even have to go to festivals to make deals. They could simply bring foreign distributors to the U.S. or send prints to distribution offices in various countries. They may change distributors if they're unhappy with a territory's promotion or accounting, but generally they consolidate old relationships. As a producer, it would be bad form not to offer first option on a picture to the foreign distributor who took your last film.

But when independent producer Peter Locke of Vanguard Releasing took his first picture, *The Hills Have Eyes*, to Cannes for broad international release, he had to establish relationships with foreign distributors for the first time. In selling his $500,000 "axeploitation" thriller, Locke discovered that "certain people try to tie up a film for their territory for the life span of the convention. They promise you a contract soon, and then they announce they have the picture. That knocks out their competition. Then they sit back on their haunches and say, 'Maybe we'll take it or maybe we won't.' What that does is stop you from making contacts with other distributors in the territory."

"But once you learn that's part of the game, you learn that you need a deal to have a deal."

On his next picture, Locke is accepting a deal with a major for worldwide rights. Why? The major is guaranteeing him production money up front. For a one-picture producer like Locke, the convenience and security the majors provide is hard to pass up, even following some success with the independent foreign route.

USE YOUR ATTORNEY?

Francis Coppola resisted giving in to a major and, following the De Laurentiis model, put together financing for *Apocalypse Now* from multiple sources, including independent foreign distributors. With only limited experience, Coppola's attorney, Barry Hirsch, assembled what is reputed to be the largest pre-financing deal ever from foreign distribution. Attorney Hirsch points out that the great benefit of using foreign monies for pre-financing is the maintenance of creative control. For a filmmaker like Coppola, such freedom is essential. Of course, to pull this off, a producer needs the right ingredients to pre-sell territories. These ingredients are said to be as follows:

A concept that works for the international market. Loosely translated, that means action-adventure and three-handkerchief melodramas. American comedies and talky, sociological dramas are out, as are costume pictures and westerns.

An internationally known director or producer.

Internationally known stars. Charles Bronson or Clint Eastwood will do nicely. Sean Connery still commands a huge salary due to his international following.

Since *Apocalypse Now* satisfied all three criteria, Hirsch was able to raise the large budget, maintain creative control for his client, and avoid cross-collateralization. However, the problem of going it alone as Coppola did, armed only with an attorney and agent, is that there's no completion guarantee to cover production costs should they go over budget, as Coppola's did. The major studios at least act as completion guarantor when a producer gives them a film. If the film goes over budget, the studio puts up completion monies. They don't like it—they'll attach penalties to the producer and director for going over budget—but they'll put up the money.

However, if the producer has merely the monies raised from multiple sources of financing (domestic distribution, private investors, foreign rights, TV rights, video discs, and the other ancillary rights), and he hasn't sold the picture for more than the budget, he may run out of money. What then? He can take the letters of credit from the various territories and cash them at a bank.

Usually, the producer receives only 15–25% up front from the foreign distributor and the balance upon completion of principal photography and delivery. If the producer cashes that balance before time, he'll suffer the bank's discount. Not that it's ever that simple. Many banks won't back foreign letters of credit, regarding them as extremely high risk areas.

Of course, rewards in film financing are often proportionate to risks. Though Coppola may have mortgaged his house to obtain completion monies for *Apocalypse*, he and his attorney clearly felt the risks were worthwhile.

Another problem arises when producers try to collect overages from foreign distributors in all the territories where they made separate deals. According to attorney-CPA Jason Brent, foreign distributors have their own problems collecting the 25–70% of the box-office receipts that the exhibitors in their territories are supposed to hand over to them. "The foreign theatre owner won't pay the independent distributor," Brent says. "He'll sit on it for six months." And, according to Warner's Myron Karlin, many of the foreign distributors keep three sets of books.

How does one sue a company in Brazil if it doesn't pay? Even attorney Barry Hirsch knew of no examples of successful lawsuits against foreign distributors. The producer's only real leverage is the foreign distributor's desire for continuity of product.

Faced with this litany of problems, the independent producer may want to throw up his hands and simply turn his film over to a U.S. major for overseas distribution. At least *they* keep honest books, right? Don't you believe it.

Collecting overages from the majors isn't an easy feat. According to Jason Brent, "Some studios provide in their agreements that you can only audit the books and records that they keep in their home offices. But they don't get full, complete accountings. Universal, which is a part of CIC, gets input from CIC headquarters in Amsterdam. When you do the audit at Universal, the numbers they report to the profit participant agree with the numbers they get from CIC, that is, distributor's gross. But you have no way of looking at theatre box-office statements." Similarly, Paramount provides in its contract that only books and records maintained at their New York headquarters may be audited.

Accountants have found that the majors *do* fudge on the overages. One example concerns foreign taxes. Perhaps they have been placed in reserve but not been paid. Or perhaps foreign taxes were taken out of the net profits of *all* a major's pictures in one country. Then the accountant must determine what portion is fair for a particular picture.

Conversion rates are another problem. At the time a picture earns money in France, the franc might be worth 20 cents, but it may vary by 10% before the picture's release. Sometimes the majors take advantage of exchange rates by truncating the last seven digits for the computer, rather than rounding up or down. When you're dealing with millions in currency around the world, that little technique can add up to a considerable amount. Needless to say, the shortcuts will never be in favor of a profit participant. Still another way for the majors to "forget" about part of a producer's foreign overages is to use up blocked currency that should be credited to your film.

THE GOLDEN MEAN

This may be the best alternative of all. Rather than going entirely with a major or entirely independent, a producer can try the golden mean: that is, first sell off the major territories, then make a package deal with a major for the remainder of the world market, all those little territories in Latin America, Southeast Asia, the Far East, Eastern Europe and Russia, and so on. The major territories—Japan, Australia, Germany, Italy, the United Kingdom, and France—will probably yield in excess of 50% of the worldwide gross. The remainder can be laid off on an American major.

A cautionary word about one aspect of overseas distribution—advertising and marketing budgets. Promotion budgets frequently exceed production costs. United Artists' release *Lord of the Rings* had an initial promotional budget of $6.5-million and a production cost of $8-million, while *Invasion of the Body Snatchers*, handled by Maslansky-Koenigsberg for producer Robert Solo, had a promotional budget of $4.5-million—almost a third higher than its production budget of $3.5-million.

How does this affect foreign distribution? According to Sandy Howard, many independent producers forget to build adequate advertising expenditures into their budgets and are in for a rude awakening down the line. Howard admits that this was a fact that his organization didn't understand as recently as a few years ago. "Now when we talk to other independents who work in conjunction with us, we want to know where the advertising is going to come from. It's something independent producers must worry about. If you're with a major, they take care of it." Howard explains that in going independent for his foreign distribution, he had to become a mini-studio and have an advertising associate supply the same promotional materials to the foreign distributors that the major would supply, but at a fraction of the cost. It isn't simple.

But then, nothing is simple in foreign distribution. "In the older days, the world was still big, things were much slower," veteran sales rep Irvin Shapiro told *Variety*'s Stephen Klain. "That was a time when product could still be saved up for one big push at Cannes. Now it's much faster. You have to sell when the opportunity presents itself, even before, and for that you need constant communication and good organization."

That's the bottom line in foreign distribution. If an independent American producer doesn't have the means to organize and communicate worldwide, he or she might as well hand over distribution responsibilities to a major. But more and more, the international producers have insured buyers for their films by obtaining market by market guarantees to recoup production costs.

The lady or the tiger? Increasingly, independent American producers are finding foreign distribution to be quite an heiress.

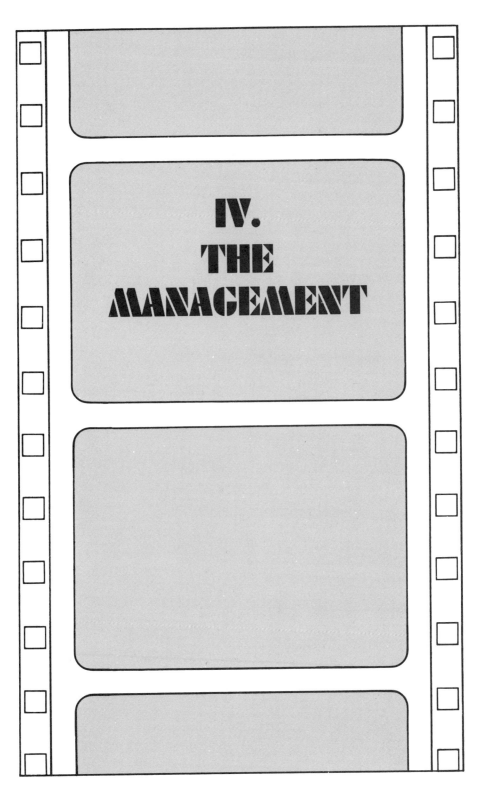

IV.
THE
MANAGEMENT

Management:
New Rules
of the Game

by **Richard Lederer,** a marketing consultant in the film industry, who has served as vice-president of worldwide marketing at American Cinema and as consultant to Francis Coppola's Zoetrope Studios in the areas of film marketing, advertising, and publicity. A 25-year veteran of motion pictures, Mr. Lederer was vice-president of worldwide advertising and publicity for Warner Brothers from 1960 to 1975, during which period he served for a year as a production executive at the Warner Brothers studio. He produced *The Hollywood Knights* for Columbia Pictures, co-produced with John Boorman *Exorcist II: The Heretic* for Warners, and has lectured widely in the field of motion pictures.

The industry is changing, but only to the extent that it always has throughout its history. It has never been static; it has always reacted in one way or another to new conditions. It has never stood still as a communication form or—to a lesser degree—as an art form.

Yet it is too easy to assume that some violent upheaval has taken place, that a new art form, a new "now" audience, and a whole new set of business rules are at hand. We must in fact observe that pictures made today—some of which are the most successful films in the history of the industry—are traditional in terms of their dramatic content. What has changed is the filmmakers' technique. New technology, such as high-speed film, very fast lenses, radio mikes, and portable cameras and lights, have given filmmakers the mobility to shoot a picture more realistically and with more visual excitement than ever before. Filmic storytelling can take advantage of an audience raised on television, and on television commercials in particular. This audience is comfortable with shortcuts in visual storytelling, allowing more information to be imparted in less time. Thus, movies move a little faster today and are more "cinematic" than they used to be, but the stories are essentially the same.

It should not detract from the expression of social concern or the aesthetic possibilities of film that major companies who have an economic interest in the business must continue to regard movies primarily as an escapist entertainment form. The management of these publicly owned companies must show a responsibility to shareholders and, consequently, to profit-and-loss statements. These are the realities a major studio must observe, and it therefore follows that they will be making pretty much the same kind of films they have always made. But this hardly implies that a slow evolution is not constantly in progress. Taste is more advanced and technique is more sophisticated than in the past. The nation has matured with regard to what it will accept and what it will tolerate in the arts and literature. Audiences have accepted, for example, a far more candid and explicit screen exploration of sexual relations. Essentially, however, the movies are simply dealing with human problems in a more realistic fashion, and the degree of realism and detail should not suggest a trend away from the basic escapist entertainment appeals.

We must not confuse, however, *what* is made with *how* it is made. Having said, in effect, that there is a great deal of stability in the fundamental nature of movies, I must now turn to the factors that set motion pictures apart from other businesses. One of the greatest of these is the uncertainty of the marketplace. Many other industries have accurate indications of their market when they set out each year. The home appliance industry can judge its potential sales and make sound business decisions regarding refrigerator styles, models and the number of units to manufacture. Unfortunately, the movie business has not enjoyed that degree of predictability in over 30 years. Before the Consent Decree, a major company owned its own theatres and consequently knew where its marketplace was. It knew how many films it could make a year and that those films would be exhibited in regular fashion. There are old-time exhibitors today who privately confess their wish that the legal action which forced the split of production companies and theatres should never have been taken; one important consequence was the lack of orderly production at any of the studios. (See footnote, p. 105.) Since the studios no longer knew with certainty where the market was—and whether their films would indeed get booked—they were unable to make judgments about how many films to make and how much money to commit to production. The number of films made fell off drastically.

A second major factor that distinguishes motion pictures from all other businesses arises from the enormous impact of individual creative talent upon production cost and upon market success. Evaluation of what the audience will accept is difficult at best and impossible at worst. This is a major aspect of the "old game," and new rules are not really changing it. The only business that comes rather close to it, I should think, is fashion, where trying to judge what styles will sell next year—how to tailor an inventory, how much cloth to buy, how much to cut, and so forth—is a bit of a guessing game. But movies are the super, number-one guessing game. Making movies, as one old-timer put it, is "not an industry, but a disease."

Let's consider the role of talent in this game. Ultimately, movies are a product, and the product comes in a package that can be more important than what it contains. The package can be more or less attractive, depending on the names that are associated with it. A producer who has a fairly good action script, for example, can make the film for $9-million with a good actor and $10-million with a top actor. That extra cost is something he must think about in terms of actual return. Is it worth the extra million? Will the film do that much more in business as a result of overinvestment in the top actor? There are, after all, only a few actors who seem capable of delivering a larger audience than the ordinary actor, and a good deal of that happens overseas. It is a fact that a good action adventure with one of five particular names attached to it will do 40% more business outside the United States than the same picture without one of those names. It is in this type of film that the industry seems willing to spend extra money for one of the "superactors." Clint Eastwood, Robert Redford, and Burt Reynolds are included on the list. Escapist entertainment is still the major attraction around the world, and although the "star system" is supposed to be on the wane in America, many a picture is made only because a certain actor will commit to do it.

To some degree, the contemporary audience dictates the type of film Hollywood will produce. It is sad but true that movies have always been an imitative—not an innovative—industry. Miscalculation abounds. Everyone reads the new demographics and learns that we have a young audience. Their immediate reaction is to plan and make films that are geared to the tastes and interests of young people. This in turn results in all kinds of unsuccessful films. It has always been that way, and I don't suspect it will ever change. Ten years ago, the most frequent moviegoers ranged in age from 15 to 25 years; then there was a sharp drop around age 28 due to marriage and the raising of children. After age 35, people went to the movies infrequently. Today, the 15–25 age group continues to attend movies on a regular basis, and yesterday's young audience, which is now 25 to 35 years old, continues its movie-going habit, with much less of a falling off due to raising families. (See audience statistics, p. 357.)

There is a new phenomenon contributed by this young generation of moviegoers: the capacity for repeat business, which is extraordinary. Repeat business is the key to the huge success of such pictures as *Star Wars*, *The Empire Strikes Back*, *Superman II*, *Airplane*, *Raiders of the Lost Ark*, and *E.T.* Proceeds from these pictures have redefined the higher limits of profit potential, and new pictures are constantly challenging those heights.

It is a fact that people in the industry, in their frantic efforts to analyze audience desires, deny the history of movie entertainment as well as their own instincts by jumping on the topical bandwagon. Management's alternative, if there is any single approach to planning successful pictures, is to try to make interesting films without regard, necessarily, to whether they really are geared to a certain type of audience. A major studio committed to doing 10 to 15 films a year should be trying to make marvelous stories—films that are interesting, different, special. Films need not necessarily be offbeat or entirely youth-oriented. If a classic Hitchcock-style thriller came along, well directed and with a tight story, it would be a tremendous success. Even if I knew it wouldn't be ready for a year, I'd bank on it.

The evidence is there. Successful films have always been well-directed, well-written, well-made films about something that a majority of the people can relate to or empathize with. But this does not mean management should avoid taking risks on what is new, fresh, and has a specialized appeal. In 1970, when I was at Warner Brothers, *Woodstock* was a gamble that worked for us. When we first committed to making the film, no one believed it would be as successful as it ultimately became. We took pride in the fact that at least two of us in the company sensed that something special was going to happen at that place. We didn't know what it was going to be. No one thought the event would take on the significance—the aura—that it did, and, of course, we hardly realized how accomplished Michael Wadleigh would be as director. His brilliant concepts about editing the film and using multiple images were unknowns, ideas too difficult to foresee at that time. We made a good, educated guess. But I also consider it to be an accident in a sense, one we cannot learn much from.

Miscalculations are possible, of course, under the best of circumstances, but I think they are even more likely to occur because of new industry developments such as the controls upon management that conglomerate takeovers introduce. In such cases, there are predictable changes, and my guess is that they usually are for the worst. We must remember that until a few years ago, the industry was still in the hands of the so-called pioneers. Good, bad, or indifferent, right or wrong, they were a unique breed in American business life. Their backgrounds were dissimilar. None of them came out of film schools. Many were immigrants, barely teenagers when they arrived in this country. With no academic training, they went into various businesses and happened to be around when movies were born. All had an innate sense of showmanship, an instinct about this country, and a prescience about the entertainment that movies would become.

These were very special people. When their kind passed on, new management or ownership replaced them, and some significant things happened. In nearly every case where the new management was a conglomerate, the company became overly business-oriented. This new breed, in the best American tradition, was made up of well-trained business-management graduates who were used to systematized and highly structured business organizations. They knew everything on the business side of how to run a company. After one look at a movie company, they found it to be amorphous and seemingly running amok.

They were aghast. Their strict sense of business training was offended, and their impulse was to systematize and structure, to make the company, in their terms, "make sense." This often led to near disaster.

It should be pointed out, however, that whatever problems "new management" had and still has in trying to fathom the mysteries of production and in developing systems that are functional, it has had extraordinary success in revolutionizing the art of film distribution. Correctly identifying the movie market as a mass market (in most cases), it moved aggressively into the area of network television advertising with heavy print and radio support. Management capitalized on this gigantic ad expenditure by having anywhere from 500 to 1,000 or more prints of the movie playing simultaneously around the country. This was not as simple as it sounds. Exhibitors who traditionally demanded and received exclusivity in major markets had to be persuaded to allow their competitors to share in the release pattern. Huge advertising budgets, which often exceeded the negative cost of the picture itself, had to be approved. The same applied to the heavy cost of release prints. This is just one example of the change in marketing technique brought about by modern management, and the results are encouraging. Successful films today are achieving film rental returns never dreamed of only a decade ago.

The old-timers were born gamblers; the new people are forced into being gamblers, and they're uncomfortable with it. They're businessmen, and no good businessman likes to gamble; rather, they like to insure their bets whenever possible. But "insurance" like high-priced stars or high-priced directors can be disastrous, as in *Sorceror* or *Heaven's Gate*.

There is an interesting cycle in management that has repeated itself recently in the movie business. It occurs when a new generation of production executives takes over a studio. They are usually somewhat unfamiliar with certain phases of the business, particularly marketing and distribution. They approach their head of sales or marketing and ask how many movies should be made this year. The answer is "If you make six successful pictures, that's all the playing time I can handle; if you make twenty failures, I haven't got enough." The insecurity that runs through this new generation of studio executives stems not from deciding what pictures to make, but how many. Because of the powerful impulse to make movies, they reach for material a more conservative management might turn down, either due to story content or the high numbers involved. But they are hungry to make movies, so they make risky, innovative decisions. In the three years it takes from making the decisions to tracking the results at the box office, this generation of studio executives usually has some phenomenal hits on its hands; the gambles have paid off. But, they are also watching some of their profits dissipate because hefty participations were built into certain artists' deals on these pictures. This executive team is now rich and successful; they're no longer the gamblers they were three years earlier. They may even begin to think they know what they're doing, which is a terrible mistake in this business. They start making tougher deals, minimizing outside participations in order to protect their profits. They're not hungry any more.

At this point, another group of new production executives takes over another studio, and they are as hungry as the first group was three years ago. An agent approaches the first group with a strong package, asking high fees and participations for his or her clients in the package. The first company refuses to make such a rich deal, so the agent goes across the street to the second studio, makes a deal with the eager executives, and the cycle goes on. Interestingly, studios that have been forced to gamble on material out of desperation or need have generally been successful. Intuition and luck play enormous roles in the business.

Unfortunately, movies are not a business in the strict sense of the word. Studios demand unique talent and unique understanding if they are to be run effectively. The successful major motion picture studio of the future will be one that manages the following: (1) a reorganization of its outdated physical structure to bring production overheads down to reasonable scales; (2) the development within its creative manpower of a "sure nose" for potential motion picture material; (3) the ability and know-how to attract the proper talent in the industry to these various projects; (4) the diplomatic skill needed to cope understandingly with the creative temperaments and excesses of these gifted producers, directors, writers, and stars while at the same time imposing upon them realistic and responsible fiscal controls. Utopia? Maybe. Admittedly, a nearly impossible set of conditions—but there are clear signs that management is slowly meeting this challenge.

Film Company
Management

by **Gordon Stulberg,** president and chief executive officer of Polygram Corporation, in charge of Polygram Group's American operations, including Polygram Pictures. Formerly a partner in the west coast law firm of Mitchell, Silberberg and Knupp, he is a member of the New York and California Bars. In 1971, Mr. Stulberg was named president and chief operating officer of Twentieth Century–Fox Film Corporation, after serving as president of Cinema Center Films, the theatrical film division of the Columbia Broadcasting System, from 1967 to 1971. Before joining Cinema Center Films, he was vice president and chief administration officer at Columbia Pictures.

. . . . it took some courage and faith on the agents' part to sell their clients to us for films and for packages when they might have gotten the same deals with more traditional companies. . . .

In the mid-1960s, the Columbia Broadcasting System began to consider the possibility of establishing a division devoted to the production and distribution of motion pictures. In 1967, after considerable research, Cinema Center Films was formed for that purpose, and the author was invited to develop the new division.

The précis that was prepared at the time outlined certain basic courses to pursue.

First, it was recommended that Cinema Center Films not own or operate a studio but rather rent studio space when necessary. Since the network owns CBS Studio Center in Studio City, California, it was assumed that the new division could utilize it for in-studio production. In the same context, it was also recommended that we should not attempt to develop a global distribution company but instead engage specialized executives who would supervise distribution. If such a group chose the most knowledgeable and experienced local distributors in all territories in the world and made deals with them, it was reasoned, there would be no major continuing annual overhead for distribution. The supervisory executives would plan the pattern of release, arrange the terms, and let the local distributor actually execute sales policy.

Finally, it was suggested that a company with limited production, distribution, and advertising operations should not attempt to supervise more than 10 films in a year. It was estimated that the average negative cost would be in the area of $3-million, and the cost history of the first 22 pictures confirmed the accuracy of the estimate. Negative cost actually averaged $2,960,000. We intended to enter the market with a desire to finance the kind of picture that would let the industry know we were serious and to test out long-held theories with respect to the elimination of large-scale fixed overhead in production and distribution. We also hoped to apply some of the more sophisticated management and financial tools that for too long had been ignored by the industry.

We began, in May 1967, adding executives somewhat more rapidly at the production level than at distribution. We moved slowly, however, bearing in mind that we were going to have only a skeleton production operation and would deal mostly with independent producers. We developed a small nucleus of highly motivated production, distribution, and sales and advertising executives. We opened sales and advertising offices in New York and a production office and a European sales and advertising department in London. Then, we engaged representatives to supervise at the local level distributors in such major territories as Japan, Italy, France, West Germany, Spain, and Australia-New Zealand (as a combined entity). The key distribution executives who were first brought in made agreements with distributors throughout the world. For United States and Canadian distribution, we turned to National General Corporation, which had formed a company to distribute the pictures they were producing.

Essentially, that was the organizational history of the company. The tradition of CBS has always been to see their ventures through, and it backed us in whatever project we felt had economic viability. This included giving permission to build up an inventory of unproduced material in full knowledge that on the basis of industry experience, two-thirds of it ultimately would have to be written off as abandoned material.

Several major business problems confronted us almost from the outset. First, we were entering at the top of the seller's market, just about the time that the million-dollar player was becoming fashionable. Everyone was scrambling for Paul Newman and Steve McQueen. If we were to become a viable company, we were going to have to meet, but not exceed, prices then being established by every company in town. That was a major problem at the time because we had to translate those prices to CBS in terms of investment.

Second, in light of the number of buyers in the market in those years, the agents—with the notable exception of the William Morris Agency—were somewhat reluctant to break their traditional lines of communication in order to deal with us. Our legal status was apparently still under examination by the Justice Department, and we had not really announced our plans for worldwide distribution. So it took some courage and faith on the agents' part to sell their clients to us for films and for packages when they might have gotten the same deals with more traditional companies. We were very thankful that the William Morris office led off in that direction; the first major deal we made was with Jack Lemmon. After that, we used Steve McQueen and others of his stature and established our credibility as a major film company.

Our next major decision involved selection of a U.S. distributor. We could have set up a distribution system of our own, to which we were opposed from the outset. We could have gone with a major distributor, which was not advisable because the majors were then making

20 to 25 pictures of their own each year, and we did not want our product lost among their films. The only logical choice, then, was to go with an independent distributor. Among available companies were the "states righters"—companies that handled franchise product from American International, whose background and tradition then was to sell exploitation pictures. There were also a few companies with five or six exchanges operating out of New York, but these would have had to expand operations to handle the type of pictures we were going to make. And then there were National General Corporation and Cinerama. Since the latter already had a contract with ABC Pictures and was therefore unavailable, we engaged National General. We were aware, of course, that NGC managed a theatre operation intelligently. We felt that since NGC was going into distribution, it would know whom to hire. Their own theatre managers and their corporate management would tell them who were the best distributor salesmen in the various regions, and those were the men NGC would be going after as they set up their own distribution company. In effect, then, we were buying their expertise with regard to the kind of salesmen who could best sell our films.

Nor did we have to make any guarantees to NGC. We did state at the outset that we planned to feed only about 10 films a year into the market, somewhat fewer than a major would offer. We helped them ease this problem by offering a deal in which the percentage of the gross that NGC collected for its distribution fee would be larger at the front end and then would, on an annual basis, drop down as more product was introduced. In other words, even though we might give NGC only two or three pictures, the distribution fee on those would be high enough to help defray a reasonable proportion of the expenses of their distribution organization. Then, of course, if we supplied more, the incremental cost of servicing additional pictures would not be as much. For our purposes, if we produced for distribution even a reasonable number of pictures—fewer than ten, but perhaps five or six—our distribution cost would be far less than it would have been had we gone with one of the major distributors. There would really be no basis for comparison.

It would be well at this point to dwell on those general decisions that can have great influence upon whether a company turns a profit or not. This is, after all, an all-encompassing concern of management. My entire experience in the motion picture business convinced me that our company was not going to survive without some great fiscal orthodoxy and some more imaginative approaches to controls in the field of sales, advertising, and production, and indeed in our relationship to CBS, a highly sophisticated financial operation. Even the most imaginative managerial techniques, however, must be grounded in the hard facts of our business. We must know how our various pictures are doing around the world before we can develop those cost-control patterns that could be applied not only to a specific picture at a given time, but to the entire annual output as it affects—or is affected by—the success or failure of that single picture.

Such knowledge came to us first through NGC, which gave us a weekly report of domestic film rentals. Similarly, each local distributor in a foreign country reported distribution income either to our local representative in the territory or directly to London or New York. The major territories reported on a weekly basis and the smaller territories bi-weekly or monthly. Major territories included Japan, the United Kingdom, France, Italy, and West Germany. Reports came in as quickly as the local distributor could send them on. Thus we had a fair estimate every week of how our pictures were doing all over the world—an important body of information with which we began "tracking" our successes and failures.

As tracking began, we could read early warning signs. If the picture opened poorly, we were in difficulty; it is a rare picture that opens badly and then builds. This building has become even less possible in recent years simply because more people are going to theatres as a result of word-of-mouth publicity. If word-of-mouth on a picture is not good when it opens, it is unlikely that it will improve.

Once a typical picture has played for from four to eight weeks, the dimensions of the problems or the prospects are clear. The tracking procedure then helped us to deal with the upside or downside limits. Any picture, for example, could open big in New York and then let down badly everywhere else in the country. Still, if we opened exclusively in New York, Los Angeles, Washington, Dallas—say seven or eight geographic areas—and uniformly performed either very well or very badly in the earliest weeks, we knew a great deal about what would happen elsewhere.

The guessing process with respect to "estimates" would then begin, particularly once we reported to CBS on revisions in full-year budgets on a monthly basis. We would track the picture as to its future opening both here and in foreign, since what happens abroad is a key factor. Sometimes the difference between success and failure lies in foreign reaction. And unlike domestic tracking, where eight or nine local engagements may tell the story, the foreign projection must wait until reactions from at least three or five major territories have been reported—Italy, Japan, West Germany, France, and the U.K. We may do spectacularly well in Japan and fail elsewhere—or succeed in Japan and Italy and fail in the U.K., France, and West Germany—and still wind up in the red. If the picture is strong enough to become a runaway success in four out of five of these territories (as did *A Man Called*

Horse, for example), you have a successful picture abroad. Then we would begin to track on a basis of comparison with other pictures that have played those territories at approximately the same time of year, in the same theatres, and under similar terms. That is how, by using a historical track, we could come up with an estimate of what a picture ultimately would do.

One might ask, where did all the financial controls fit in? If everything is boom or bust, why were we so preoccupied with management skills and techniques in controlling sales? The answer is that skilled financial management applied to three out of every ten pictures made can minimize the effect of boom or bust. What was important was to concentrate upon the fact that there were pictures whose losses could be dramatically minimized and pictures whose gains could also be maximized.

If the difference between being in the red or the black on an annual divisional accounting could turn on a swing of as little as $100,000 a picture, management asked itself, What factors in handling each film could we control so as to effect the divisional statement in this manner? Where could we save costs or stimulate the added business that could so impact the P & L statement?

First, we kept our annual operating overhead under constant scrutiny. The number of people kept on the production, sales, and advertising staffs on a year-round basis was often reviewed. Since we attributed a portion of our annual costs to each picture, the smaller that portion was, the less, in the aggregate, the total cost of the film would be.

Next, we examined our pre-production and preparation costs. How much is spent on development deals? If we assumed that over half of development money never results in a picture, then obviously we had to do as much as we could to avoid this expense and more aggressively seek "packages." If a script, a budget, and a producer already exist, the chances of a film's not being made are reduced. Our business affairs department kept close track of the costs of acquiring and developing material and expressed these costs as incurred rather than permitting them to be carried in inventory. In addition, we would submit a budget for development expenses in advance of each year and require production to track its costs against that budget every month.

Another area of cost protection was found in the constant review of spending on the picture while in production. We exerted pressure to budget realistically in advance to keep cast costs down, to reduce location moves, and eliminate "protection" personnel and equipment. The same thing was true in the post–principal photography stage. The longer we held onto the picture while it was being edited, the longer we had to pay interest. The sooner we got the film into release, the sooner we returned our investment, and the less the interest charges against capital we had frozen in production.

Assume that the trimming of production, post–principal photography, and project development costs on any picture saved $100,000. Multiply that by seven or eight pictures, and we were suddenly considering a $750,000 item in our annual profit-and-loss statement.

Management can also initiate savings in the sales area, especially in terms of advertising dollar commitments. An early decision to foreclose advertising if it looks as if the picture is not going to perform can save a great deal. Shifting media expenditures or trimming the size of the advertising buy if it looks as though the picture is going soft can effect real savings. In this connection, we insisted that *advertising is a function of sales* and that the amount of expenditures must be directly responsive to sales estimates of the potential revenue from any engagement.

Finally, we tried to negotiate better distribution deals as we went along. We tried to neutralize the exhibitor's bargaining strengths by negotiating for advantages that would ultimately keep more of the theatrical income in the hands of the financing-distribution companies. Until 1948, the exhibitor was also the distributor, and the contract between exhibition and distribution was just a matter of bookkeeping. Since divorcement, however, we have had to establish arm's-length negotiations between distributor and theatre owner, and we must continue to rid the industry of practices that grew up when the left hand was negotiating with the right hand.

Nearly every criterion we established for viability at Cinema Center has been adopted by almost every major company in the last several years. They have eliminated the studio; they have tried to eliminate large production staffs; they have sought as small a distribution overhead as possible; and they have contracted advertising campaigns out—which we did from the start—thereby eliminating an in-house advertising overhead ranging in the millions of dollars.

Since the closing of the company in 1972, I have looked back with satisfaction on the subsequent life of the Cinema Center product. Those 32 films, I have been advised, have been evaluated in the current marketplace at well over one hundred million dollars for their network and syndication uses alone, so that the latent economic value to CBS for the 32 negatives is quite extraordinary.*

When I was asked in 1971 to become president of Fox, it was a good opportunity to take the Cinema Center experiment one step further by utilizing my prior experience to plan and execute fundamental changes in a traditional motion picture studio. The single most impor-

---

* Editor's Note: In 1979, CBS returned to the big-screen market by establishing CBS Theatrical Films.

tant step was to convert the studio into a profit center, as an independent rental studio, which is now how the Burbank Studios acts on behalf of Warners and Columbia. The idea was to eliminate the studio as part of the operating overhead chargeable against the feature and television operations; let it run itself as a profit center and have the production operations rent from it. The immediate result was to free the studio from the grip of the theatrical production office, which was putting holds on stages that were never utilized. We soon welcomed long-term renters to the lot, such as Spelling/Goldberg and the ABC Circle Theatre.

The next important step was to merge production and distribution into the same facility. At the time, the distribution operation was based in New York, along with those of the other majors. Since the distance and time change reduced communication, I decided to move the entire marketing operation base to the Los Angeles studio, close to our production personnel. Since then, other majors have followed suit.

The third step was to reduce the cost and extent of the overseas distribution network. I had learned from Cinema Center that it was possible to produce large film rentals from foreign territories without a vast foreign sales organization. I sat down with the head of foreign distribution, David Raphel, a bright, progressive, and knowledgeable executive, and developed a plan to reduce our overhead by working through subdistributors in less lucrative areas. For example, in Japan we maintained our staff in the top six cities, but decided to subdistribute through Towa in the provinces. In Italy we maintained our presence in Rome, but turned to subs in regional exchanges. This reduced costs substantially. In Canada, we went out of business and made a deal with a subdistributor; in the years I was at Fox, we grossed more in Canada with a sub than we had with our own distribution company. In some other territories we joined with other American majors to share distribution, among them Columbia and Warner Brothers.

What was accomplished by reorganizing foreign distribution was to change, in large measure, from a fixed to a variable overhead. While we had previously maintained full-time worldwide operations at a staggering annual overhead cost, we were now charged by a subdistributor for 15 or 20% of our gross on specific films producing revenue in certain territories at certain times. We were now paying specific overhead for the actual product serviced. A second value of this approach was to avoid labor costs, which were inflating all over the world. If we had maintained a fixed organization, we would have had to bear these increased costs. A subdistributor got paid on the basis of our volume and was responsible himself for foreign labor increases, like the massive ones of the mid-1970s in countries such as Italy and Japan.

Next, it was important to turn to attracting filmmakers, since their work is the lifeblood of the business. When Mel Brooks had *Young Frankenstein* at Columbia and they did not want to make it because of the budget figure, we invited him and the result was a multiple-picture deal. Paul Mazursky and *Harry and Tonto* were brought to Fox after that project had been turned down at other studios. In 1973, we bought *Star Wars* after Universal declined, although they had first call on the material resulting from their distribution of *American Graffiti*. If there are any lessons here, they are to avoid trends, to try to be first in the marketplace with a fresh, inventive project, and to have the courage of your convictions (as we did with *Poseidon Adventure,* the first of the large "disaster" pictures).

There is one very interesting element that characterizes the business recently: the gradual elimination of the downside risk in films. Fifteen years ago, it was possible to make a picture for $3,000,000 and lose the entire investment because ancillary rights were unimportant. Today, on a picture costing $8,000,000, a large return on that investment is possible from nontheatrical distribution sources alone from the "ancillary rights." For instance, pay-television rights can be sold for $850,000, based on 10 cents or more for each of the 8,500,000 or more pay-TV terminals available around the country, with upward escalation based on the strength of the picture in the theatrical market. Network television sales, which produced revenue for an average feature ten years ago of about $500,000 for two runs, can now pay as much as $10,000,000 or more for two runs. Television syndication rights domestically and around the world have escalated over the years. After the syndicator is paid for selling the picture and residuals are paid to people in the film, it's possible to produce net revenue against the picture of $300,000 to $800,000. Sales to airlines for showings in-flight can deliver between $60,000 and $150,000 per picture. Navy sales, covering one branch of the military, can produce from $25,000 to $60,000 in revenue. Sixteen-millimeter sales to colleges can be important, as well. *Little Big Man* grossed over $1,000,000 in college rentals alone. Motion picture soundtrack albums and singles can mean huge revenues, as proven by *Saturday Night Fever* and *Grease.* Once a successful song is established, the ASCAP or BMI performance revenues increase. There is also a lot of money to be made in the exploitation of book-publishing rights in the form of novelizations of screenplays, picture books, calendars, or reprints. Merchandising is also a lucrative ancillary right. Because all of this potential income from non-motion picture sources adds up, it becomes clear that revenue from ancillary rights can produce a figure covering half or more of the entire $8,000,000 production cost. To this extent, the "risk capital" flowing into the movie industry is not as risky as it once was.

The Film Company as Financier-Distributor

by **David V. Picker,** an independent producer who has served as a top-level motion picture executive for years. A graduate of Dartmouth, Mr. Picker held various executive positions at United Artists Corporation before being named president and chief executive officer of UA in 1969. Later, after a period of producing pictures independently, he was appointed vice-chairman of Paramount Pictures Corporation and president of the motion picture division in 1976. Mr. Picker resumed his producing career before being named executive vice-president of Lorimar Productions in 1979, a post he held until 1981. Among his production credits are *Lenny, Smile, The One and Only, Oliver's Story, Bloodline, The Jerk, Dead Men Don't Wear Plaid,* and *The Man With Two Brains.*

Since 1950, the major studios established in earlier years have had to seek new roles and functions for themselves within a changing industry. United Artists created what may in many ways be regarded as a blueprint for film companies that sought to combine an already-existing enterprise with the skills of successful financing and distributing of motion pictures.

In order to understand how this new identity was established, we need to begin when Arthur Krim and Robert Benjamin bought control of United Artists from Charles Chaplin and Mary Pickford in 1951. The company had been losing money. But by late 1952, United Artists was in the black, and Krim and Benjamin were in a position to consider financing their own productions. Their plan was to finance pictures by dealing directly with the creative forces who make them. Their initial concept involved the extension of creative autonomy and a percentage of profits to the filmmaker. The company's interest was to secure all distribution rights and a share of the profit in the film. This *modus operandi* clearly was contradictory to the policy of the major studios that owned all their films and—by keeping editing powers to themselves—did not relinquish creative control to individual filmmakers.

This idea could not be given any real test, of course, until United Artists built a strong financial base. But as a result of a succession of good pictures, the concept that Krim and Benjamin had initiated became a way of life for the company. Such early successes as *High Noon, The African Queen,* and *Moulin Rouge* resulted from deals with filmmakers. By the mid-1950s, they had also initiated production programs with various film companies, one of which was Hecht-Hill-Lancaster, and this resulted in such remarkable films as the Academy Award–winning *Marty, Trapeze,* and *Sweet Smell of Success.* Later, they established a relationship with the Mirisch Company that lasted some 60 pictures.

Throughout its history, the management of United Artists gave creative filmmakers the right—within various approved frameworks of budget, script, cast, and director—to make films as they wanted to make them. In exchange for that right, which was revolutionary for Hollywood, UA was able to attract many of the top filmmakers in the world.

Other companies eventually caught on because there was nothing essentially unique in what UA offered, with the exception of its own management techniques. The Krim-Benjamin philosophy of extending creative freedom to the filmmaker in 1952 led to the general industry approach of today.

It may be informative to consider in some detail the way this philosophy has been translated into operational realities for other financier-distributors. We can usefully examine what happens to a dollar that comes in at the theatre box-office window, following its course backward from there in order to see how a company makes its money.

Let us assume that the financier-distributor has arranged a 50% deal with the theatre, which means that half of each dollar is retained by the exhibitor and half is turned over to the distributor of the film. That company does not share in the receipts from concessions in the theatre, which are exclusively the exhibitor's (see "Refreshment Sales and Theatre Profits" by Philip M. Lowe, p. 343). The $.50 that comes to the distributor represents 100% of *film rental*. When a picture has "done $20-million," that does not mean its box-office gross is $20-million, but that the film rental earned by the distributor is $20-million. The figure in fact represents, depending on various deals in various theatres throughout the world, the sum that comes to the financier-distributor.

A percentage of this money is charged for distributing the film: 30% of the gross for the United States and Canada, more overseas. Out of each dollar of film rental paid to the distributor domestically, $.30 is retained as its distribution fee. In addition, distribution costs are deducted, including prints, advertising, and interest as well as other expenses. From the "film rental dollar" then, $.30 is taken as distribution cost and another $.20 is taken to cover prints, advertising, interest, taxes, and distribution expenses. (These figures are approximate.) What is left is known as the *net producer's share*, which is used to pay off the loan secured to fund the negative cost of the picture. If a picture costs $10-million to finance and distribute, then the $.50 returns that constitute the net producer's share must add up to $10-million, before the picture theoretically has broken even.

At this point, all profits are split between the financier-distributor and producer on a basis that can vary from 50/50 to 80/20, usually favoring the financier, and depending upon bargaining power. Because of the great delay in reaching profits (if any), many more "gross deals" are being made, wherein gross participants get money "off the top," without any concern for what the actual profits are. Various formulas may find a director or star receiving a percentage of the gross from first dollar, a percentage of the gross after an agreed-upon, fixed break-even formula is reached (but before profits are divided), or a percentage of the gross after a multiple of the negative cost is reached. In these cases, "gross" is the distributor's film rental, not the theatre gross. For example, a certain actor might be given $200,000 cash against 10% of the gross. If the film rental on the picture totals $8-million, that actor will have received $200,000 in advance against the total $800,000 he will earn on the film without regard to distribution costs, prints, advertising, or any other costs. A *percentage of the gross* deal, it might well be said, is a favorable deal if a picture does well.

If the net producer's share always equals the cost of the film, then there are never any loss pictures. Of course, it does not always work out that way. Some pictures make a lot of money, and a lot of pictures make no money. Where does the distribution/financing company look for money to repay loans if films cannot gross enough? The only available source is the distribution fee. They get 30% of the gross as the distribution fee and have to maintain their business with proceeds from that. Some measure of profit also has to be built into that 30% simply to assure survival. They have to use the profit built into that distribution fee to pay off bank loans on pictures that do not independently earn money.

To summarize: If the entire net producer's share equals the amount of overall production risk, the company is in good shape. If it falls short, and losses can be recouped from the distribution fee without threatening a basic financial position strong enough to carry on the organization, then they are also in good shape. Where they can get into trouble is with a motion picture that costs a great deal of money and grosses nothing at all. This is why it is so dangerous for any company to sink an enormous amount of money into one picture. If the picture fails, they not only have lost the distribution fee that keeps their establishment going but also have no distribution fee profit to pay off the loan against the picture. And, of course, they lose the net producer's share as well.

In 1967, Transamerica Corporation acquired UA in an effort to diversify into the leisure-time field, just as Gulf + Western had acquired Paramount a few years before. The move gave United Artists an umbrella of enormous importance, since it was now part of a corporation with over a billion dollars in assets. With the advent of non-movie corporate management, the gap between executive and filmmaker and between corporation and filmmaker became increasingly wide. In the case of the Krim and Benjamin team, certain policies set down by the parent company were so unsettling that, in 1978, they left United Artists and established Orion Pictures Company, releasing product through Warner Brothers.* In the following year, the management team led by Alan Ladd, Jr. similarly left Twentieth Century–Fox and set up shop as The Ladd Company, also releasing through Warners. Filmmakers are attracted to these mini-majors because they get to deal directly with a small group of creative executives rather than the large-staff studio operation.

It's a seller's market, and because of this there are no longer any deal terms that are sacrosanct. If a seller has a project that is in demand, companies such as Columbia, Paramount, and Fox can step up to competitive deals. Issues such as overhead, viewing of dailies, final cut, and the net profits definition can favor the seller if his project is desirable. Bargaining power decreases if the project is something the financier-distributor would be willing to develop on a less-competitive basis. In this case, the seller will face tougher terms and definitions.

A producer faces the same basic dilemma that confronts any financier or distributor. What an audience is going to want to see, how they will respond to a given motion picture, and all the variables that take place while a picture is in production—these factors are beyond analysis. One difficulty in this regard is the lag between the time the decision is made to finance a script or go into production and the time the picture is released. In addition, there has been a polarization in taste. In practice, this means that the successful picture is more successful than ever, but the unsuccessful picture is more unsuccessful. There used to be a base audience; you knew you could count on certain numbers for almost every picture. That audience simply does not exist anymore. How can we know that the $8-million that is going to be spent is being invested in a product the mass audience will want to see a year hence?

In closing, I might say that we are in a time that is more precarious, but at the same time more exciting, than ever before. Audiences are extremely unpredictable, and their decisions often have nothing to do with a film's merit. When millions are being risked in an effort to choose those few pictures that audiences will decide to see, it can become a pretty scary business. The trouble with our business is that nobody trusts anybody in it. The distributor doesn't trust the ex

---

* Editor's Note: United Artists was acquired by MGM Film Company from Transamerica in July, 1981, and later the combined entity was renamed MGM/UA Entertainment Company. In early 1982, the principals of Orion Pictures joined with other investors to take over Filmways (formerly American International Pictures), including the company's distribution organization, film library, and TV production operation.

hibitor. The exhibitor doesn't trust the distributor. The producer doesn't trust the creator. The creator is sure the distributor is putting in invalid charges against his picture. The financier is positive that the creator has spent 43 unnecessary days in shooting the picture. Despite all this, somehow or other, we wind up with films that people sometimes go to see.

Studio Operations

by **Roger L. Mayer,** vice-president in charge of administration for Metro-Goldwyn-Mayer Inc. (now MGM/UA) since March, 1975, and executive vice-president in charge of MGM Laboratories since January, 1974, joined the company in 1961 as assistant general manager of MGM Studios. He later served as both vice-president in charge of MGM Laboratories and assistant secretary of the corporation. Before joining Metro, he was an attorney for Columbia Pictures from 1952 to 1957 and a corporate executive there from 1957 to 1961. He is a graduate of Yale University and Yale Law School and has been both trustee and chairman of the Directors Guild and Producers Guild pension plans.

MGM studio facilities in Culver City include 24 working sound stages and extensive pre-production and post-production facilities, such as a full motion picture production and release laboratory. In the 1930s and '40s, on a given day, the MGM plant population would consist of a large number of writers, directors, and producers on year-round weekly salaries. They would be working on stories for a production schedule of between 30 and 50 features a year. A great volume of scripts would be turned out from which the material for production would be selected. There would be four to six pictures in active production, involved in budgeting, location scouting, scheduling, and casting. Another three to six would be in actual photography. Six to fifteen films would be in post-production, including editing, rerecording, and scoring.

Most exteriors of theatrical motion pictures are now shot on the actual location of the story. Consequently, the use of studio stages for exteriors is variable because of the emphasis on using locations. This does not mean that studios are not used on occasion, particularly for films of a period nature or with special physical effects in them. A typical day currently, in contrast to the one described in the 1930s or '40s, would show at least half of the stages being used for photography and several stages being prepared through construction for future use. Unless a company immediately needs to use a particular stage, the tendency is to leave the set standing after a production has finished with it. Construction costs are so high that television films cannot be made economically unless they use a set that is already built or build a set and reuse it often in other shows. The cost of building the reused sets can then be *amortized,* or spread over many episodes. For example, if a series calls for the construction of a $50,000 interior set, and it runs for twenty episodes, each episode would be charged $2,500 for that set; the $50,000 figure would be amortized or spread over the set's useful life of twenty episodes, rather than having one $50,000 cost in the first episode.

All the studios that are considered part of today's Hollywood (though Burbank and Universal City are located in the San Fernando

Valley) are now at practical capacity. Their stages are being used either for construction or shooting or are holding for specific pictures; the films using the stages are either studio pictures or are independently financed. The stages in Los Angeles are so busy today that the old Columbia Studios on Gower have been reactivated as rental studios. The Burbank Studios (housing Warners and Columbia) and Universal have added new post-production facilities, and we've built a new film storage and handling structure and are adding extensive postproduction facilities as well as a new parking structure and office building. The general business of running a studio is today a reasonably successful one.

Our first contact with a company that will be working on the lot is generally when the production manager visits to plan the use of facilities. If it's an MGM picture, all services will be available for the standard studio overhead charge, which varies from 15 to 25% of the negative cost of the picture (depending on the studio and on negotiations) and is included in the budget of the picture. If the company is independent, the production manager can choose from a chart of basic studio facilities rates, ranging from $1,800 to $2,100 or more per shooting day, depending on service.

Studio overhead charges that are added to a production budget are frequently cited as contributing to the high cost of making films. The term *overhead*, however, is widely misunderstood. Many people believe that overhead is not actual cost. They have the notion that it is a charge just tacked on to a budget to give the studio a little more income at the expense of the production. In fact, overhead does represent the actual cost of innumerable studio operations. These services are varied and sometimes not easily identifiable. Therefore, instead of trying to figure what part of what cost is applicable to a specific production, the overhead is computed as a percentage of the total production costs. This amount is then charged by the studio against that film. It covers services from preparing legal contracts, researching copyrights, making out payroll and accounting for production and distribution to simple janitorial and maintenance services. Most studios also provide cameras, lights, grip equipment, editorial and transportation equipment, offices, and projection facilities for the overhead charge. The cost of acquiring and maintaining the equipment is chargeable to overhead. All of the commissaries, a desirable service to production, run at a loss. There are expenditures for police protection, plant engineering, plumbing, air conditioning, the mailroom, messengers, telephones, salaries for department heads involved in running the studio, and an overall planning department in the production area. All of these services and more are provided by the studio from income it receives for overhead and the rental of facilities.

159

As for independent pictures, instead of overhead, they are charged for simply renting studio facilities and are offered a choice of packages featuring certain services. For example, a full service and equipment package charges $2,100* per day for the use of two stages and includes these features among others: no charge for the use of standing sets; two free days for each three shooting days for holding or constructing sets prior to photography; $100 per studio day allowance for camera equipment; no charge for normal sound, grip, and electrical equipment (up to $1,250 per day on the rental value); two free editorial rooms; one free hour in a projection room per shooting day; six offices at no charge; free local phone calls; six dressing rooms at no charge; free use of makeup, wardrobe, and hairdressing rooms as available; striking costs at 20% of construction labor and materials; power at a fixed rate; studio-owned special effects at no charge; fringes payable at 40% of labor costs. Costs for scoring, dubbing, recording, and other post-production charges are computed on a separate rate card. This full-service package is a popular one. Certain areas within it are negotiable; after all, our interest is to keep the studio fully active.

When people talk about the studio being obsolete, what they really mean is that it is not necessary to have a studio in order to make a motion picture. This is true. But it is necessary to have some kind of corporate headquarters for activities that involve financing and distributing. There is surely a need for some kind of post-production headquarters. And, to varying degrees, there needs to be some kind of production headquarters. All of these needs add up to the viability of the studio as a central physical plant. Other activities that can take advantage of a centralized studio location are estimating and budget control, accounting, and payroll. Union agreements have grown more complicated, in part by requiring residual payment not only for television films but for theatrical films when they are shown on television. A studio computer helps to keep track of such an extensive financial operation.

Because it has become more desirable to shoot pictures on location rather than in a simulated environment on the back lots, MGM sold most of these back-lot facilities and eliminated the traditional standing outdoor sets. At the same time that the land upon which these sets stood grew more valuable, their utilization became less frequent. This combination of factors rendered it economically unsound to keep them.

The main expenses added to location shooting arc transportation and room and board for the cast and crew. These expenses can sometimes be offset by not having to build elaborate, expensive sets.

---

* Editor's Note: The reader should take into account inevitable, periodic price increases.

Construction costs have risen so much in the past ten years that often the kind of set required would not be feasible to build in any event. In fact, the overall below-the-line cost of producing a film in the United States has doubled in the past eight years. The increased cost of production is being offset by increased revenue from higher sales to network television and by increased grosses in theatrical and television markets worldwide.

Feeling that there should be some kind of library collection of all the films it has had an interest in, whether feature, short, or cartoon, MGM spent several years and many millions of dollars preserving its film library. Prior to 1952, most pictures were made on nitrate stock, which disintegrates with time. Since that year, pictures have been made on durable safety stock. Fortunately, it was possible for the nitrate negatives to be converted to safety negatives, thus preserving one of the most important assets a motion picture company has: a record of its productions. In addition to insuring this heritage through a studio library collection, the company has second copies of everything stored in underground vaults in Kansas with ideal temperature and humidity controls, giving double protection should a disaster occur at one location.

With our full-service studio fully active and our schedule of feature and television production, MGM/UA is maintaining itself as a major force in the entertainment industry.

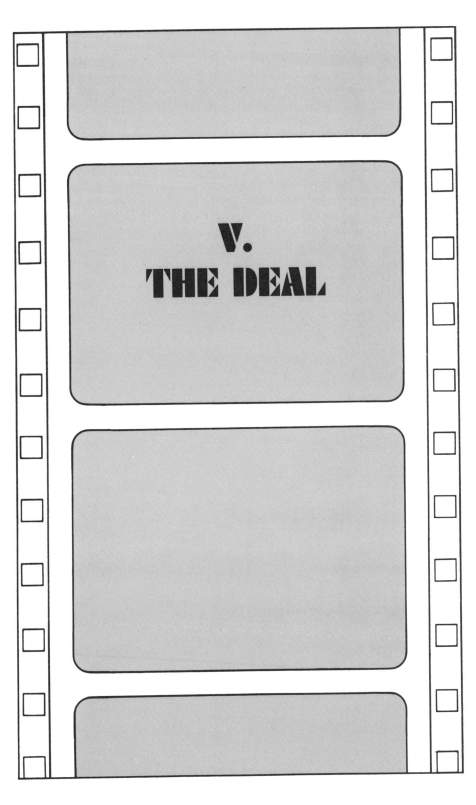

V.
THE DEAL

The Entertainment Lawyer

by **Norman H. Garey.** For a biographical note on Mr. Garey, see page 95.

> *A lawyer in the entertainment field must . . . get along with people under difficult circumstances, and sometimes . . . know the client perhaps better than he or she knows him- or herself. . . .*

An entertainment lawyer's practice and his relationships with clients may differ significantly from those of other practitioners. The emphasis is on servicing an individual and thus on the relationship between an individual lawyer and an individual client. These relationships are often lifelong or at least career-long and go deeper than traditional lawyer-client relationships in other areas of legal practice.

The clients an entertainment practitioner has are typically creative, volatile, and quixotic. A lawyer in the entertainment field must have the ability to adjust and adapt to disparate personalities, to get along with people under difficult circumstances, and sometimes to know the client perhaps better than he or she knows him- or herself. Many clients realize this and often ask for or expect advice that is not, strictly speaking, legal advice.

In the feature motion picture business, there are several individuals besides the lawyer who typically influence the client's life and career. A performer will usually have a business manager–accountant responsible for financial counseling and planning, an agent, perhaps a public relations counselor, and sometimes a personal manager as well. It's interesting how these interpersonal relationships overlap and how they affect one another in the decision-making process that goes on for each issue in the client's life; it often seems that an actor's life is run by committee. A producer will usually have only a lawyer and a business manager or accountant; a director or writer will have a lawyer, business manager, and in most cases, an agent.

If the client is a performer, a writer for hire, or a director for hire—somebody who simply renders services for compensation—it is the primary function of the *agent* to seek, find, and negotiate the basic terms of employment for that individual; it is not (and should not be) a lawyer's responsibility. The lawyer should be working closely with the agent, and ideally they should have a good personal relationship with each other. The lawyer (and the business manager) should be kept apprised by the agent of the client's career prospects, including what possibilities are being explored and what the status of each of these explorations or negotiations is; in other words, it should be very much a team effort.

However, if the client is a producer, an "entrepreneurial" or "promoter" producer, the lawyer's involvement generally should be primary. Frequently, the agent doesn't have the formal background in business organization, accounting principles, economic theory, or literary rights in the legal sense that a lawyer has. And all of these areas of preparation are necessary for effective representation of a producer or of an entrepreneurial writer or director who also acts in a packaging or producing capacity.

If a client simply renders services for hire, it's not necessary that the lawyer hear from the agent until the agent has struck the basic deal for the employment of the client, whether as writer, director, or both. When that is done, the lawyer becomes involved in the negotiation to assist in refining the deal, particularly in developing the formulae that relate to the net profit or other contingent compensation position and definition. A lawyer generally shouldn't have to get involved in the up-front negotiation, which includes such major terms as cash fee, services to be rendered, time periods involved in the rendition of those services, and the basic rights to be granted (if there are rights to be granted). All of the selling and positioning that it takes to get a client a job in the first place, to create the "want to buy" on the part of the buyer, are an agent's function. Upon the lawyer's entry into the negotiation, he should learn the history of the negotiation from the agent and then generally speak to the business affairs person with whom the agent has been negotiating—the buyer. The business affairs vice-president is usually the primary negotiating representative of the buyer, if the buyer is a studio financier-distributor or a major independent production company (see article by Richard Zimbert, p. 175). If the buyer is an individual producer, the attorney in question may deal with the buyer-producer's own outside lawyer. In any event, the buyer's representative and the lawyer will then refine the deal further, and the documentation will commence. The lawyer generally ought not to get involved in the negotiation until he has seen something in writing, whether it has come from the buyer's representative in the form of a deal memo or from the agent for his client in the form of a deal letter that informs him rather clearly where things stand at that point. It's part of the agent's task to memorialize in writing the basic terms that he has negotiated.

If the creator-writer client wants to buy the rights, for example, to a magazine article on which to base a story in a script, it is his lawyer who will typically supervise the buying activities, such as acquiring the rights and checking and clearing them. But when it comes to selling the completed screenplay of the pure creator, that more properly is an agent's role. If the agent is experienced, knows the buyers, and will listen to a lawyer when it comes to constructing price, he will then perform the primary selling function.

In the case of a screenwriter selling his writing services to adapt a novel for a producer-buyer or studio-buyer, the documentation would be generally in the form of an *employment agreement,* in which the writer-client is acting as a writer for hire; or a *loan-out agreement,* in which case he has his own internal corporation formed for various corporate and tax purposes, which loans his services to the buyer. However, if that same writer plans to render writing services in the adaptation of the magazine article he's already bought, the documentation would characteristically take a bifurcated form. There would be an employment agreement prepared with respect to the rendition of his future services, and there would be a rights option and acquisition agreement prepared with respect to the property rights being conveyed; in this case, the rights to the existing magazine article.

For any pure creator, whether writer, actor, or director, there are employment agreements that focus on the nature of the services to be performed. These agreements include a definition of the responsibility assumed; the period of time during which the client is expected to render his services; whether and, if so, to what extent he's to be exclusive during that period of time (i.e., whether he can engage in work on other projects); and the money involved. A myriad of questions can arise within those general categories. If he's not to be exclusive, what is his availability? Does he have to be on first call, giving first priority to this project? Are there options in favor of the employer-buyer for any further services? How much is to be paid for the services? How, and over what period of time, is the guaranteed compensation to be paid? Regarding contingent compensation, is there a *deferment,* meaning a fixed amount of money paid on a contingent basis if a certain time event, profit event, or other event comes about? How does the deferment relate in order of priority to any other deferments? Is there a contingent participation (gross receipts or net profit)? If there is a gross receipts participation, when does it accrue? If it's a net profit participation, how are net profits defined and determined? Is there a reducibility factor; that is, is the client's participation reducible by participations granted to others?

Then there's the important area of controls. This isn't quite as important in an actor's or writer's deal, because writers and actors generally are considered under the control of the producer or director for whom they work. The director generally is considered to be under the control of the producer, but not always. The director's control may supersede the producer's in certain areas and under certain circumstances. For example, the director's cutting rights may be superior to anybody else's; he may in fact have "final cut." But a "star" writer, for example, may have the equivalent of the Dramatists Guild covenant for his protection: "thou shalt not touch my work." That's very rare, but there are a number of top writers who have the exclusive right to perform personally whatever changes are requested to be written and to be paid for doing so. In this fashion, a writer is able to exert a degree of control over the progress and integrity of his work.

The actor is typically not in a much different position than a writer for hire or a director for hire from the standpoint of controls—he's going to be rendering certain services under the instruction of others. But there are certain rights that arise out of an actor's services that are unique to an actor. Merchandising happens to be one of them. The actor has a face. If it is well-known, people will want to put it on box tops, sweat shirts, T-shirts, book jackets, and record labels; it's a valuable right that has to be negotiated for an actor client with some attention. If he is an important actor, his image carries with it a certain dignity that must be preserved. This is also a valuable asset, which must not be merchandised in a denigrating fashion; controls must be negotiated and employed. It isn't just a matter of how much money will be paid and whether it will be in the form of a gross piece ("gross" in the merchandising business is generally represented by royalties) or a net profit piece.

Another negotiable item is the way in which the actor's performance can be used in other presentations: in sequels, in remakes, in television presentations, or in audio-visual presentations. There are certain actors who will not allow these uses, and their contracts prevent them. There are others who will permit their representatives to deal that right out, piece by piece, for additional compensation payable in cash, in contingent compensation, or both.

An important issue arises with respect to whether and when an actor may be paid off without his services having been used. What is the talent losing by not being used if he's been paid? The answer is credit and billing. Credit and billing have a value in this business far beyond just seeing a name on a marquee because credit and billing may get an actor his next job or the opportunity to advance his career in various ways. In the early days of the film business, if an actor was fired and a jury had to assess the damages which arose from the employer's breach of contract, they would often determine that the actor was guaranteed the salary he'd lost and should in fact be paid. But since he also wasn't used in the picture and didn't get the billing or the enhanced reputation that might have resulted, the jury placed another value on that. The sum might be astronomical because the issue is so amorphous. So the producers and financiers, in order to protect themselves, developed what is called the *pay or play clause*, which says in effect, "We can pay you off, we don't have to use you, and if we do that, all we owe you is your guaranteed compensation. Don't look to us for anything else; you don't have the right to." That has become the almost invariable custom of the business. But today the term *pay or play* is frequently used as a shorthand method for saying simply that there is a firm financial commitment under a deal. The distinction, however, is whether that firm financial commitment also requires the financier to use the person's services, which means it's more accurately pay *and* play (in which case the loss of credit may be compensable in damages) or whether it doesn't require the financier actually to use the actor's personal services, in which case it's pay *or* play, based on what has become the custom.

Producers' controls are many, and the negotiation of controls between a producer and a financing entity occupies a great deal of time because not only artistic and creative controls, but financial controls as well have to be worked out between financier and producer in great detail. Attention also has to be paid to a producer's credit because he'll get not only the "produced by" credit, but also in most cases some kind of entrepreneurial, proprietary, presentation, or production credit. Questions arise: Does it go above the title or below the title? In what kinds of ads must it appear? These are negotiable points. When getting into directors', writers', or actors' credits, the lawyer can refer to the relevant guild contracts on the subject, which stipulate order and size. Beyond that (and this is particularly true of producers, whose credits are not regulated directly by guild contracts) credit is mostly a matter of prestige, stature, and precedent, a question of who comes before whom. What is the placement? Must the credit appear in paid advertising? (*Paid advertising* is all advertising, as distinct from screen credit, issued by or under the control of the distributor—in print campaign ads, display ads, television ads, etc.) Most lawyers leave credit negotiations (except for producers) to the agent.

A director differs in one respect from an actor, writer, or producer who renders services for hire. He has an interest in protecting the integrity of his work that goes slightly beyond the interest of the others because the director is generally considered to be responsible for the total creative rendition of the product, and his reputation rides on the overall result. The writer, for example, is responsible only for the literary contribution, as opposed to the visual and audio contribution made by the director. The actor is responsible for the performance of his role. The director is held responsible for all of the performances in the picture. Therefore, the director's cutting rights—the right to protect the integrity of his work—have to be negotiated with some care. Who gets to perform the television cut or supervise it? Who gets to do the foreign censorship cutting or supervise it? How many cuts does the director get? How many previews? When do they have to take place? Who has the right to select the preview sites (an important item, since audience reactions may differ widely from site to site)? Does a particularly important director's right to final cut depend on budgetary, marketing, or other financial or commercial considerations?

In all of the foregoing matters, the agent and lawyer ideally function as a team. But if a client is an entrepreneurial producer, the lawyer, and usually only the lawyer, will be involved from the very beginning, from the very moment the movie idea is conceived. First, there will be a rights question. If the entrepreneurial producer is planning to acquire a piece of published material, a title search is conducted. The lawyer should have one or both of the major organizations that perform this function do so at the copyright register in Washington, D.C., to find out whether the idea or material has been exploited before and, if so, to what extent and by whom. This has a definite bearing on how much should be paid for it. Second, it must be determined that the rights are indeed owned by the person who is planning to purvey them and, if they aren't, it is important to know who else owns any of them. Third, are there any further title problems? Can the title be used? Can it be used only in connection with this material? Can it be used in adaptations of this material? The lawyer will usually conduct the negotiation for the acquisition of the rights on behalf of the producer or entrepreneurial creator (which would include an entrepreneurial director, writer, or, sometimes, actor who acts in a producing capacity).

When the rights have been secured, there is then the necessity (unless the client is also a writer) to have the material developed into screenplay form. A negotiation must take place with a representative of the writer who will develop the material if the producer client is going to finance the development himself. There may be still another negotiation, this one with a development-financing source, if it is not the producer client who will finance the development of the material.

There is one situation in which no negotiation takes place up front; that is where the client is an entrepreneurial writer who has conceived the idea and is also going to write the screenplay and ultimately sell it for financing or set it up for financing. In this case, there won't be any negotiations until some time later, but the rights-checking process still has to occur. The lawyer may have to learn whether the writer's idea is as original as his client thinks it is, or whether he will perhaps be infringing on somebody else's rights if he develops this project in the way he wishes.

An early issue that arises is the establishment of price. From the standpoint of an entrepreneurial creator, what are his cost factors? What's his out-of-pocket expense, what is it for, and what commitments have to be assumed by somebody else or discharged by him and then made whole with somebody else's money? That's bedrock. Next, what kind of speculative risk has to be taken? How much of the creator's time, energy, and services are at risk for no money? What is the return to the financier likely to be if this project is exploited successfully? All these factors must be taken into account. Finally, as a marketplace matter, there has developed over the years a whole set of percentages of the estimated production cost of a theatrical motion picture that apply to various creative services as guidelines to their relative value. For example, 5% of the direct cash budget is a fairly standard wage for screenwriting services.

The price of services is influenced very greatly by the factor of sales strategy or positioning. How do you make something seem more than it is? How does synergism develop through the uniting of several different elements? These are intangibles. Selling is the function of an entrepreneurial producer or creator or of an agent; it is not a lawyer's function. But, sometimes, when the entrepreneurial creator is engaging in packaging and the lawyer is assisting in this effort, the lawyer can usefully participate very directly in the politics necessary to get people together and then to create excitement around them. In this connection, is the entertainment lawyer acting as more than a lawyer? Is he allowed to do this? The California Labor Code and Business and Professions Code lay out the requirements for licensing on the part of those who solicit employment opportunities for people in the entertainment industry and the rules of professional conduct for lawyers. The codes, and the regulations adopted under them, as well as certain Bar Association rulings and opinions support the proposition that a lawyer (or an accountant) who performs such services incidental to his professional practice may do so without a separate license. Thus, it is not unethical or inappropriate for a lawyer to engage in the kind of activity that real estate brokers, loan brokers, or insurance brokers engage in as long as it is incidental to the performance of his services in his professional practice. Certainly, these functions extend beyond what most lawyers would consider traditional legal practice. On the other hand, there are lawyers practicing in real estate, in the insurance industry, and in the financial community who perform functions above and beyond the traditional law practice. Entertainment lawyers are no different from those people, they are just more visible.

In any negotiation, it's important to know the psychology of the buyer with whom one is dealing and to have a very real sense of the value of the elements within the package one is representing. Frequently, the entrepreneurial creator who is in touch with the marketplace has a better sense of the situation than the negotiating lawyer himself. Therefore, a lawyer negotiator has to stay in very close contact with his entrepreneurial client during negotiations. That may mean from one to twelve phone conversations during the course of any single day because frequently the lawyer will be negotiating with the business affairs vice-president whose authority is limited to devising mechanical ways of shifting money to accomplish a certain result. This vice-president doesn't have the authority to commit more than a certain amount without going back to his creative principal, who is usually the production head of the studio. Frequently that studio head and the entrepreneurial creator (the client) will be talking at the same time; thus the negotiation often proceeds simultaneously on two levels.

Once a transaction has resulted in a signed document, problems may arise in the administration or implementation of the deal. If it's a legal problem, then the lawyer had better become involved promptly. Frequently the problem will not at first be a legal problem, but rather a relationship problem. Perhaps communication has broken down between the creative people involved, and it's simply a battle of egos about whose creative views should prevail. Rather than expressing it in just that way, the creative people will often start looking for business reasons to further the dispute. This kind of problem can often be solved just by counseling and mediating. On the other hand, sometimes it is genuinely a legal problem. Perhaps something has come up that makes performance as originally contemplated more difficult, more expensive, or in fact impossible. Circumstances may have changed; expenses may have exceeded what was originally estimated. In these situations, lawyers obviously have to step in. Lawsuits are filed in some cases, but most are settled. There is more contention and less completed litigation in the entertainment business than in most other industries. However, there are some problems that cannot be solved by mediation or negotiation; arbitration and litigation are the only way to solve them.

There are a number of matters for the entertainment lawyer who is administering a career that are more financial than they are strictly legal in nature. For example, there is an important function to be performed in the area of tax planning and general financial planning and implementation. The matter of auditing net profit participations or gross receipts participations in connection with motion picture or television product is a very important function. It is imperative that the distributors who are responsible for the payment of these participations be policed because they do make mistakes both from an accounting and from a contract-interpretation standpoint. In all of these areas, it is important that the lawyer and the business manager or accountant maintain an effective working relationship.

There is also the matter of organizing the personal affairs of a client. People in the entertainment business engage in politics, get married and divorced, have problems with lovers, spouses, and children, pay taxes, buy and sell property, and do all the things other people do, but often with more flair and a great deal more visibility. The entertainment lawyer frequently has to serve as a liaison between the client and the other partners or associates in his law firm who are performing the more traditional legal functions for that client and often he must simultaneously monitor publicity (wanted or unwanted) that may be attendant to the legal matter at hand.

Finally, the lawyer in many cases may be asked to perform a kind of psychological, rabbinical, or personal-counseling function in addition to his business function. Advice sought is frequently personal advice about how to conduct not only one's career, but one's life. Lawyers in many cases may have neither the formal training nor the temperamental inclination for these kinds of counseling. It is always possible, however, for the lawyer to consult and involve others who do have the requisite background and either to use their advice in counseling the client or to involve them directly when the occasion requires it. One danger of the close working relationship between lawyer and client is the lawyer's temptation to assume the persona of the client. There is sometimes a seductive sense of power to be derived from those acts of guidance and decision making, both personal and professional, that shape a prominent client's life. As exhilarating as this can be, it can also take a toll on the practitioner's own sense of self. If one is sensitive to this danger, the practice of entertainment law can be fascinating, rewarding, and satisfying.

Business Affairs & the Production/Financing/Distribution Agreement

by **Richard Zimbert,** senior vice-president and assistant to the president of Paramount Pictures Corporation. He joined Paramount in April, 1975, as vice-president in charge of business affairs and, in April, 1977, was promoted to senior vice-president in the Motion Picture Division. Earlier, he had served as vice-president and general counsel of American International Pictures (April, 1971) and, before that, he had been executive vice-president of Aaron Spelling Productions (1970) and vice-president in charge of business and legal affairs for the American Broadcasting Company (1964–1970). Mr. Zimbert is a graduate of the University of Illinois and a member of the California and Illinois Bars and is admitted to practice in the Supreme Court of the United States, the United States Court of Military Appeals, and various other courts.

Since the movie business boils down to one thing, money, everything in the deal revolves around that. . . .

Editor's Note: *These comments attempt to place a relatively unique function, namely business affairs, in the framework of key agreements underlying theatrical motion pictures. They are intended as general comments for nonspecialists being introduced to the area.*

From the late 1920s to the late 1940s, major motion picture companies (of which today's survivors are Fox, Universal, Warners, Columbia, Paramount, and MGM/UA) kept important creative talent under contract. These contracts specified the employer's right to direct or order activity and the employee's duty to perform as directed to get paid. Except for the amount of compensation, most contract terms were considered standard. Studio legal departments and law firms developed forms to expedite much of this contract work.

Later, under the combined impact of television, government intervention (in the form of antitrust consent decrees), availability of investors from other fields, heavy income taxation, a diminution of the importance of movie-going in society, and the availability (via playing off one film company against another) of substantial profit-sharing arrangements, most creative talent found it more expedient to make one-time or limited-term arrangements. These contracts created in effect what were picture-by-picture, company-by-company relationships, rather than the previously applicable long-term contracts with a single employer.

The complexity of these new arrangements gave rise in the entertainment-oriented law firms to lawyers who are deal makers as well as lawyers. These individuals possess the knowledge and experience to weave creative, business, legal, and tax aspects of a deal in a manner most advantageous to their client. (See article by Norman Garey, p. 165.) Some agents have also become heavily involved in deal-making as their traditional role of merely getting someone a job and negotiating the price has expanded under the changed conditions of many employers competing for a limited and unique talent pool. Thus, the traditional studio lawyer method of using a form contract on an essentially "take-it-or-leave-it" basis became insufficient. Deal-making expertise has developed on the studio side as a professional skill of which

176

legal expertise is just a part, though an important part. These professional units, many of which were and are staffed by personnel with studio legal department or law firm training, are called *business affairs departments*. They are headed by a vice-president and include several negotiators as well as numerous administrative support staff.

In today's motion picture business, and within a fully structured company, business affairs (or deal-making) ranks as one of the five key management-level decision-making sections immediately under the chief operating officer. The other key departments are distribution (or sales), advertising, finance, and production.

Business affairs is brought into a situation as soon as the company (for our purposes, the studio financier-distributor) finds itself interested enough in a project to want to work on it for possible production as a movie. If the proposed deal involves important personnel and significant dollars, then the top management of the company, such as the president, sometimes the board chairman, the head of production, and the head of business affairs, are generally involved in establishing the basic structure with the representatives (lawyers and agents) of the project. Frequently management deals with the filmmakers themselves, many of whom have learned the desirability of having a direct hand in arrangements affecting them. Deals of less complexity or less initial importance start on other levels, but all deals involve a representative of the business affairs department as an active participant and frequently the point man in the company negotiation team. Of course, business affairs calls in the studio legal department and tax, finance, production, and other areas as the circumstances of the specified deal require.

The actual instruction or authorization to "make a deal" generally comes from the president or vice-president in charge of production. The head of business affairs evaluates the importance or complexity of the deal and decides whether and to what extent he should become personally involved in the negotiations. Since there are literally scores of negotiations going on at all times, obviously assignments and delegation are important. As working relationships evolve, more informal procedures are developed, and in the press of daily activities, who gets the job done is more important than following rigid chains of command.

The first stage of discussions is generally to try to reach agreement on the most basic elements of a proposed deal. Since the movie business boils down to one thing, *money*, everything in the deal revolves around that. The effort is to achieve agreement on the basics: who will do what for how much; what the options, rights, or opportunities of each party are as the project develops and their cost levels; and finally the accounting for and division of receipts from the distribution of the picture, if it's made.

If basic agreement has been reached, the studio legal department (as opposed to the lawyers for the other party) will usually prepare the contractual documentation appropriate to the circumstances. This ranges from an exchange of telegrams to an 80- to 100-page "formal" agreement, with every possible variation in between. However, there are no rules in the motion picture business, and frequently the studio business affairs department will itself prepare and secure the execution of a binding *deal memo*. This in essence is a short-form agreement covering those matters deemed most important by the parties. Usually, if this route is taken, formal contracts are not signed until unresolved issues have become moot through the passage of time. After the signing of a deal memo, the motivation for resolving minor issues is not high, and they are often more sensibly resolved by circumstances rather than by lawyers' agreements.

As is frequently the case in a real estate transaction, the buyer—the studio in the motion picture business—wants as many rights and protections as possible for his money. The seller—the filmmaking or creative entities—frequently wishes to give as little as possible. To expand on the real estate analogy, there are people perfectly willing to sell the house without the land (in the picture business, a project but no services) or the land without the house (services, but no project) if they could, and if buyers with cash could be found.

Everyone in the picture business moans about the length and complexity of agreements. Generally, the less one knows about the business and the people in it, the more willing one is to use short-form agreements. New managements are particularly susceptible to this view and may even require short agreements entered into rapidly. Then, when there is trouble (and there almost always is), and the trouble is not contractually covered, all concerned insist that protection on that point be secured in the future. So generally the short-form agreement slowly balloons up into a long form, until new people come in and forget (if they ever knew) why the agreements are long, and the cycle begins again. The essential tragedy of the massive documentation attempted in the picture business is that it reflects lack of trust between the parties compounded by a tradition of corporate instability. The writer of this article knows many filmmakers with whom a three- or four-page memorandum agreement would suffice; but the filmmaker then says, "What if you and your colleagues leave? I'd be stuck; therefore, I need protection . . . ," and away we go back to the long-form agreements.

There are many types of agreements, and each type has an almost infinite number of variations. Since they are entered into on a per-project basis, the filmmaker in effect chooses to do a project by making

178

a deal—and since no one can force someone to make a deal, creative freedom begins with this up-front commitment.

Most agreements involving personal services are still essentially employment agreements though some are treated as *loan-out agreements*. Loan-out agreements involve, for example, a star who has an agreement with a company controlled by him; that company, as the star's nominal employer, loans his services out to the real employer who, of course, is not designated as such so that tax advantages can be secured by the star where possible.

Basic writers' agreements run the gamut from those covering an idea purchase, to securing rights on a published book or an existing speculative script, to those for a script written for hire to be owned by the employer, to agreements solely for rewrites and polishes. In addition, there are agreements that must be reached with other individuals—the executive producer, producer, director, lead actors, cast, and various technical personnel, such as the cinematographer and production manager.

There are also contractual arrangements relating to shared financing. So-called tax-shelter deals have been the most prominent. These have been virtually eliminated in the United States, but they can be a tremendous spur to motion picture production, as the recent developments in Canada illustrate. Another basic type of agreement is the *pickup deal*. Pickup deals have various permutations, but the essential element distinguishing them is that the picture to which the pickup deal refers is, to some extent, financed independent of the major studio system. As a result of differing financial risks, the treatment of receipts and the rights granted and reserved depart from a normal studio deal. Sometimes this type of deal is better for the filmmaking party, although the ratio of pickup hits to total hits is quite small.

There are still a few people who have long-term, multiple-picture agreements. These arrangements, generally called *overall deals*, bear mentioning. In overall deals, the people involved are concerned with several added factors, and one that bothers many is *cross-collateralization*. The point is negotiable, but in essence, it is intended to deal with a situation where a filmmaker under an overall contract makes two pictures, one a hit and one a loser. Without cross-collateralization, on a loser, the studio would lose 100%. On a winner, the winnings would be shared with the filmmaker. Cross-collateralization, which can take many forms, is an attempt to treat films in groups so that the studio and its filmmaking partner both win or lose together on the group, with losses fairly shared rather than loaded 100% against the studio.

Finally, the most basic agreement of all is called a *PFD agree-*

ment—short for production, financing, and distribution. It usually contains all the elements of the individual types of agreements outlined above and is, in a sense, the spine of the movie production contract area. Since the PFD agreement is most basic, a tour through its key elements may be useful.

The first section of a PFD agreement usually deals with the development process. It states the form in which the project exists: as an outline, treatment, and so on. Then, it identifies the roles of the people tied to it. If the deal is with a producer, that will be clearly stated. If there are writers involved, the writers will be identified, along with the terms of their responsibility: Are they writing a new script? Are they rewriting it? Other questions must be answered relating to the development period. Is the project being budgeted? Is the producer supposed to find a director or only if certain events occur? What is the basic monetary commitment on the part of the studio, and what payments are required as the project progresses? This is all contractually spelled out.

Development deals within the PFD structure are usually referred to as *step deals* because the development process itself is based on a series of steps. For example, the rewrite of a script could be considered step one when there's an existing script. Securing a director prior to a second rewrite could be step two. Preparing a budget and production schedule based on the rewritten script could be step three. This process is spelled out in the development section, with every project having cutoffs at certain steps to give the financing entity various "outs."

During the development process, the PFD agreement usually requires a producer or director to supervise the writing and rewriting of the script, assist in the preparation of the budget and shooting schedule, and furnish suggestions for casting. "Suggestions" is a word of art. Contractually, it means the producer is responsible (with the aid of the studio) for furnishing talent willing and able to perform required services in the proposed picture at a certain price.

The producer's compensation is also generally tied to steps. If the producer is responsible for a rewrite only, that's one fee. If he's taken a project from an idea through a first draft script, a second draft, rewrites, budgets, and so on, he generally would be entitled to greater compensation because he's performing more services over an extended period of time. Writers' deals follow a similar pattern. Generally, producers work on a number of development projects at the same time and are thereby considered nonexclusive. Writers may also work on a number of development projects but are usually required by contract to finish one specific project before starting another; this, however, is not often the reality. Many writers concerned with developing one project spend part of their time trying to set up their next one, and contracts are gradually changing to reflect this reality.

After the development of a project is completed, the point is reached where a decision can be made by the financier-distributor as to whether the picture will go forward. The time frame of development usually ends upon the furnishing of elements so that a decision to make the picture can be made with full consideration of a developed script, budget, cast, director, producer, and any other key elements. The theory of a time frame is to give the producer a trigger to keep the project from forever being hung up in the air—to force a yes or no from the studio. If the answer is no, another studio should be given the opportunity to say yes, which often results in the first studio getting its money back, through a procedure called *turnaround.*

Turnaround is the effort, after an abandonment, to set a project up elsewhere, repay prior investments, and get the picture made. The vast majority of hit pictures in recent years have been in turnaround in one form or another; somebody passes, somebody else proceeds. *Star Wars* was abandoned by Universal; *Heaven Can Wait* was in turnaround; *The Goodbye Girl* was abandoned by Columbia; United Artists turned down *American Graffiti.* One key point that should be recognized regarding turnaround is the "changed-element" clause. The studio that is abandoning a project is abandoning on a set of facts: a particular director, particular script, and particular budget. If, for example, a project was presented to Paramount starring me and then goes to Fox after the producer gets Robert Redford, Paramount is going to feel aggrieved and will say, "How come we didn't get Robert Redford?" Generally, there's an obligation on the producer's part to come back to the original studio if an element has significantly changed. It's a clumsy clause, hard to write, hard to agree on, but necessary from the studio's point of view. Most people conduct themselves with reasonable good faith in this turnaround area, in part because they will have to deal with an abandoning studio in the future on a new project: Hollywood's a small town.

If the studio elects to proceed with production of the picture, the PFD agreement specifies what, how, and when the key people get paid. The "when" can be a complicated question because suggesting a cast or getting an approved budget doesn't actually mean that the cameras are going to turn. Usually, it is the studio position that most people should not be entitled to get paid until the cameras turn (stated as "the start of principal photography"), even though a special element, such as a star, may be committed in one form or another. In one case, the *pay or play deal,* the money is due whether or not the picture is made, as long as the star (or director) is ready, willing, and able to perform during a stipulated period. The degree of financial commitment prior to commencement of principal photography and at various stages thereafter is usually a result of leverage. For example, if there is no approved cast, the producer and director may not receive full picture fees even though they are ready, willing, and able to proceed.

PFD agreements all contain sections applicable when development is completed and the project is not abandoned, typically starting with a "producer's obligation to produce picture." The language is reasonably standard—it must state what the producer is going to do, but if Bob Evans or Warren Beatty produces a picture, it means years out of their lives; for some other so-called producers to produce a picture may mean a minute away from a poker game. Yet, both types have a contract saying they'll produce the picture, and both types get a producer fee and credit. Of course, individual deals do vary depending on each person's leverage, but sometimes ability is far from the sole or even most important aspect of this leverage, and control of an "element" becomes the heart of the negotiation.

The production section also contains other requirements and obligations connected with the picture. For example, is the picture to be in black and white or in color? This clause could be left out, one might think, but what happens when after two years of work and hundreds of thousands of dollars spent in development and preproduction costs for a color picture, the director decides it should be in black and white? Thus, the issue has to be settled up front. There also are paragraphs included that say the picture must be made on certain locations approved or designated by the studio and that refer to the running time of the picture, when it is to be delivered, the rating of the picture, studio consultation requirements relating to casting, music, and similar matters, and creative and business approvals during production. The technical requirements are placed together in a schedule as an exhibit at the end of the agreement.

Production manager approval is part of the group of clauses that relate to studio approvals. Generally, the studio will allow the most responsible picture makers to select their own crew subject to union requirements and EEOC hiring and other governmental regulations, but for certain personnel, such as the production auditor or the production manager, the studio generally retains the right to designate or approve them because they really are responsible for watching the money.

Legal fees must be negotiated. There is a mass of contracts required during production, and some financier-distributors find it easier to use the producer's own lawyer if he's competent to do that work rather than have it done in-house; this involves the producer and his counsel more in the project and gives them a vested stake in its being done properly.

"Takeover of production" is a remedy that in many contracts is an anachronism because, if the producer or director is an employee and you can tell him what to do, why does the studio need the right to take over? But since judges are human beings and sometimes don't seem to focus on this point, lawyers have found it better to spell out the studio's right to step in, take over, and throw a person off a picture. A recent case involved Dustin Hoffman and First Artists. Even though Hoffman is a part owner of First Artists, he claimed his own company took the picture *Agatha* away from him and didn't let him finish it during post-production. The company claimed, of course, that he would never have finished the picture if they hadn't taken over.

One production element that deserves separate comment is the MPAA rating. (See article by Jack Valenti, p. 362.) The director, producer, and studio try to reach an agreement as to the rating they want for the finished picture. They can't be sure that the rating board will rate it accordingly, but if they seek or need a particular rating, that provision would be spelled out together with what happens if the rating board doesn't agree.

An extremely critical area is "television coverage." What this means specifically in terms of reshooting or redubbing should be spelled out so it is clear what the parties expect. It's easy to cover language unacceptable to TV, but what if scenes the filmmakers do not plan to reshoot are needed to provide a suitable television version; who pays and who decides what's to be done? It's preferable to have the people making the theatrical picture also put together the television version at the same time. Again, this is an effort to encourage the filmmakers to make their own picture, barring catastrophies such as going over budget or failing to make timely delivery.

A sensitive area is the studio right to view dailies. Some directors go crazy at the thought that a studio executive is going to view *their* dailies. Others are perfectly happy to show dailies. It all depends on the players and what their respective interests are.

Where the film is to be processed and what laboratory is to be used are also usually covered by contract. There are some laboratories that are better than others for some filmmakers. In the old days, this was an important point because there were kickbacks from the laboratory to the producers and the studios. Today, as far as Paramount is concerned, we let the producer and director go to whatever lab they choose, but they must secure rates no higher than those the studio itself would pay. Availability of technical skill, not kickbacks, is the sole determining factor.

The pictures financed by Paramount are required to comply with our union agreements. Studios are signatories to dozens and dozens of union agreements and are required to comply with them, so we impose these obligations on the people making the pictures.

It is important to specify the rights of the parties in the production section of the agreement. There is a producer who is producing, a director who is directing, and a studio that is financing; ultimately, who is in charge? The agreement must provide whose decision is final. One of the sensitive areas here is the right of "final cut" or the various degrees of that power. In most PFD agreements, probably the studio decision is made final under the theory that the studio's money is being used and money speaks loudest. But, once again, the practical reality is often far from that because it is often imprudent for a studio to intrude on a creator's finishing touches and so risk negative publicity.

The start date is another important contractual matter. Some pictures are authorized for production because they're scheduled for release at a particular time, such as Christmas. Somebody thinking about production would say, "To release the picture at Christmas, working backwards, we must start production in the next four months." In such circumstances, meeting that schedule can be critical.

Overhead costs must also be dealt with. Basically, Paramount doesn't have a studio overhead charge to motion pictures. Although overhead is simply a way of grouping charges in a percentage arrangement so that, from a studio standpoint, the parties don't have to argue about whether a pencil costs a penny or a nickel, Paramount found (and United Artists was really the forerunner of this) that the percentages were sometimes unfair. Rather than saying, "The pencils are free, but you pay an overhead percentage instead," the parties agree that if a picture uses a pencil, it's charged for that pencil; if it doesn't, there is no charge. That's the way Paramount operates; no percentage overheads in the feature area.

Next, there are concerns about contract breaches. What happens if the producer or director gets drunk, disorderly, doesn't show up, or doesn't perform? This can be complicated in a number of ways; for example, when the producer has done a lot of work before the picture starts but dies or breaches or gets drunk or does whatever producers do before going further. This does not necessarily mean that he loses everything or that the picture doesn't get made. But, as a counterweight, studios don't want to encourage people to breach. Therefore, even though someone may have completed 90% of his work before the picture starts, if he's breached, nobody is going to pay him 90% of his money; the payment vestings or settlements in this connection become negotiable points.

That's an overview of the production part of a sample agreement—the *P* of the PFD agreement.

The financing part of the PFD agreement today doesn't need, in my opinion, more than a few paragraphs to set out exactly how production money is allocated. This can be covered in a very simple way by stating there'll be a production schedule and a production board and a budget—and whatever costs are based on those items are paid.

Securing an outside guarantee of "completion" is a great scam, it seems to me, that is generally used by insecure executives to fool their bosses that their investment is covered. If a studio is financing a picture, it's financing a picture and must finance until completion. Whenever a picture is completed, it's completed, and never before. Sometimes outside completors are used. In the vast majority of cases, the outside guarantor of completion will never in a practical sense be permitted to make good on that guarantee. No one will allow him to touch the picture, because of the fear that he would just take scotch tape, paste the celluloid together, and say, "Here's the picture." The situation involving *Meteor* was the classic illustration. Going in, the financing entities had a completion bond. The picture went millions of dollars over budget. The completion bond holder was perfectly willing to finish the picture, but none of the financiers involved would dare accept such a picture finished by a banker. In the end, they had to put up more of their own money to complete it. The result was that the completion guarantor got his fee and did nothing, and the investors ended up carrying the picture. It's not that guarantors are fools or knaves; it's just that if you spend $10-million for a picture directed by Ronald Neame and it goes over budget, you do not want Sam Smith, the completion guarantor from an insurance company, finishing your Ronald Neame picture.

In the distribution section, the first important point in our sample agreement deals with the specificity of credit given to the producer, director, writer, actors, and author of the book (if applicable), both on the screen and in paid advertising. This relates to size, color, type, and relationship to other credits. This part of a negotiation can take more time and create more frustration than the rest of the agreement. Paid advertising is at the core of the problem. Today, half an ad can be taken up with names many of which have no meaning at the box office, where the money is. When discussing credits, people seriously spend hours and hours on whose name goes first and on which line, if anyone else's name goes on their line, or whose name is bigger. Studios and other distributors do not object to crediting people or to the recognition of abilities or performances. What the advertising people for a distributor object to is trying to sell a picture using an ad wherein a name must be placed in a particular size and location according to contract, regardless of how this may affect the aesthetics or impact of the ad campaign. Of course, some names have a positive box-office effect, but this judgment should be left to the advertisers, not the agents and lawyers. Kellogg's would probably be vexed if, as they try to sell their cereal, they had to put the name of the inventor of cornflakes on every box, ad, and commercial. But this is a battle that the studios have long been waging with the Hollywood creative and union community, and wasting a third or more of purchased ad space or time for legally imposed credits doesn't seem to bother those groups and individuals that require it.

Now we come to money in relation to distribution, and this is the heart of the PFD agreement. Here, the agreement must define *gross receipts,* which is the money that is received from the theatres— not the money the theatre grosses, but the money the theatre turns over to the distributor (in this case, the studio financing entity). This is called *film rental* or *distributor's share of gross receipts.* From this the distributor takes a distribution or sales fee, which is for his costs of selling the picture. In Paramount's case, sales costs include 300 staffed offices throughout the world. A 30% fee is charged for the U.S. theatrical distribution fee, but other media and areas have different fees. One fee that is a problem is the 25% fee for network sales, which is frequently objected to by producers because they think a network license is obtained with just a phone call. (Producers often learn to their sorrow what a network does to them when they want to make an independent deal and try to make that phone call themselves.) The various distribution fees relate to the costs of selling in particular media, and over that range of activities some fees appear unfair to one party or the other. Competitive factors also exert a ceiling. On balance, these fees are the lifeblood of the production/financing/distribution business.

Distribution fees cover not only theatrical but also nontheatrical outlets: television, merchandising, soundtracks, book publishing, and music publishing. There may be different fees or fee scales for the same function in different territories because it may be more difficult to accomplish something in one country than in another. For that reason, the distribution fee for the United Kingdom is 35% and for the rest of the world is 40% since it is somewhat easier to distribute in the U.K. than in Germany or France. One obvious difference is that the latter require dubbing or subtitling, which are distribution expenses.

Further comment about distribution fees is perhaps appropriate. Sometimes a studio can make money on its fees, depending on a variety of circumstances. Fox made so much money with *Star Wars* that the one picture carried the entire distribution organization; any fees they received from other pictures were "profit." But, if a studio has 20 pictures that all do $10-million, it could lose money because the production and marketing costs would be enormous and the distribution fees would not be enough to cover them. People run around saying the studios always make money on distribution fees, but sometimes we don't—sometimes there is a loss in distribution fees.

After subtracting distribution fees, the remaining funds are applied for recovery of advertising, the cost of prints (today a broad domestic release can cost $900,000 or more just for prints), shipping, inspection, insurance, and delivery. Next in the PFD agreement is the studio's right to market the picture in any reasonable way—in two theatres or two thousand theatres, or anything in between. The studio's ultimate control of advertising follows, frequently with an obligation to consult with the director or producer on the size of the advertising budget and the conceptual advertising campaigns, which comply with credit requirements.

The next item in the distribution section covers recoupment of negative cost and interest on the negative cost. *Negative cost* is a concept that is unique to the picture business; what it really means is the cost of physically making the picture before the cost of prints and advertising charges are incurred. Assume that the studio went to a bank and borrowed the money to make the picture. That money must be paid back, plus interest. That is the next step of the money flow from the box office—the recovery of this loan or investment from what is left of film rental.

Up to this point, all of this effort is simply trying to get money back that has already been paid out. Once the picture recovers its costs, it reaches the rarefied realm of breakeven or "net profits." Then, in our model, these profits are split, generally 50% to the financing entity (the studio) and 50% to the participants. Variables apply to special talent in superior bargaining positions, such as a top director or actor who might receive percentages of proceeds at stages defined somewhat differently and falling earlier than others in the revenue flow. For example, major stars like Clint Eastwood, Robert Redford, or Warren Beatty are likely to receive money ahead of other participants.

Included in the distribution section of the PFD agreement is the accounting portion, which is critical. When are statements due? Who checks accounting statements? How much detail is provided in statements? What is their frequency? What are the audit rights? What effect does an audit have? How much time is there to audit? How much time is there to object?

Then, a whole series of relatively standard provisions follows dealing with the ownership of the picture, including the right of the financing entity or owner to copyright it in order to secure the investment tax credit; the right to settle or file lawsuits; the right to settle with theatres and exhibitors and, as mentioned earlier, to make deals with television networks. Basically, this group of clauses is intended to state that the financing studio is the owner of the picture and that though the filmmakers are entitled to certain monetary interests, they are not the owners. Insurance requirements are also spelled out and if there is an insurance loss, how it is applied. For example, normally a studio wouldn't take a distribution fee on an insurance recovery, but somebody could suggest it, and the producer could be silly enough to agree to it.

Another area covered here refers to sequel, remake, and television rights. (In recent years, the new term *prequel* has been added to this category.) In normal good-faith dealing, regardless of the contract (though it should be in the contract), people involved in a successful picture should have the right to do a remake, sequel, or television series based on that picture. If they choose not to do so, there's some argument as to whether they're then entitled to money from the derivative work for the act of making the original, even though the derivative work has its own creators and filmmakers. Today, due to the high risk and cost of the feature business, sequels become more and more tempting. There's already an audience that has seen a particular picture like *Star Wars*, and, if something decent is produced as a sequel, they are likely to come back for more. For these and other reasons, sequel, remake, and TV rights, and the obligations of picture makers and the studio to one another in these areas, are bitterly fought-over issues.

Naturally, all of the related agreements, such as those of the director, actor, and other key creative personnel, must mesh with the PFD agreement and its provisions.

The work of business affairs is completed when the negotiations and documentation are final. We can only hope that we've protected the studio so that, when a picture makes money, there is enough to please the stockholders and to finance more pictures.

Over–Budget Protection and the Completion Guarantee

by **Norman G. Rudman,** a member of the firm of Slaff, Mosk & Rudman, who has practiced law in Los Angeles since 1956. He was educated at UCLA and the Boalt Hall Law School (U.C. Berkeley). He has written and lectured on a variety of subjects including constitutional law, bankruptcy, divorce, and the development, financing, and production of feature films. Involved as counsel in many motion picture productions, he has also served as executive producer of several films.

. . . the essence of a completion guarantee is that the investors will get a finished picture for the budget amount they have financed. . . .

The motion picture business is a risky, highly speculative business. Only affluent and sophisticated investors should be involved in it. The investors take risks on many factors: on the creative capabilities of the writer, producer, director, and actors and on the ability to secure distribution and compete in the marketplace, to name a few of the more obvious. But the single risk that any investor will find intolerable is the risk that a picture will not be completed. In the production of any motion picture, whether a studio project or an independent venture, the need is always present to assure that what is started will be finished. That is where the issue of "completion" enters into the structuring of a motion picture deal.

If a studio-financed picture goes over budget for whatever cause, there is reasonable certainty that the studio has the financial strength to cover the extra costs. For undertaking the risk of over-budget costs, the studio will probably add to the budget or retain a contractual right to recoup a cost item in the area of 5 to 6%. Further, the studio may invoke contractual penalties against the producer and/or director for any excess costs unless such costs result from studio-approved enhancement (that is, content not found in the approved screenplay prior to shooting).

Assume a studio picture budgeted at $8-million. In addition to the producer's fee and overhead allowance, the producer's deal with the studio would typically give him a share of the net profits of the picture, say one third, reducible for profits paid to other talent to a floor of perhaps 20% of 100% as defined in the studio's standard PFD (production, financing, and distribution) agreement. (For details of a sample PFD agreement, see article by Richard Zimbert, p. 175.) Assume this is a generous studio that allows the producer a 10% contingency over the going-in budget so that he is not penalized if the picture comes in at a negative cost of up to $8,800,000. What happens if the cost reaches $8,900,000? One of the consequences may be that the producer's profits are, by contract, delayed while the studio recoups not only the $8,900,000 (plus, of course, all distribution expenses, interest, and distribution fees), but also double the over-budget costs, or an additional

$100,000, before profits are deemed to have been reached. Or the producer may be required to agree that part of his fee be payable on a deferred basis and that, to the extent he goes over budget, such deferment is paid to the studio to cover the excess costs, rather than to him. Or the studio may take profit points away from the producer: the deal that gave him a floor of 20% of 100% of profits may begin to shrink on a formula whereby he may forfeit a point of profits for every, say, $50,000 of over-budget costs.

The specifics will, of course, depend on the producer's bargaining power vis-à-vis the studio, and what has been said with regard to the producer's deal might, in certain cases, apply to the director's as well. The point is that the studio will take the budget seriously; hence, if the costs run over, the studio is likely to believe either that the budget was false to begin with or the producer did not manage the production competently. In either event, it will likely want to make him pay for his sins.

In independent production, the need for completion protection can be fulfilled in a variety of ways. A producer may be capable of meeting excess costs out of his own pocket; the deal with investors may permit an over-call; a standby commitment may be in place for over-budget financing on certain terms; or a producer may deal with a company whose business it is to provide a completion guarantee.

A producer who is strong enough financially to sign his own guarantee of completion is generally strong enough on the line to assure that the picture comes in without invading his personal resources. This type of completion assurance can be as simple as the producer informally assuring his investors that he will complete the picture.

A second form of completion assurance is simply an over-call from investors. For example, if investors are organized into a limited partnership, the partnership agreement may permit going back to the investors for an extra 10 or 20% of their investment in order to meet over-budget costs.

A third approach might be a standby commitment to invest over-budget costs as called for. Assume an independent picture is budgeted at $2,500,000. The standby investor, for a negotiated cash fee or other consideration, might commit to provide an additional amount up to, say, $1,000,000. If called upon to put up any of that money, he might be entitled to take over production. (The completion guarantor, the fourth general category of completion assurance, is also likely to reserve takeover rights.) The principal distinction between the standby investor and the completion guarantor is that the standby investor will normally obtain a recoupment position prior to or at least equal to the people who put up the $2,500,000 for the principal budget, and a profits interest in the picture besides. The profits interest is likely to be cal-

culated at a better rate (perhaps double) than what the original investors would receive. (That profits interest would normally come out of
the producer's share rather than the financiers' share of the profits.) If
the original investors were receiving 50% of the profits for their
$2,500,000, each would have one percentage point of profit for every
$50,000 of money invested. For example, if an investor put up
$250,000, he would be entitled to 5% of the net profits of the picture.
Let's assume that $250,000 of the standby investor's money is used. On
the standby deal hypothesized above, he would be entitled to ten
points of profit for that $250,000, but out of the producer's end, not that
allocated to the principal financiers.

I distinguish between a standby investment and a completion
guarantee because the standby investment dilutes or postpones the recoupment position of the original investors while the completion guarantee does not. Further, the completion guarantee rarely requires the
producer to give up any profits for the use of the guarantor's money. On
the other hand, the standby investor may be willing to pay for the costs
of enhancing a picture. The completion guarantor will not. The
standby-investor format might provide acceptable completion assurance to equity investors. It would not satisfy a bank if a bank were putting up any of the production money, because the bank would not accept any position other than first recoupment. For the same reason, it
would not satisfy most distributors putting up production money in the
form of negative pickups of distribution licenses.

As another example, assume it actually cost $3,000,000 to make
the picture budgeted at $2,500,000 and that the standby investor ad-
vanced the $500,000 over-budget costs. Assume further that the distrib-
utor has collected film rentals that, after deduction of distribution fees,
print and advertising costs, and other distribution expenses, leave
$800,000 of "producer's share" to be devoted to recoupment of produc-
tion costs. If the picture had been brought in on budget, or as is explained below, if the over-budget costs had been paid for under a typical completion guarantee, that $800,000 would be divided pro rata
among the investors who funded the budget. Each would receive
roughly one third of his money at this point. But if a standby investor
put up $500,000 (because the picture actually cost $3,000,000 to complete), under a deal calling for his recoupment prior to the original
investors, the first $500,000 of that $800,000 goes to him. That leaves
only $300,000 to be divided among the original investors of $2,500,000,
who would get back roughly 12% instead of closer to 33%. Similarly, if
the standby investor's deal calls for recoupment pro rata with the principal investors, then the $800,000 recoupment is divided among
$3,000,000 of investors, making a return of roughly 27% of investment.
Thus, the standby investment commitment is not a completion guaran-

tee because *the essence of a completion guarantee is that the investors will get a finished picture for the budget amount they have financed.* If their recoupment is subordinated or diluted by the concurrent (even if pro rata) recoupment by a standby investor, they have not had the benefit of their original bargain in that respect.

My fourth category of completion assurance is the only one properly entitled, in my view, to be called a completion guarantee.

The typical completion guarantee is a three-sided transaction among bank, producer, and guarantor. The guarantor guarantees to the bank the producer's performance of the conditions of the loan agreement. It is not uncommon that completion guarantees are issued in two-sided (producer–guarantor) transactions, where the production financing comes not from bank loans but from equity investment or direct studio financing that is circumscribed by direct studio involvement in production. Here the guarantor may in effect be guaranteeing the performance of the producer to the producer himself or to a party so closely allied with the producer as to be chargeable with the producer's actions. The differences between three- and two-sided transactions are most clearly seen in the framing of issues in disputes over whether a guarantor is responsible for an over-budget cost.

To illustrate how a three-sided completion guarantee works, let's turn to an example of an independent picture budgeted at $4-million. To raise that money, assume the producer makes a pickup deal with an American distributor for theatrical rights in the United States and Canada for $1-million, payable on delivery of the picture. A foreign-sales representative may sell distribution rights in 25 territories in the world and come back with as many contracts, some for $5,000, some for $100,000, making a total package of $1,500,000, all payable on delivery. The producer may take the project to a network and negotiate a presale for two network runs for $1-million. And a pay-cable company may commit $500,000 to license the picture to its subscribers. Ignoring, for ease of illustration, such complicating factors as interest, discounts, fees, commissions, compensating balances, and the like, these numbers round out the $4-million budget. With the exception of relatively nominal down payments, these contracts will usually be payable not on signing but only on or after delivery of a specifically described picture. The contracts will not be collectable if the delivered picture does not meet specified conditions, such as that it must be based on a specific screenplay, directed by a certain director, have specific stars and running time, meet first-class technical requirements, and be delivered by a specific outside date. The producer takes the contracts to one of the few banks that deals in motion picture transactions and "discounts" them, that is, tenders them as security and the source of repayment for the $4-million production loan he needs.

What is the bank going to require in order to make that $4-million loan? All the bank can look to for payment is the fulfillment of the conditions set forth in the various (often numerous) distribution contracts. If it is assured that those conditions will be met, it may make the production loan. Furnishing such assurance is the function of the completion guarantee. Naturally, it is the bank's burden to satisfy itself as to the creditworthiness of the paper against which it is lending. But the delivery conditions that must be fulfilled to make notes collectable, letters of credit draftable, or contracts enforceable are what the completion guarantor guarantees.

As earlier observed, banks will make loans against distribution contracts only if they, and only they, have recourse to those contracts until their loans are repaid in full. For this reason, the completion assurances of a so-called standby investor will not be acceptable to a bank if he has a recoupment position ahead of or even equal to the bank's. Professional completion guarantors, such as Film Finances of London or Completion Service Company of Los Angeles, have accepted this fixed truth. They offer a standard completion-guarantee format involving subordinated recoupment that will very likely be acceptable, depending, of course, on the bank's assessment of the specifics of the guarantor's contract and financial responsibility. Professional completion guarantors have learned to live with having recoupments of their advances, if any, subordinated to the bank or distributor recoupments or, if need be, to entire budgets.

The producer in search of a completion guarantee has several, but not many, markets to explore. The guarantors are highly competitive. Their costs range in the area of 6% of approved budget. What they will ask to see for purposes of qualifying a picture for a guarantee includes the screenplay, budget, shooting schedule, rights and major employment agreements, and any and all supporting materials that help to verify and authenticate the budget and production schedule.

To a completion guarantor, a screenplay is a legal document, analogous to what the plans and specifications for a building are to a construction firm. The guarantor regards the screenplay not merely as a story to be told on film but as the definitive description of the qualities and characteristics to be embodied in that film, including specific action, sets, props, locations, costumes, and effects, among other elements. The guarantor's objective is to bring the picture in within the budget and on schedule, thereby fulfilling the delivery requirements of the various distribution contracts. Therefore, it is the specific proposed picture disclosed by the screenplay and production plan that becomes the subject of the guarantee, just as it is the subject of the distribution contracts and the production loan. The difference between the guarantor's objectives and those of the bank and the distributors in this respect is that the latter normally have no responsibility for costs beyond their loan or pickup commitments. They can hardly be expected to object if the picture's cost zooms far beyond budget. The guarantor, however, has such responsibility provided it is the cost of the specific guaranteed picture that escalates. He will, therefore, resist being charged for cost escalations that are voluntarily or incompetently incurred by the producer. Changes in script, new locations, unscripted effects—all such things in the nature of enhancement of the picture will be outside the guarantee.

In reviewing a proposed picture to be guaranteed, the guarantor will want, among other requirements, to see the budget *proved*. He will be suspicious of round figures and will find the word *allowance* in a budget intolerable. The budget will be closely analyzed in relation to the screenplay, the shooting schedule, and the professionalism of the principal creative, production, and business personnel.

The completion guarantor will have to be satisfied with the director, cinematographer, production manager, location manager, production designer, and stars, among others. Does the cinematographer take too long to light every shot? Does the director show up on the set without a shot list so that there is down time between setups? If the same person is going to star in and direct the picture and the director must be replaced during shooting, will the star show up on the set? Is the director married to the star?

Another issue the guarantor is wary of is a "sweetheart deal" whereby the producer is acquiring some essential service (such as post-production facilities) on a better-than-prevailing-rate basis. If the "sweetheart" nature of the deal is what brings the budget down, then the completion-guarantee fee may be reduced, but the picture is almost certain to go over budget if the sweetheart deal falls out. All of these issues and more must be resolved to the satisfaction of the completion guarantor before the guarantee will be issued.

Aside from a fee of about 6% of the budget, what does the producer "give up" to the guarantor? Guarantors normally require that they be vested with certain powers to police and oversee the course of production toward the end of keeping it to schedule and budget. Included among such powers may be the right to co-sign production account checks; to observe on the set during shooting; to screen all the rushes; to sit in on all production meetings; to review the books; to receive on a timely basis copies of all production reports, such as camera, sound, production manager, and script supervisor reports; to demand and receive answers to questions; and to become co-insured under all the production's insurance. This way, the completion guarantor can review the financial status of the picture on a daily or weekly basis, in partnership with the production company, to anticipate and correct potential over-budget incidents. In case of trouble, the completion guarantor can exercise the right to take over the production and, if need be, to fire personnel whose performance is below par (subject, of course, to the requirements of distribution, collective bargaining, and other relevant agreements).

The typical completion-guarantee transaction contains many documents including a complex one between the producer and the completion guarantor that details the completion guarantor's rights. The guarantee itself is likely to be a simple and straightforward document in favor of the bank, whereby the guarantor undertakes to assure completion of the picture. The guarantee may also provide that, in the event the guarantor is impelled to declare a production hopeless and abandoned, he will simply repay the bank its production loan. Abandonment is rarely invoked because it is simply too expensive.

There are certain areas of controversy characteristic of completion guarantees. The most common issue in the area of claims is the difference between a legitimate over-budget cost, part of making the picture as contemplated and guaranteed, versus enhancement. In the three-sided transaction, the guarantor usually has no choice but to finish the picture. If he has failed to police the production, and the producer has thereby succeeded in raising the cost of the picture by enhancing it, the guarantor is still obligated to the bank to make delivery notwithstanding over-budget costs. He may have to advance these costs and then bring an action against the producer to collect that portion of the extra costs occasioned by enhancement rather than by legitimate over-budget contingencies. In a two-sided transaction, the issue may also arise in the context of a lawsuit by the producer (or a closely allied financier) against the guarantor, wherein the guarantor raises the defense that the costs in question are enhancement costs rather than legitimate over-budget costs.

Another source of dispute may be diversion of a picture's budgeted production funds to some purpose other than payment of the production's expenses. The possibilities are limitless. They include the charging of travel to the budget where the travel actually related to another project or a personal frolic of the producer; concealment of personal debt repayments in checks to vendors ostensibly for materials or equipment for the production; and purchase of long-term capital assets out of the budget rather than renting them for the limited period of production. While the completion guarantor's watchword is always vigilance, such occurrences will have different ramifications in the two-sided as against the three-sided transaction. If, in the two-sided transaction, someone on the production team has succeeded in diverting funds from the production budget to some other purpose, resulting in a need for additional cash for completion, the guarantor may simply refuse to put it up. The guarantor could rely for a defense on the producer's own default in failing to devote the production budget solely and exclusively to the production of the picture. But this wouldn't be so if the guarantor's obligation is owed to a bank. Here the guarantor still must finish and deliver the picture and look to his own devices to attempt to retrieve any diverted funds from the producer.

The remarkable fact, considering the complexity and scope of feature film production, is that there are few such disputes. The guarantees of the established guarantors are rather routinely accepted, relied upon, and performed, and guarantors make payment of substantially more money to producers or investors in the form of "no-claim bonuses" or rebates than on over-budget claims.

The completion guarantee, as developed in the industry, is only one of several possible ways of assuring that a picture will be finished. It is probably the most satisfactory approach for independently financed pictures. The concept of the completion guarantee is very much in the minds of bankers considering entrance into motion picture work, securities brokers as they review movie financing through public issues, and investment counselors as they give advice on private placements. Since even the most competently prepared budget is at best an estimate of what it will take to bring a picture in, pictures do go over budget, notwithstanding the best intentions and efforts of all involved. For that exigency, the completion guarantee provides a significant measure of protection.

The Talent Agent

by **Barry J. Weitz,** who joined the William Morris Agency after graduating from New York University in 1962. He was transferred to the Beverly Hills office of the agency and worked as a member of the motion picture department there until 1971, when he became an independent producer. His producing credits include the feature *The Seven Ups* and television series such as *Movin' On*.

The aim of all negotiations is, of course, to secure the best possible deal for the client. . . .

The stength of a talented individual lies in his ability to continue to create. Whether it be a performance, a book, or a screenplay, creating is where the energies are. Often, creators do not want to cope with business decisions or career guidance. An individual who must sell himself or negotiate terms in his own behalf might well be less successful than if another individual were taking care of these matters for him. Therefore, the commission that is paid to an agent—10 or 15%—is often the best investment an individual can make in his career. An agent generally receives 10% of the gross fee that an actor receives. For instance, if an actor is to receive $100,000 for a role, the agent will receive 10% of that fee, or $10,000.

In the triangle of buyer, seller, and agent, the agent performs two important functions. First, he sets up a very clear delineation between the buyer and the seller; second, he gives the buyer a professional person to deal with on a consistent basis and in a business atmosphere. Thus a freedom from emotion is established, allowing the parties to cut to the core of the negotiation and agree upon what each party considers essential. The presence of an agent is certainly a great aid to the buyer, since he does not have to become too closely involved with the artist during the negotiations. The buyer can deal with the artist on a creative level and with the agent on a purely business and career level. For these reasons, the talent agency is a very real part of the entertainment business.

There are two ways for a talent agent to obtain clients. He can, through his connections or aggressiveness, bring the individual client to the agency on his own. He may also be assigned a specific client because of his experience, seniority, or a personality that complements the client's. Because human lives and livelihoods are so closely involved, the goal is to find the right kind of combination between agent and client. It is most important that the client be satisfied with his specific link to the business world, the individual who must communicate his thoughts and aspirations to the marketplace.

When an agency takes on a new client, he is required to sign an authorization contract. The contract calls for the agency to represent him in all areas for a stated period of years. Depending on the stature of the client, the agent will plan different approaches to potential buyers. If he is representing a relatively young, less-experienced actor, the agent may feel it necessary to have him meet casting directors and other individuals who are active on a daily basis in casting film and television roles. The agent has a fairly good idea of what his new client's abilities are, so he may decide to move him into the area of dramatic television for the purpose of getting a certain type of role that will show a young actor in a certain light. Of course, he may make the same decision merely in order to get the actor to work immediately. There are a great many more employment opportunities in TV episodic dramas than in feature films. An agent may feel that it is best to move into TV at the outset, assuming that if the venture is successful, he and his client will be provided with the type of sample reel that can be shown to producers and directors in both the feature film and television areas.

Dealing with a new, young client requires a certain experience. The agent must take maximum advantage of the client's talents and expose them effectively in a fair atmosphere with a proper sense of direction. The agent's plan should be to move the actor along to various important roles while increasing his salary so he is making steady advances in both areas. For instance, if an actor earns $1,250 a week in a supporting role for which he achieves proper acclaim and notice, the agent may then be able to move him further along, perhaps to a costarring role where he can make as much as $25,000. If this level is successfully mastered, the agent may well have a young talent who will, as few actors can, move into major starring roles. Either because of a lack of opportunity, improper combination of role and actor, or various other indefinables, these ideal situations may never present themselves. In any event, assuming success along the line, the agent may have an actor who can move from $1,250 a week up to a very high six-figure category that also involves a percentage of the profits or a percentage of the gross on a given film.

An agent must be vary cautious with an actor, however, and move properly to keep him working at good roles. Continuity of employment is an extremely important aspect of client development. The creative lives of many performers are generally not as long as those of other professionals, such as lawyers or doctors. The best-earning years of their careers may be very few, and certainly during that time they have every right to try to make the most of their talent. The agent has the obligation to try to extend their creative life.

There is the danger of an agent becoming so deal-oriented that he or she may be more concerned about making a deal (and collecting a commission for the agency) than about the client's career. It's sometimes tempting to make, for example, a long-term television series deal for an unknown client that will effectively lock him up for years. The talent's only recourse is to renegotiate for higher salaries each year.

In an actor's career, there may be a time when an agent has to decide whether to pursue employment or hold back from it. For instance, an actor may have completed a feature film in which his performance has a great impact. However, the picture is in the can and will not be released for six months. If he is immediately cast in a subsequent picture, his salary will be higher than for his yet-to-be released picture but will not reflect the heat and attention that will result when that picture is released. Should the agent make the deal or wait until the release of the big picture, with the offers and resulting bargaining power that are sure to come? One alternative is for the actor not to take the new deal unless the salary reflects what the agent believes he will be worth after the big picture opens. This kind of decision must be made on an individual basis, as part of the ongoing trust between client and agent.

Contract negotiations are probably the most time-consuming as well as important aspect of an agent's workday. Some agents like to think that there are certain secret methods that enhance their ability to negotiate, but there is no standardized formula or checklist that can be relied upon. Each negotiation is individual and unique. The aim of all negotiations is, of course, to secure the best possible deal for the client. Every agent, I am sure, has walked out of a negotiation assuming he has secured the absolute last penny only to discover later that the buyer was prepared to offer more than was finally paid.

There are times in an agent's life when he is working with an actor who is "hot"—one who is in demand throughout the industry because his popularity in earlier films indicates that his presence in a film will insure a degree of success from the outset. The agent's responsibility in this situation is to exercise great care in analysis of screenplays that are being submitted to him. He must choose scripts that will have an important influence in the film business in the next year or so, thus exposing his client in a well-rounded fashion that will insure greater career longevity. In these moments of great demand, the agent must take care to resist any tendency to overplay his position. Work and creative contribution are still the most important aspects in the performer's life.

If a client is not an "in-demand" actor, the agent must go out and strongly hustle for his sales. If the talent is there, and if various reviews have not overlooked that talent, then the agent has some sort of "hook" to use in selling his client. If, however, the performer has little motion picture ability—if he had the opportunity but has not been able to prove himself—then the agent must reevaluate his client's career. There are many clients, for example, who have not been able to succeed in features, but who have starred in their own television series. There are also clients who have not been able to succeed in either motion pictures or television but have become major stage performers. A great deal depends upon the talent finding his own medium. The agent certainly should assist in the search and give proper guidance to a client in this endeavor.

If, for any reason, the client should not be satisfied with the progress he is making in the agency, or if he is simply not happy with the way he is being represented, he can discharge the agency. The unions and guilds generally allow a period of 90 days after he signs a contract, or one beginning 90 days after he has received his last offer, in which he is able to terminate his agency relationship. The client is always able to discharge his agency, but if he is not able to show cause, then he is obligated to pay any commission due the agency until the termination of the agreement.

Packaging has become an important part of the talent agent's work. Agencies such as International Creative Management (ICM), William Morris, Creative Artists (CAA), and Ziegler-Diskant will assemble feature packages, usually consisting of the material, the writer, the director, perhaps the producer, and perhaps the star, and present them to a financing source in exchange for a profit position in the picture and/or a packaging fee. In television, series are often created in such packages by agencies who receive a packaging fee in return.

The concept of stars wanting a degree of ownership and creative control over their product really goes back to the formation of United Artists in 1919, founded by Douglas Fairbanks, Mary Pickford, Charlie Chaplin, and D. W. Griffith. Today, stars are putting together their own packages, using material that is submitted to their own companies, and are being financed by major distributors. They give the studios the benefit of their talent, their box-office draw, and an exclusive call on their pictures. In exchange, the stars receive very high guaranteed compensation, low overheads, the most favorable distribution fee possible, the most favorable definition of net profits possible, and a share in the ownership of the pictures. Stars such as Clint Eastwood, Robert Redford, Barbra Streisand, Jane Fonda, and Sidney Poitier have enjoyed great success as owners of as well as stars in their pictures. But along with the privilege of sharing profits or ownership of a picture comes the responsibility of sharing the risk of financing the picture in the event that it goes over budget.

Often, business-oriented studio types do not concern themselves with a creative environment for the client. They may be more concerned with getting the project released or getting the return on their dollars. The agent's problem may very well start, then, after the deal has been made, when the buyer and seller start to "live together."

Keeping the relationship alive and viable—and keeping the creative juices flowing—may be the most important aspect of the agent's work.

After he has closed the negotiation and the contracts have been signed, a different phase of the work begins. An agent must now live with his deals and not expect someone else to follow up. I think if an agent does not emerge from behind his desk, his relationships with his clients are going to fall apart, and his relationships with buyers, producers, directors, and studios are going to deteriorate. The studio looks to the agent to be there at times to help solve his client's problems. The agent, of course, may have to walk a thin line between asserting himself in his client's behalf and meddling in matters that don't concern him. Generally, however, the studio is open and receptive to the agent. They feel his behavior and presence will, in the final analysis, be of help in easing difficulties.

One can easily see that a good agent will raise a business relationship to a human relationship, a circumstance that is difficult to find in any industry outside the entertainment business. The relationship can be a very personal, intimate one. An agent is a diplomat, negotiator, salesman, friend, and a very real part of the performer's life. To review, the agent's responsibility includes careful shaping of the client's career, sound negotiating for the right kind of deal, awareness of what the trends in the market are, and the ability to anticipate what the market will be like after a film has been completed. It is difficult, however, for an agent to generalize to a client about this responsibility. He can put his finger on it only after he has found the right kind of project and has negotiated a deal offering a specific dollar amount for his client to perform in that project.

The agency will always be an integral part of the motion picture business because there will always be a need for the creative middleman—the buffer—who is in touch with the changing business, and who can bring together various creative and business elements for the mutual satisfaction and reward of those who participate. Since many agencies continue to have training programs for qualified men and women, the level of professional expertise will be maintained.

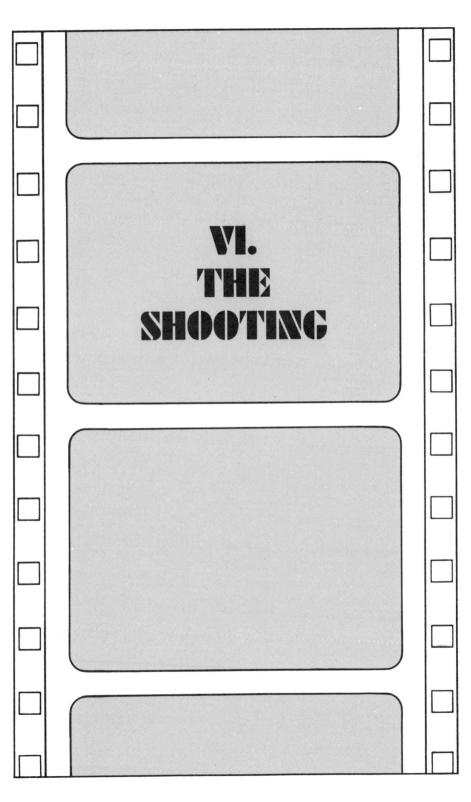

VI.
THE
SHOOTING

The Line Producer

by **Paul Maslansky,** one of the most active line producers in the business, who has made motion pictures around the world. Before turning to producing, he served in production capacities for Columbia Pictures and United Artists in Europe. Notable among his producing credits are *Race with the Devil* for Twentieth Century–Fox; *The Blue Bird,* a Fox co-production with Lenfilm Studios, Moscow; *Damnation Alley* for Fox; *King,* the award-winning 6-hour drama for NBC; *Hard Times* for Columbia; *When You Coming Back, Red Ryder?* for Melvin Simon Productions; *The Villain* for Rastar; *Hot Stuff* for Columbia; *Scavenger Hunt* for Mel Simon Productions; and *Love Child* for the Ladd Company.

The line producer is the man hired by the financiers or producers of
a picture to be directly responsible for the money. He's in charge
of the day-to-day physical production of the picture, planning and ap-
proving costs, hiring and firing personnel, and the many intangible requirements of maintaining a film crew on schedule. Although his
screen credit may vary from executive producer, co-producer, producer, or associate producer, it is the line producer who has the extensive background in physical production that makes him a key person
on a picture, second only to the director and bridging the gap between
management and the technical crew. If the director has creative control
during shooting, the line producer has financial control.

A line producer can be hired by various parties: by a writer
who wants to produce his screenplay and have the creative control, but
who has no experience in physical production; by a new producer,
bearing the title because he or she has acquired the most important element in a film deal—the property—but who may be a former agent, perhaps, with no production experience in the field; by an independent
producer-financier, such as Melvin Simon Productions, who will em-
ploy his services on a specific picture that they are financing; or by a
studio that may be financing a picture on which they need someone to
oversee their money, someone with whom the buck stops.

A project is already in the works, usually, when the line producer is hired. There is a completed screenplay, and there is financing
(the line producer is a paid employee). When I join a picture, the first
thing I do is read the script thoroughly and estimate how much it's
going to cost. I start asking myself whether certain scenes should be
shot on location or in a studio. Shooting on location is going to cost extra not only for travel but for per diem expenses for the cast and crew.
At a studio, there's a five-day workweek; on location there's a six-day
workweek. A six-day workweek on a seven-week picture on location is
42 days; a seven-week picture in a studio is 35 days. Time is of the essence, and you want to finish shooting at the earliest possible time
without sacrificing quality.

If I am taking on the responsibility of bringing in a picture at a certain figure, I must approve the budget. This means I would take the existing budget, analyze it very closely along with the screenplay, discover the problem areas, and make the appropriate changes.

A budget is divided into two main areas, above-the-line and below-the-line. The below-the-line is broken down into three sections, production period, post-production period, and "other charges." Different studios have different forms, and I would support an industry effort to settle on one standard form for all theatrical feature budgets. The top sheet is a summary of each area in the budget. (Please refer to the sample budget top sheet, p. 210–11.) The budget body can run from 20 to 30 or more pages, depending upon the complexity of the picture.

In analyzing a budget for production, the only figures that would be difficult to change are the above-the-line figures. *Above-the-line* costs refer to fixed costs of key creative commitments and personnel made before shooting starts, including the cost of story and other rights connected with the acquisition of the underlying literary material; screenplay (scenario) costs; the producer's unit, covering salaries for the producer, co-producer, associate producer, plus their secretaries; director costs, meaning the salaries for the director and his secretary; and cast, referring to the acting talent in the picture, including stunt people. For a location picture, add the traveling and daily living expenses (per diems) of all those people. Above-the-line costs may also include a finder's fee for someone who might have discovered the property and brought it to the attention of the producing entity, and maybe a production fee to the company that represents the original owner of the material (who was bought out).

Next, add the *fringes*, meaning the pension, health, and welfare costs that are tacked on to the various guild members in the above-the-line area, such as those in SAG (Screen Actors Guild), DGA (Directors Guild of America), and WGA (Writers Guild of America).* When we hear that a director gets $100,000 to direct a movie, it's deceptive because the figure is really closer to $120,000 of actual cost, adding the various fringe payments required by the guilds. Fringes add between 20 and 30% of labor costs.

The *below-the-line* accounts cover the costs incurred to physically make the picture. Whenever a budget has to be cut, it can only be trimmed in the below-the-line area, where strategy must be applied to

---

* Editor's Note: For information regarding current SAG minimums or other questions, contact the Screen Actors Guild, 7750 Sunset Boulevard, Hollywood, CA   90046 (phone 213–876–8030). Inquiries as to the content of the current DGA Basic Agreement should be sent to the Directors Guild of America, Inc., at one of these addresses: 7950 Sunset Boulevard, Hollywood, CA   90046 (213–656–1220); 110 West 57 Street, New York, NY   10019 (212–581–0370); or 40 East Oak Street, Chicago, IL   60611 (312–787–5050). For information on the Writers Guild, please see footnote on p. 68.

TWENTIETH CENTURY-FOX FILM CORPORATION

REV. FORM A450 4/79

PRODUCTION BUDGET

Starting Date _____
Finishing Date _____
Production Days _____

Production No. _____
Producer _____
Director _____
Title _____

Ratio _____
No. _____

RELEASE TITLE _____

1

ACCT. NO.		PG. NO.	ACCUMULATED COST TO	BUDGET		ACTUAL COST	OVER OR (UNDER) BUDGET
					TOTAL		
101	Story Rights	2					
102	Scenario	2					
104	Producer	2					
106	Director	2					
110	Cast	3					
	TOTAL ABOVE-THE-LINE						
111	Extras	4					
112	Staff	5					
114	Art Costs	6					
115	Set Costs	6					
115	Light Platforms	6					
115	Set Strike	6					
115	Set Costs – other	6					
116	Operating Labor & Materials	7					
117	Miniatures	8					
118	Camera	8					
119	Production Sound	9					
120	Electrical	10					
121	Special Effects	11					
122,3	Set Dressing, Drapery	12					
124	Animals & Action Devices	13					
125	Wardrobe	14					
127	Makeup & Hairdressing	15					
128	Process Shooting	15					
131	Props	16					
140	Production Rawstock & Processing	17					
141	Stills	17					
147	Transportation – Cars & Trucks	18					
148	Tests	17					
160	Location Expense	19					

	TOTAL PRODUCTION PERIOD					
113	Music	20				
129	Post-Production Sound	21				
130	Special Photographic Effects	21				
143	Titles	22				
144	Post-Production Film, Processing	22				
146	Projection	22				
149	Editorial	23				
	TOTAL POST-PROD.PERIOD					
170	Miscellaneous	24				
179	Rental Charges & Fees	25				
	TOTAL OTHER CHARGES					
	TOTAL BELOW-THE-LINE					
	TOTAL ABOVE & BELOW LINE					
	OVERHEAD					
	GRAND TOTALS					

	ACTUAL
Date Compiled	
Starting Date	
Finishing Date	
Production Days	

REMARKS

BUDGET CERTIFICATIONS

Estimator	Producer
Head of Estimating Dept.	Sr. Vice-President, Finance & Administration
Manager, Production Accounting	Vice-President, Worldwide Production
	President, Feature Film Division
Vice-President Prodn. Mgmt.	Chairman of the Board

* Copyright © 1980 by Twentieth Century-Fox Film Corporation.

reduce the physical costs and cut shooting time. Below-the-line costs are divided into three areas. The production period refers to every cost directly related to making the picture during shooting. All the departments are represented here: art, construction, camera, sound, electrical, special effects, set dressing, wardrobe, makeup and hairdressing, props, and transportation. In each department, the personnel costs include salaries, living expenses, travel, and fringes. Add on the cost of the film, the processing, all the physical equipment used, catering, first aid, costumes—everything involved in the actual making of the picture during the production period.

Another part of the below-the-line costs is known as the post-production or editing period. This area in the budget concerns itself with the editorial crew (an editor plus assistants) and any laboratory work directly related to the editing period. (The rushes and development of the film during shooting are budgeted in the shooting period.) This area also covers reprints, opticals, black and white dupes, and titles, right up to making the answer print. Add to this the cost of scoring the music and post-production sound, such as looping and mixing the dialogue and sound effects. Fringes based on labor costs in this period are usually an added 30 to 40%. If the editor is making $1,500 a week, his account is charged perhaps 30% more, or an added $450, for a gross total of $1,950 per week. He will receive his $1,500 salary and the $450 will be contributed to the editor's pension, health, and welfare funds.

The third area of below-the-line costs, "other charges," can include publicity costs (during production only) and travel and living expenses for people who might be connected with the picture from the distribution company or financiers. If we're shooting in San Antonio, and one of the financiers who's put up 10% of the budget wants to visit with his wife, that's an expense that must be found somewhere in the budget. Next, there are miscellaneous costs, for example, insurance costs, since the picture must be covered from the moment the first employee goes on payroll. Generally, that person is the director. If monies have been spent but the director has to be replaced due to illness, insurance would compensate for those costs. It's also essential to insure the fact that you have the rights to the story. "Errors and omissions" insurance covers the possibility that the story's not original or that someone else owns it. It insures title, like title insurance for a house. Add the total above-the-line and below-the-line costs for the grand total of the budget.

If it is an independent production, I may have to arrange for a completion bond on the picture, which would mean making a deal with a financier, called a *completion guarantor*, who will insure that the picture is completed if it goes over budget. (See article by Norman G. Rudman, p. 189.) Generally, a completion guarantor gets 6% of the budget for that service, which becomes a budget item. A completion guarantee is written in such a way that the penalties are very severe; the guarantor can take physical control of the movie if it exceeds the budget plus a cushion. For example, on a $4,000,000 movie, the guarantor will want a 10% contingency, or cushion, which would require him to start paying if production costs go over $4,400,000. There's rarely a picture that runs *under* budget; usually, such a picture was overbudgeted and overscheduled in the first place. On a studio picture, there is no completion bond. Instead, there is overhead, which varies from studio to studio but averages about 20% and is part of the *negative cost* (literally the cost to deliver the negative, or production cost) of the picture.

Now, let's follow my procedures on a picture financed on an independent basis. Assuming the director has been chosen, the first person I would hire is the production manager. He's my right-hand man, along with the accountant. They're going to provide the fiscal control over the picture. The production manager will approve daily costs, and I will oversee this. The accountant feeds the daily costs, what each department is spending, to the production manager. It's important to select a production manager who has a good reputation from previous pictures.

Let's say we have a $4,000,000 picture independently financed, and I have approved the budget. In order to plan the shooting schedule, I'll sit down with the production manager and break down the screenplay scene by scene. We'll specify which characters are involved in each scene, the description and location of each scene, whether it's day or night, interior or exterior. Each scene will be so described on a strip of cardboard about three quarters of an inch wide and sixteen inches long. These strips will be juggled in various orders to determine the fastest and most economical sequence in which to shoot. Once this sequence is determined, the strips will be fit into a breakdown board and divided into shooting days. This becomes the road map for the shooting schedule. (For examples of production paperwork, see article by James Bridges on page 222.)

Part of this scheduling will be dictated by where the money is. Usually, the most money is found in the cast. If I have Paul Newman for four weeks and the picture's to be shot in eight, I may want to finish with him early, so that his expense is behind me. I would take all of Paul Newman's scenes and place them in a sequence so that he's gone in four weeks. I also try to schedule all my exteriors early, because they involve the intangible of weather. If there are weather problems, it's better for them to affect us early in the shoot when we can move to an interior cover set. Later in the shoot, waiting for clearing weather means losing time and money.

I will present the proposed shooting schedule to the director, and he will evaluate it, knowing how he works and making changes accordingly. The ideal would be to shoot a picture in continuity, that is, in order. But if the first scene of the screenplay is set in Macon, Georgia, the second scene in Snellville, Georgia, and the third scene back in Macon, it's economical to shoot the two scenes in Macon together, eliminating travel time back and forth.

Now, the breakdown board and shooting schedule have been agreed upon, which gives us the number of shooting days. This helps us finalize the budget, since each shooting day represents an amount of dollars. What are some ways to save money? One way is to shoot seven pages of the screenplay on a given day rather than four, but that puts the company under tremendous pressure. A better way to save money is to cut out days by combining or even eliminating scenes, since time is money. Saving money usually means making compromises. Making movies generally is a series of compromises.

With every scene now locked into a shooting sequence, I know which sets are required on which days, so I can hire an art director (or production designer). After consulting with the director, the art director goes out to search for locations. Sometimes we'll send out letters to the various state film commissions with a list of locations needed and their descriptions. They will send back assorted photographs, since they all want us to come to their state and make the movie. This helps in location scouting and saves a lot of footwork.

Next, there is other crew to hire, and each department is responsible for hiring some of their own. For example, the costume designer will hire the wardrobe master (or mistress), who actually takes care of the handling and cleaning of the garments.

On a six-week shoot, pre-production will last about six weeks. In the first week, I've done the board and worked on the budget with the production manager and accountant. In the second week, the art director has left to search for locations, and casting is going on, since we've hired a casting director. The accountant has some payroll to contend with and sets up the books and the picture's bank account. Next, the balance of the hiring is done, including the assistant directors, director of photography, other heads of departments, and their staff.

Once we start shooting, the director runs the show. He has a department that includes the first assistant and second assistant or assistants. These people are responsible for running the floor logistically, keeping order, and handling the background action so that the director can concentrate on the principals in front of the camera. The second assistant generally does the paperwork, such as the *call sheet*, which announces the subsequent day's work schedule and is ready for distribution to the crew before the end of a shooting day.

The head of the camera department is the director of photography. His men are the camera operator, who actually looks through the camera, and two assistants: one to follow focus and one to load the camera and use the clapboard. The director of photography is responsible for the photographic look of the picture, so lighting falls in his domain. The chief electrician is called the *gaffer;* he's on the floor with the director of photography, helping set the lights. The chief electrician's assistant is called a *best boy.* There are two best boys on a picture, best boy to a gaffer and best boy for the chief grip. The chief grip is responsible for moving the camera to the place where the director wants to shoot and for moving the boards and panels that shade off lights. The construction crew is usually not around during shooting. They've been there, finished their work, and gone to work on whatever construction is needed on the next location. The only construction person who remains is there in case we have to float (or move) different walls. To review the departments: production, art, construction, photography, sound, electrical, special effects, props and set dressing (both generally part of the art department), wardrobe, makeup and hair as one, transportation, and editorial.

Very early in pre-production, I ask each department head to provide a breakdown of their department budgets after I've made an initial budget estimate from the screenplay. This avoids a situation where I may have estimated wardrobe on a picture to cost $50,000 but the costume designer comes in very fancifully with wardrobe designs that cannot be delivered for less than $200,000. Or perhaps I don't know that the price of filigree has gone up 200% because Taiwan's having a political problem or that the cost of lumber in Houston is far more than in Oregon. Each department head confers with the director in preparing this breakdown figure, so they are expressly following the director's requirements. Generally, a department head's figure and my estimate are close. If there's a real discrepancy, I make it known that I'm very distressed that a reasonable figure can't be met. If there's a lack of communication and that wardrobe figure, for example, is still not practical, I'd better find some extra money elsewhere in the budget or find another costume designer.

When the art director returns from the location search, he will sketch out thoroughly his concept of the sets and supervise the drafting of the construction blueprints by a draftsman. The result is the art director's vision of what the sets should look like, after collaborating with the director and producer, and guided by the screenplay. The art director works with a set dresser, who is responsible for bringing in furniture, giving the set life. The set dresser has a lead man working with him as well as other laborers, called *swing gang.* The art department also includes the prop people (prop master and assistant prop master),

215

who are responsible for the hand props used in the picture, as well as the cars and sometimes animals. If it's a western, livestock would be handled by a wrangler.

The photography department consists of the D.P. (director of photography), camera operator, first and second assistants, and still man, who takes all the still photographs used in publicity. The sound department is generally composed of two people: the *mixer*, who sits with earphones at his portable console, and the *boom man*, who holds the microphone. Sometimes a cable man is added to this crew. The mixer is responsible for proper sound levels and for clear sound; his quarter-inch audio tape runs at a speed exactly synchronized with the film in the camera. During pre-production, the director, production manager, and D.P. agree on what camera equipment to rent. This equipment is reserved, as is the raw film stock.

Wardrobe, which is self-explanatory, is headed by a costume designer who conceives of the garments, goes out with the wardrobe master, and rents certain wardrobe from companies such as Western Costume, or else sees that costumes are constructed. The wardrobe master cares for the cleaning of costumes and makes sure that each garment is tagged so each artist knows on what day he wears what garment. They know that on day 15 Jane Fonda is going to be wearing the blue gown and on day 13 it's the green gown. In estimating budget items, the areas where one can go most wrong are the art department (covering set construction), wardrobe, and transportation.

The transportation captain supervises the work of between eight and twenty drivers and other personnel, charged with the logistics of moving the entire company from hotel to set and back to hotel every day. A driver gets paid $700 to $1,500 a week and is responsible for maintenance of his equipment.

When we start shooting, there are two elements I have no control over: weather and health. There's no way to protect against bad weather except to have an interior cover set handy so that some shooting can be accomplished. In order to protect the health of the artists and key technicians, it makes sense to stay at a comfortable hotel so they are mentally and physically prepared to put in 12-hour workdays and 72-hour workweeks. I won't work a crew over 12 hours unless I'm losing a key artist the next morning because of a stop date, or unless there's such a good roll on a scene that stopping the scene will lose the dynamics that have been building creatively. Morale is an important intangible. Management and labor must have an open relationship on a movie because the crew becomes a family. It's pretty tough to get up at six every morning six days a week for twelve weeks and not slow down after a while. Motivation is not found only in the money: there has to be a good spirit created, too. That's important for management, such as the production manager, line producer, or financier, to understand.

Now we are entering the production period, the most intensive of the three stages, when money is being spent at the rate of $4,000 to $5,000 an hour. How is this organized on location? During pre-production, a local bank will have been selected because of its reputation and its convenience to the location. The bank is usually delighted, because having a movie company's account is glamorous and means $1,600,000 to $2,000,000 worth of activity circulating through the bank over six weeks of shooting for our $4,000,000 picture.

A checking account is opened through the use of signature cards after we have demonstrated to the bank the validity of our corporation. There are two signatures necessary on each numbered check; I generally sign on one line, and the accountant signs on the other. As backup, one of the financiers at home can sign in my place, and the production manager can sign in place of the accountant. We order books of numbered checks, and the accountant opens a master ledger in the production office that will account for each check in detail.

Checks are used to pay for physical equipment and wages. In the purchase of equipment, our company works like any small company. If a department member needs a piece of equipment, he will tell the department head, who will make out a purchase order for each item, approve it, and get the production manager to approve it. When the bill comes in, the accountant will refer to a copy of that purchase order bearing the two approvals and make out a check for payment, which the production manager approves. One of them signs on one line of the check, and it's entered into the master ledger. Then, I will review this check along with many other checks, study the backup paperwork, and sign it on the other line before it is mailed out. If the item is a certain antique lamp to be rented for two weeks so that it can be in the scenes of a certain living room, the set decorator will have selected it from a dealer and negotiated the rental price approved by his department head. The set decorator will then hand in a purchase order for the rental of that lamp, approved by the art director and production manager. The company will use the lamp for two weeks and be billed accordingly.

As for wages, each worker on the picture has a payroll folder kept by the accountant and a weekly time card that indicates his starting time each day, when the lunch break was, what time he resumed work after lunch, the time he wrapped, and the time he returned to the hotel. Each week, the accountant figures the cumulative number of hours, multiplies by the hourly rate, and notes the amount due the worker. The production manager cross-checks each rate card against the production reports, which verifies that the worker's crew did in fact work those hours that week. As an example, the production manager, reading a grip's time card, can verify that he did work 12 hours every day and six days that week, so he's entitled to be paid for a 72-hour week. The production manager approves all the time cards and returns them to the accountant, who prepares the payroll checks. Generally, the accountant begins preparing payroll on Monday, and the checks are ready by Thursday, payday, covering the previous week. I sign every payroll check.

The only item that does not have all this formal backup paperwork is petty cash, used for many small purchases where checks are not practical. In order to minimize problems, I issue only $1,000 of petty cash at a time, and each $1,000 must be returned in the form of receipts. Each week I get an accounting of how much petty cash is out to whom. If one particular department is negligent in returning receipts, I will speak to those people. It's an incestuous business, and the crewmen who are hired have reputations to uphold. There are two aspects of reputation: skill and attitude. If someone is very skillful but unwilling occasionally to give an extra 20 minutes or so necessary to complete a job without putting in for overtime, for instance, or if someone else is suspected of stealing, this affects their reputation in the business. After all, other productions will follow this one, and other line producers will do hiring based on the crew's previous reputation.

The production period is very concentrated, with a high, intense energy level demanded at all times. Tremendous amounts of money are being spent in a short period, so it's important to be constant in terms of cost control. At the end of every shooting week, on Saturday, I meet with the accountant and production manager and review all the accounts to verify whether we're on budget or behind. If we're behind, we must either find more money, cut down in certain departments, shorten the script, or find a more efficient way of working.

Each week during shooting, a cost report is prepared for the financier. This compares the amount spent for each item from a budget top sheet against the original budgeted figure, gives a "cost to complete" figure, and shows in one column to what extent these figures are over or under budget. The completion guarantor also receives this weekly cost report, as well as the call sheets and production reports.

During production, the daily paperwork is prepared carefully to memorialize the progress of each day's shooting. The script supervisor or continuity person sits by the camera during the entire picture. Every night he types up notes itemizing every take, recording script or dialogue changes, comments from the director, details such as what lens was used, what f-stop (for the lab to refer to later to match the shot), and what takes were to be printed. He also keeps a diary as to the times we start work, break for lunch, and the time any accidents might have happened. This diary is given to the production secretary at the end of every shooting day, and he fills out the production report from the data provided by the script supervisor and from other data from the second assistant director, who then verifies and completes the report.

On the set, the first assistant director has his hands full with the actual functioning of the set; he also approves the production report completed by the second assistant. The first assistant ultimately signs production reports (as does the production manager) and call sheets (the itemized schedule for the next day's shooting), but most of the paperwork is initiated by the second and the production secretary.

By the last day of shooting, I've given notice to most of the department heads. I don't need the photography or sound departments anymore, but I need people from wardrobe, props, and set dressing to return articles that have been rented and to resell the items we've bought. Makeup and hair personnel are gone, unless there are some wigs to return. The continuity person or script supervisor stays on for at least a week to type up all the production notes. The production secretary, production manager, and accountant remain until all invoices are in and all bills are paid. When bills are paid, all the time cards are in, the last payroll is done, and adjustments are made for lost or damaged equipment, the production manager has completed his job and can prepare a final accounting. Generally, this is two to six weeks after shooting ends.

It's helpful to make a list early in the picture of all items purchased outright by the department heads. Transportation may buy cars, generators, jacks, tires, and tools. I'll take this inventory at the end of the picture and put the remaining items up for auction to the cast and crew. The production manager runs the auction, and the items go to the highest bidders as a cash sale. The money goes back into the production for use during the post-production period.

According to the Directors Guild, the director has a minimum number of days to deliver his cut, roughly one day of cutting for every two days of shooting. Usually a cutter is assembling the best takes during shooting, so that soon after the last day of production, the editor has a roughly assembled picture to show. This would be an assembly of the specific takes chosen by the director during the daily viewing of rushes and usually runs longer than our target length for delivery.

The picture is then turned over to the editor and the director for the director's cut. When the director delivers this cut, the producers, the studio, or the financial entity can take over, if they have the contractual right to do so.

A post-production period can stretch out unless somebody places certain limits upon it. Pressure is brought to bear either by the studio or financier-distributor because of a contractual delivery date or an impending release date. Generally, the first instincts of a director and editor in cutting a picture are close to what the final cut becomes, though it's tempting to refine a picture infinitely. Since interest continues to be charged on the money being used, the picture should be cut as efficiently as possible.

During pre-production planning, certain bookings of facilities for post-production have been made. For recording the musical score, a studio and an orchestra have to be scheduled; the composer may have just so much time before his next commitment. Rooms have to be rented for the recording of sound effects, looping, and mixing. For the two to four weeks it takes to mix a picture, the mixing room must be reserved months in advance. For example, if this is August and I'm in pre-production on a picture, it would go into post-production facilities in February. I must reserve the room now, because February is a rush period; pictures are being prepared for summer release then.

Let's assume we now have a final cut approved by the financing entity. Next we have to loop (or dub) the picture, which is redoing some of the audio to improve the quality. For this, we may call actors back to rerecord dialogue in a studio, matching in perfect sync with the dialogue on the screen.

During looping, sound editors start building the effects track. If a scene includes a motorboat, and the audio during shooting sounds like a tiny engine rather than a powerful one, the sound editor will either search for the right effect in a sound effects library or go out and reproduce the sound on location.

Since we've cut our picture to its final length, that half of the film is locked in. Now our composer and director view the cut and discuss where musical bridges are needed and where musical cues and stingers will help. The composer will create this music over a period of weeks and return to a recording studio to record the music after it is orchestrated, which requires the hiring of musicians and copyists.

The optical work to be done, such as titles, fades, dissolves, or other effects, will be given to an optical house. Black and white prints, called *scratch prints*, are made for the sound, music, and optical people to view while they're planning their work. At the same time, the negative is being cut in the laboratory. All negatives bear numbers on the edges. By referring to these edge numbers, laboratory technicians conform the negative to the final cut, frame by frame, in a delicate process.

The sound track (including dialogue, music, and effects on separate tracks) is then brought into a mixing room for the final mix. The chief mixer, who runs the dials that govern the dialogue tracks, is joined by a sound-effects mixer, who controls the pots and faders for the sound effects to be added to the picture. He may control ten different sounds at once: wind, cars, natural ambiance (the "presence" of a room), sirens, footsteps. A third person controls music, with separate dials for the different recorded music tracks, such as percussion and strings; that person is a virtuoso in himself. The fourth person is the director, who makes sure the mixing achieves what he has in mind. This is a great process to watch, because at last the picture is coming together, joining final sound to picture.

Once the mixing is complete, everything is turned over to the laboratory. Miraculously, four or five days later, there is an answer print, the first marriage of picture and sound on the same reel of film. Between the first answer print (or married print) and the first release print, there may be several efforts to correct color in various reels The director of photography may come in and supervise the coloration of the picture scene by scene, involving the losing of color or infusing of color into different scenes.

Contractually, my job on a picture is generally completed when the first release print is delivered to the financier-distributor; emotionally, I follow a picture throughout its exploitable life.

"The China Syndrome:" Shooting Preparation and Paperwork

by **James Bridges,** a writer-director who began his Hollywood career as an actor in over 50 television shows and several features. He then turned to writing such feature films as *The Appaloosa, Colossus: The Forbin Project*, and *Limbo* before becoming the writer-director of *The Baby Maker*. Bridges earned an Academy Award nomination for best screenplay adaptation for *The Paper Chase*, which he also directed. He has since written and directed *September 30, 1955, The China Syndrome, Urban Cowboy*, and *Mike's Murder*.

During physical production, huge amounts of money are spent daily for the one-time-only opportunity of capturing performers on film within the environment created by the artistic and technical members of the crew. Although the director is intimately involved in the meticulous preparation that precedes the first day of shooting, once shooting has begun, the crew basically takes over the details of physical production. This frees the director to concentrate on performances, the look of the picture, and the telling of the story.

The director's immediate family during shooting includes the producer, production manager, first assistant director, second assistant, cameraman, and script supervisor. The extended family includes the cast members, heads of departments, and crew. Each film is different, with a unique set of problems, and each director develops a personal style in solving such problems. On *The China Syndrome*, I was given great support by first assistant Kim Kurumada, associate producer/production manager Jim Nelson, executive producer Bruce Gilbert, actors Jack Lemmon, Michael Douglas (who also produced), and Jane Fonda (whose company co-produced), second assistant Barrie Osborne, cameraman James Crabe, and script supervisor Marshall Schlom.

In order to trace preparation and paperwork, one scene has been isolated and will be followed from the pages of the screenplay, written by Mike Gray, T. S. Cook, and me, through to the production report. All materials are furnished courtesy of Columbia Pictures.

SCREENPLAY

The screenplay is the blueprint of the picture. Every bit of physical planning and each commitment of money flows from the screenplay. The screenplay form separates dialogue from description and is divided into scenes in a way that allows space for notations so that every department head can focus on specific needs of each scene. This example covers scenes 247–251, which are the last scenes of the picture. Reporter Kimberly Wells (Jane Fonda) and cameraman Richard Adams (Michael Douglas) are outside the nuclear power plant confronting co-workers of Jack Godell (Jack Lemmon) who has just been killed inside.

                         SPINDLER
          It's over -- it's stable ---

Kimberly looks down at Godell. Richard is beside her.

                         KIMBERLY
          He's dead.

DeYoung looks up at MacCormack who leans back from the
window.

                                        CUT TO

EXT. POWER PLANT - NIGHT - MATTE   247

The outside is all lit up. More reporters have arrived.
More television stations have moved in. Gibson moves out
of the plant with MacCormack, DeYound, Spindler and join
the reporters as Kimberly and Richard follow. The two look
at the crowd and start for the truck. Some cameramen
shooting 16mm, others on tape. There is the gangbang
of reporters clustered about the group. There are lights,
obviously. The various vehicles are parked about.
People rushing.

                         REPORTERS
          1. What's happened?
          2. What's going on?
          3. Get out of the way!
          Etc, etc.

                         GIBSON
          If I can have your attention please.
          I'd like to make an announcement.
                    (beat)
          A few minutes ago, the situation
          inside was resolved. The Ventana
          Nuclear Plant is secure. I'd like to
          emphasize that at no time was the
          public in any danger.

                         REPORTERS
                    (overlapping, interrupting
                    each other, shouting)
          1. How was the situation resolved?
          2. What happened in there?
          3. What can you tell us about the
              armed man who siezed the plant?
          4. Who's this guy Godell?

Kimberly and Richard arrive at the truck. Churchill is there.

                                        CONTINUED

                         KIMBERLY
          Did any of it get on the air?

                           MAC
          Enough to make Godell look like a
          lunatic ---

Kimberly, Richard, and Churchill watch the TV monitor.

                         GIBSON
          Gentlemen -- we'll have a prepared
          statement in just a few minutes --
          again, I want to stress at this time
          that the public was in no danger of
          any kind -- the emotionally disturbed
          employee was humored only long enough
          for us to get the situation under
          control ---

                        REPORTER
          Had he been drinking?

                         GIBSON
          I've been told he had been drinking.

Kimberly, watching on the monitors, has had enough. She
moves closer, looks off at MacCormack, DeYoung, Spindler
etc., as they stand behind Gibson, listening.

                         GIBSON
          Unfortunately he did cause some
          damage to the plant itself, but that
          damage was completely contained ---

                        REPORTERS
          1. What kind of damage?
          2. What happened to him?
          3. Has he been arrested?
          4. Were there any injuries?
          5. How did you get into the control
              room?

Kimberly moves toward the group. DeYoung and Spindler are
being brought forward by MacCormack and others.   248

                         GIBSON
          Gentlemen -- this is Mr. DeYoung and
          Mr. Spindler -- Mr. DeYoung is in
          charge of this plant and Mr. Spindler
          was in charge of the operation through-
          out ---

                                              CONTINUED

The reporters start asking DeYoung and Spindler questions.

> REPORTERS
> 1. How did you stop Godell?
> 2. What was he doing?
> 3. What happened to the tele-
>   vision signal?

> SPINDLER
> We crossed some wires ---

Kimberly moves into the crush of reporters, elbowing and
fighting like the rest. They are all shouting. DeYoung
and Spindler are being interviewed as there is mass
confusion, everyone talking.

Kimberly has managed to get herself up in front with her
mike. Her cameraman right behind her, adjusting. The
others turn and see her. Their cameras on her, their mikes
being thrust forward at her.

> KIMBERLY
> Let me ask a question! A few minutes ago
> Jack Godell was shot to death in front of
> me. Why was he killed?

> DeYOUNG
> The man was emotionally disturbed --
> he was ---

> KIMBERLY
> Who ordered the SWAT squad into the
> control room?

> DeYOUNG
> I told you, he was disturbed -- the man
> was dangerous ---

> KIMBERLY
> Mr. Spindler, do you believe Jack Godell
> was emotionally disturbed? Do you
> believe that?

Spindler looks at Gibson and at DeYoung.

> CUT TO

INT. KXLA TRAILER - NIGHT   249

Mac is in the van with Richard, watching the monitors.
Spindler is looking over at MacCormack and DeYoung. He
hesitates.

> CONTINUED

> KIMBERLY
> Do you believe that? Do you believe
> he was disturbed?

> RICHARD
> Get him, Kimberly ---

                                        CUT TO

EXT. PLANT - NIGHT   250

Kimberly questioning Spindler. The other reporters around,
sensing that something very dramatic is about to happen.

> SPINDLER
> I don't know ---

> KIMBERLY
> How do you explain his behavior
> tonight? What did he say to you?

> GIBSON
> That's enough -- thank you. Mr.
> Spindler -- DeYoung ---

> KIMBERLY
> What did he say?

> SPINDLER
> He said he thought that this plant
> should be shut down ---

> GIBSON
> That's all -- thank you ---

Gibson takes Spindler by the arm and starts to lead him
away. MacCormack and his men trying to stop the reporters.
Kimberly in the crush, fighting to keep questioning, pushing
after them.

> KIMBERLY
> Should it? Should it be shut down?

> SPINDLER
> It's not my place to say ---

> KIMBERLY
> If it's not your place, Mr. Spindler,
> whose is it?

Spindler stops and looks at her.

                                        CONTINUED

> GIBSON
> Let's go, Mr. Spindler -- we have to
> go ---

> KIMBERLY
> If there's nothing to hide, <u>whose</u> <u>is</u>
> <u>it</u>? Let him speak ---

> SPINDLER
> Wait a minute -- Jack Godell was my
> best friend -- these guys are trying to
> paint him as some kind of looney -- he
> wasn't a looney -- he was the sanest
> man I ever met ---

> KIMBERLY
> You believe he had reason to do what he
> did tonight? Was this plant unsafe?

> SPINDLER
> He shouldn't have done what he did if
> there wasn't something to it -- Jack
> Godell was not that kind of guy ---
> (looking at Kimberly)
> I don't know all the particulars -- he
> told me a few things -- but I'm sure
> there's going to be a big investigation
> -- the truth will come out -- and when
> it does, people will know that my
> friend, Jack Godell, was a hero -- he
> was a hero and not some kind of looney
> -- I've said too much already -- I --
> got to go ---

> CUT TO

INT. TV CONTROL ROOM - NIGHT   251

Kimberly can be seen on the monitor. ON AIR. She turns
away from the crowd and to another camera. They are
controlling what is being fed to the audience. Jacovich
very moved by her reporting, standing back, watching,
thinking. The technical staff are barking instructions.

> KIMBERLY
> Pete -- I met Jack Godell two days ago
> and I'm convinced that what happened
> tonight was not the act of a drunk or

CONTINUED

                    KIMBERLY (cont'd)
        a crazy man. Jack Godell was about to
        present evidence that he believed
        would show that this plant should be
        shut down. I'm sorry I'm not very ob-
        jective. Let's hope it doesn't end
        here -- this is Kimberly Wells for
        Channel Three.

On the monitor we see Richard move up to Kimberly and they
embrace as the technical staff cues Pete to appear.

            PETE   DIRECTOR
Thank you, Kimberly, we'll   Spectacular!
be back with more on the
Ventana Power Plant take   JACOVICH
over by one of it's   Good job -- she did a hell
employees right after this --- of a good job -- I must
                               say I'm not surprised.

The commercial continues in the ON AIR monitor. Richard
and Kimberly move through the crowd. The music of the
commercial rising and interestingly enough, it tells us
to buy more electrical appliances.

                                        FADE OUT

On the basis of the screenplay, a preliminary budget is prepared, the shooting schedule is estimated, major casting commits to the
project, and all of this ideally leads to the producers securing a deal
with a financier-distributor. *The China Syndrome* was financed and distributed by Columbia Pictures.

Early in pre-production, there were two problems that were
faced on *China Syndrome.* One was the set; enough lead time had to
be afforded to production designer George Jenkins (who had won an
Academy Award for *All The President's Men*) to construct the elaborate
control room of the power plant. Second, the shooting schedule had to
be planned to free Jack Lemmon to honor a prior commitment to the
Broadway show *Tribute.* This meant that all of Jack Lemmon's work
had to be scheduled first so that he could be released.

A lot of time was taken to assure that the technical aspects of
the picture were accurate. The technical adviser, Greg Minor, was a
scientist and the designer of nuclear power plant safety systems who
had left the industry saying that such systems weren't working. He
worked closely with the production designer and staff.

Informal meetings were held with certain heads of departments
who had to reserve equipment for shooting. For example, the cinematographer, James Crabe, and I discussed the ratio we would shoot in,
the kind of light the picture would use, and the overall visual style of

the picture. Then, he reserved the necessary equipment, including dollies or cranes. He also worked closely with the production designer to consider lighting and physical movement on the set, such as which walls need to be wild (movable). The cameraman also met with the matte artist to plan how matte shots would be framed. In the case of our example, the basic exteriors of the power plant were matte shots, combining live action with the artist's rendering on glass.

Location selection and principal casting occurred very early in pre-production. When it was decided to use the outside of a power plant at Playa Del Rey as our nuclear plant (when we were close enough not to need a matte), I knew that I would want to have a big crane shot from above to establish all of the activity and news coverage outside, as well as an actual helicopter within frame to heighten the action. I was casually blocking the action of this scene when we scouted the location, and this would be carried over formally when it came to actual shooting.

The casting director, Sally Dennison, worked closely with Jane, Michael, Bruce Gilbert, and me to fill the supporting roles, and we would not cast anyone who Jack Lemmon thought might be wrong for the part. We had one reading with all of the actors together during pre-production. Out of that reading I went away and did some rewriting because I felt strongly that Jane's character didn't have enough to do in the piece. I spent two weeks rewriting in the mornings and working with the production people in the afternoons.

BREAKDOWN SHEET

A budget figure is not meaningful until it conforms to the specific breakdown board and shooting schedule prepared by the production manager and first assistant director and approved by the producer, director, and financier-distributor. Budget figures up to this point have been speculative; these are for real, prepared and approved by those people who are being paid to fulfill their own planning during physical production.

The whole process begins with breakdown sheets. The first assistant director takes the screenplay and isolates each scene or piece of complete action to a new breakdown sheet. The sheet lists all personnel and equipment necessary to shoot the scenes on that set, along with one-line synopses of action that correspond to specific scene numbers and lengths. Our example follows scenes 247–251, covering the exterior set of the nuclear power plant. Each cast member is numbered for easier identification and cross-reference. The police helicopter envisioned is listed under "props."

BREAKDOWN SHEET
"CHINA SYNDROME"

| SET | EXT. NUCLEAR PLANT | DAY NITE SHEET | N6 |

| SEQ. | SC. NO. | | |

		DAYS	
247	1 2/8 pages	PAGES	4 7/8
248		STAGE	
249	3 5/8 pages		
250		LOCATION	
251 (pt)			

SYNOPSIS	MUSIC—SOUND

247
Kimberly, Richard, Gibson, MacCormack, DeYoung, Spindler exit. Kimberly & Richard move to their truck and begin to watch Gibson make his statement to the press.

248 249 250 251 (pt)
Kimberly moves to Gibson, interviews Gibson and Spindler, then gives her wrap.

Note: Mini cams to feed live and record all takes for later coverage.

SPECIAL EFFECTS	VEHICLES—ANIMALS	PROPS
	1 Godell's car	1 Flying police Helecopter
	1 SWAT Truck	w/search light
	1 Fire Truck	1 Waterwagon
	1 Rescue Truck	1 Crane
	1 Ambulance	1 Extra Generator
	4 TV News Vans	1 CGE Helecopter
	3 TV News Cars	
	2 Motorcycles	
	4 Sheriff Cars	
	4 Police Cars	
	1 Coroner's car	

CAST	BITS	EXTRAS
1. Kimberly	4 KXLA Tech.	20 News co-workers
3. Richard	8 Control Rm. Tech.	12 FBI Men
5. Churchill	6 Plant Sec. Guards	12 Sheriffs
7. Spindler	8 News Reporters	8 Policemen
8. DeYoung		8 Firemen
9. Gibson		4 Paramedics
10. MacCormack		30 Plant Workers
14. Tom		30 Spectators
30. Cameraman		
39. Reporter 1		
40. Reporter 2		
61. Reporter 3		
62. Reporter 4		
63. Reporter 5		
60. SWAT Chief		
61. Mrs. Spindler		
46. Barney		
49. Tommy		
44. Donny		

BREAKDOWN BOARD

All of the information from the breakdown sheets is then transferred to a breakdown board—a large wooden headboard (five feet or longer) on which the actual sequence of shooting scenes is determined. Each unit of shooting is represented by a cardboard strip containing descriptions and requirements from the breakdown sheets. These strips can be juggled so that a proper sequence of shooting can be arrived at. The strips can vary in color (distinguishing day from night shooting) and follow the same numbering system referring to cast members as noted on the breakdown sheets. Each cast member is listed in a column on the left side of the breakdown board. The board itself accommodates the scene strips, divided into shooting days.

One priority in preparing the *China Syndrome* board was to place all of Jack Lemmon's scenes first because of his play commitment. The director, producers, production manager, and first assistant all work on the breakdown board in planning exactly how many scenes can be shot in one day, bearing in mind all of the logistics involved. Once there is agreement on the board—the sequence of shooting and the number of days—it is presented to the financier-distributor. Generally, their response is to reduce the total number of days, in which case the board must be redone (generally adding strips to each scheduled workday), making the picture harder to shoot. Once the breakdown board and budget (both reflecting final decisions regarding equipment and personnel) are approved by the financier-distributor, the shooting schedule can be prepared.

SHOOTING SCHEDULE

Since the sequence of shooting and number of days have been approved from the breakdown board, all of these data can be transferred to a shooting schedule. This is prepared by the first assistant and approved by the production manager. The shooting schedule records in order the intended scenes to be shot each day and the sequence of shooting days, along with the necessary cast members, equipment, personnel, props, and sets to be used, again following the information set down in the breakdown sheets.

Because of the logistical requirements of *China Syndrome*, the picture could not be shot in order. The scenes that ended the picture were actually shot around the middle of the schedule, on days 43 and 44, at night.

DAY & DATE	SETS-SCENES-DESCRIPTION	CAST	LOCATION
	END OF 42nd DAY		
43rd and 44th shooting days Tue., Mar 16 and Wed., Mar 17	Ext. Nuclear Plant Scene 147 -- Nite for Nite (N6) 1 2/8 pages Kimberly, Richard, Godell, others exit. Gibson begins interview to the press. Extras & Bits Approx. 200 extras Picture Cars 1 Godell's car 3 TV News Cars 1 SWAT Truck 2 Motorcycles 1 Fire Truck 4 Sheriff Cars 1 Rescue Truck 4 Police Cars 1 Ambulance 1 Coroner's car 4 TV News Vans Props Police guns News Team Props, cameras, etc. Hardhats Work Tools Note: Live mini-cams to work throughout the sequence.	1. Kimberly 2. Richard 5. Churchill 7. Spindler 8. DeYoung 9. Gibson 10. MacCormack 14. Tom 30. Cameraman 29. Reporter 1 40. Reporter 2 41. Reporter 3 62. Reporter 4 63. Reporter 5 60. SWAT Chief 61. Mrs. Spindler 46. Barney 49. Tommy 44. Donny	Scattergood Power Plant 12700 Vista Del Mar Playa Del Rey
	Scene 248 thru 251 (pt) -- Nite for Nite (N6) 3 5/8 pages Kimberly interviews Spindler, gives wrap up. Note: Film and video footage to be later used for Sc. 251 complete Int. News Room. Trans., Props, Bits Same as Sc. 147	See Above	
	END OF 43rd & 44th DAY		

Once there is a shooting schedule, the producer, director, and first assistant sit down with each department head to formally go over the requirements of each shooting day. For example, the transportation captain and I review the need for a SWAT truck, fire truck, ambulance, and other vehicles for shooting outside the plant on days 43 and 44. The prop master will know that we'll need police guns, news team equipment, hard hats, and various work tools for the actors on that location. Naturally, all of this is to review what had been discussed earlier in pre-production, when each department head prepared a budget figure and began renting necessary material or equipment. Now, these elements can be secured for specific shooting days.

It would be nice if the actual shooting of a picture followed the shooting schedule exactly, but this is not the case. The reality is that pressures of time, money, weather, temperament, and other contingencies generally throw a production company off the first shooting schedule, forcing them to revise constantly. This calls for real flexibility and imagination on the part of the staff, particularly the first assistant, production manager, and producer. Restructuring the shooting schedule and planning around contingencies of weather and ill health are ongoing responsibilities of this collaborative mix.

CALL SHEET

The call sheet—prepared by the second assistant director and then approved or changed by the first assistant and finally by the production manager—is issued each day to the cast and crew for the following day's shooting. Any departures from the shooting schedule or changes in equipment or personnel requirements will be listed in the call sheet. The call sheet lists the times the actors must report to makeup and what time they must be on the set. It also lists the reporting time of crew members, stand-ins, extras, and certain vehicles.

This example of a call sheet was prepared for the 43rd day of shooting *The China Syndrome* at the Scattergood Power Plant location. Most crew members and vehicles were to be in place by 5 p.m., with extras and stand-ins in place by 5:30. Cast members were to be on the set by 6:30, and there is a provision for 215 dinners to be ready for cast and crew by 11:00 p.m. This call sheet covers the first of two nights at the location, which was the time allotted to shoot our sample pages.

Most of the daily paperwork during shooting is done by the assistant directors in order to free the director to focus on the actual shooting. Each director prepares for a shooting day in his or her own style, and every style is different. I get up every morning, make myself some coffee, and go directly to the typewriter. I'll retype a scene some-

EYEWITNESS LTD.

SUNSET-GOWER STUDIOS · 1438 No. Gower St
Hollywood, Ca. 90028 · (213) 466-3295

PRODUCER: Michael Douglas
EXEC PROD: Bruce Gilbert
DIRECTOR: James Bridges

COMPANY WILL REPORT TO
LOCATION, RD. TRIP:
52 MILES

CALL SHEET

Prod No. 132441

Day THURSDAY, MARCH 16, 1978
43RD   48+1HOLI
Crew Call   5PM HAVING HAD
Shooting Call 6PM
SCATTERGOOD POWER PLANT
12700 VISTA DEL MAR – PLAYA DEL REY

SET	D/N	SCENES	CAST	PGS	LOCATION
EXT. PLANT	N5	247,248,249pt,		3	(see above)
EXT. PLANT	N5	250,251pt,253A,			" "
		254pt		2 5/8	" "
INT. KXLA TRAILER	N5	249pt,251pt		5/8	" "

NOTE: 5:00PM REHEARSAL SCENES: 247, 248, 249pt !   TOTAL PAGES: 6 2/8

CAST & DAY PLAYERS	PART OF	MAKE UP	SET	REMARKS
1 Jane Fonda	Kimberly Wells	5P	630P	Courtesy PU 430P
3 Michael Douglas	Richard Adams	5P	630P	Courtesy PU 430P
4 Daniel Valdez	Hector Salas	HOLD		
5 James Karen	Mac Churchill	5P	630P	
6 Peter Donat	Jacovich	HOLD		
7 Bill Brimley	Spindler	5P	630P	
8 Scott Brady	DeYoung	5P	630P	
9 James Hampton	Gibson	5P	630P	
10 Richard Herd	MacCormack	5P	630P	
13 Khalilah Ali	Marge	HOLD		
14 Jack Smith	Tom	5P	630P	
15 Stan Bohrman	Pete	HOLD		
26 Reuben Collins	Sportscaster	HOLD		
39 Frank Cavesani	Reporter #1	430P	630P	ND Meal
40 Terry House	Reporter #2	430P	630P	ND Meal
61 Chris Woods	Reporter #3	430P	630P	ND Meal
62 Val Clenard	Reporter #4	430P	630P	ND Meal
63 Mark Carlton	Reporter #5	430P	630P	ND Meal
60 Clay Hodges	SWAT Chief	5P	630P	
Trudy Lane	Alma Spindler	5P	630P	Recalled for added scene
46 Ron Lombard	Barney	5P	630P	" " " "
49 Tom Eure	Tommy	5P	630P	" " " "
44 Dan Lewkowitz	Donny	5P	630P	" " " "

ATMOSPHERE AND STANDINS		SPECIAL INSTRUCTIONS
3 SI (Gary, Jerry, Jim)	5PM	PROPS/SET DRESSING: News mike & equipment, guns,
4 SWAT	530PM	SWAT, stretcher, recorders & notebooks, plant
30 Plant Techs/15 F.B.I./4 Guards	530PM	blueprints, hard hats, walkie talkies, plant
4 Firemen/2 Fire Rescue/2 Medics	530PM	cushman cart, tools, plastic explosives &
12 TV crew/4 Reporters	530PM	blow torch, beer
2 Coroners/10 Sheriffs	530PM	FX: wet down exterior/practical red lites, all
6 Police/2 MC Cops/Own Ward.	530PM	POLICE: 2 @ 5PM vehicles
6 Wives	530PM	VTR: Playback in KXLA Trailer - scs. 249,251,
		254
		1 Security Cars 5PM

CREW

1 Cameraman	5P	4 Grips	5P	1 Mixer	530P	1 Make Up– Fonda	448P
3 Operator	530P	6 Electricians	5P	1 Boom Man	5P	1 Hair– Fonda	448P
3 1st Asst Cam	5P	1 Gen Op–Loc 40	5P	1 Cable Man	5P	1 Costumer– Fonda	PU 415P
1 2nd Asst Cam	5P	40 man		2 VTR Crew	5P	3 Make Up	418P
Loader		2 Sp Effects	5P	1 Painter	5P	Hair	
1 Stillman	530P	3 Props	5P	Greens		1 Men's Costumer	418P
1 Script	5P	1 Craft Service	430P	X Set Dress	Per Art	1 Women's Costumer	5P
1 1st Aid	5P					1 Xtra Costumer	418P

TRANSPORTATION

PICTURE CARS/SPECIAL EQUIP					MOTOR HOMES/CARS	
1 SWAT Truck	Catering:		Cam Tk	Loc	1 Mot Hom Fonda Loc	430P
2 Fire Tk & Fire Rescue	30 Nd Meals Rdy	515P	1 Prod Van	Loc 5P	1 Mot Hom Douglas Loc	430P
1 Ambulance	X Gal Coffee Rdy	515P		Loc	Mot Hom Lemmon Loc	
4 Minicam Trucks	Doz Donuts Rdy		Effx Trlr	Loc	Mot Hom Bridges Loc	
1 Coroners Wagon	Lunches Rdy		1 Utility Tk	Loc 5P	1 Prod Car PU. Bridges	345P
3 TV station wagons	215 Dinners Rdy	11P	1 Prop Tk	Loc 5P	Staff Car	
4 Sheriff & Police Cars				Loc	Key Car ⟩ Per Craig	
2 Motorcycles (Police)	Busses:		1 M/U–Ward Trlr Loc	4P	Trans Car /	
1 Police Helicopter	1 Titan Crane & Arm		3 HoneyWgns 18 DR	4P	Fonda Car PU Dot	415P
1 CG&E Helicopter					Cost Car PU Douglas	430P
1 Water Truck						

ADVANCE

Fri., Mar. 17 - complete above - total pages (6 2/8)

times to get it in my head. Then I'll type a diary of thoughts and images for myself and place this opposite the screenplay pages that I'll be shooting that day. I'll also make a list of shots needed for each scene and perhaps sketch out drawings of a scene, including camera placement and movement.

When I arrive at the set, I go to the first assistant and to the cameraman with my list of shots. We discuss the scene and review the shot list in terms of movement, style, and content. The cameraman will cover the plans for the day's shooting with his staff, along with the lighting and sound crew. Then I am free to work with the actors.

PRODUCTION REPORT

The production report is a document that states what has been accomplished during a day's shooting. It notes exactly what time the first shot was made; the number of scenes shot; the number of scenes to be shot in order to complete the picture; the status of the production (ahead or behind schedule); how many feet of film were shot, printed, and wasted; the exact time players reported to the set, ate meals, and were dismissed for the day; and any explanations of injuries or delays. The script supervisor, one of the key people around the camera, supplies the first assistant with the time of the first shot, time of camera wrap, number of scenes completed, number of set-ups, and the total and daily timing of scenes. All other information, such as the company's status and how time was spent, is prepared by the first assistant. The first assistant confers with the production manager at the end of each day to determine how the picture is doing in terms of cost and what changes need to be dealt with in allotting additional time for shooting, thereby affecting scheduling, contract changes, and rental agreements. The information on the production report is prepared by the second assistant, checked and approved by the first assistant, and approved as well by the production manager who is responsible to the producer and to the financier-distributor for the cost of that day's shooting. The production report is a documented account of time spent, and therefore of money spent.

What I find exciting about making a movie is that every day I hold the entire picture in my head—constantly arranging, rearranging, and working as it takes on a life of its own. *The China Syndrome* posed a specific cinematic problem, and I was determined that it would be resolved. With the support of the creative and technical team, the picture was completely realized. Good directing, to me, involves hiring the very best people in all departments and creating an atmosphere

NO. OF DAYS ON PICTURE INCLUDING TODAY					
Holidays	Idle	Travel	Rehearsal	Work	Total
1				43	44

PRODUCER: Michael Douglas
EXEC PROD: Bruce Gilbert
DIRECTOR: James Bridges

PRODUCTION REPORT
PROD. 132441

DATE: THURSDAY, MARCH 16, 1978

48 + 1

Date Started 1/16/78   Est. Finish Date 4/4/78   No. Days Estimated HOLIDAY   Status 7 DAYS BEHIND

Location & Sets:

EXT. PLANT, FINALE
SCATTERGOOD POWER PLANT - 12700 VISTA DEL MAR - PLAYA DEL REY, CA.

Crew Call 5P   Shooting Call 6P   Lunch From 11P Til 1130P   Dinner From — Til — Finished 440A
First Shot 855P   First Shot After Lunch 1230A

SCRIPT	SCENES	PAGES	MINUTES		SETUPS		SCENE NOS. 247
Total in Script	258	129 3/8	Prev.	81:15	Prev.	428	
Added Sc. (Credits)			Today	1:10	Today	13	
Shooting Total	258	129 3/8	Total	82:25	Total	441	
Taken Prev.	157	84 1/8	Added Scenes/Retakes Other Pictures:				
Taken Today	1	1 2/8					
Total To Date	158	85 3/8					
To Be Taken	100	44					

	PICTURE NEGATIVE				SOUND		FILM INVENTORY	
	Exposed	Print.	No Good	Waste	Prod'n. Rolls	Footage	Tt'l drwn	209,310
Shot Prev.	149,010	83,630	65,000	16,130	75		Rec'd.	0
Shot Today	4,110	2,110	2,000	800	1		Used	170,050
Total To Date	153,120	85,740	67,000	16,930	76		Bal. O.H.	39,260

No.	CAST	CHARACTER	W/H S/F R/T TR	Report	Dismiss	1st	2nd	Leave for Location	Arrive on Location	Leave Location	Arrive at Studio	REMARKS
1	Jane Fonda	K. Wells	W	515P	440A	11P-1130P						
3	M. Douglas	R. Adams	W	535P	440A	11P-1130P						
4	D. Valdez	H. Salas	H									
5	J. Karen	Churchill	W	5P	440A	11P-1130P						
6	P. Donat	Jacovitch	H									
7	B. Brimley	Spindler	W	5P	310A	11P-1130P						
8	S. Brady	DeYoung	W	5P	310A	11P-1130P						
9	J. Hampton	Gibson	W	5P	310A	11P-1130P						
10	R. Herd	MacCormack	W	5P	310A	11P-1130P						
13	Khalilah Ali	Marge	H									
14	J. Smith	Tom	W	5P	320A	11P-1130P						
15	S. Bohrman	Pete	H									
26	R. Collins	Sptscaster	H									
30	D. Arnsen	Cameraman	W	430P	315A	11P-1130P						ND Brkfst
39	F. Cavestani	Reporter #1	W	520P	315A	11P-1130P						
40	T. House	Reporter #2	W	430P	315A	11P-1130P						ND Brkfst
61	C. Woods	Reporter #3	W	430P	315A	11P-1130P						ND Brkfst
62	V. Clenard	Reporter #4	W	430P	315A	11P-1130P						ND Brkfst
63	M. Carlton	Reporter #5	W	430P	315A	11P-1130P						ND Brkfst
60	C. Hodges	SWAT Chief	W	5P	315A	11P-1130P						
	T. Lane	Alma Spindler	W	5P	320A	11P-1130P						RECALLED FOR ADDED SCS.
46	R. Lombard	Barney	W	5P	310A	11P-1130P						RECALLED FOR ADDED SCS.
49	T. Eure	Tommy	W	5P	310A	11P-1130P						RECALLED FOR ADDED SCS.
44	D. Lewkowitz	Donny	W	5P	310A	11P-1130P						RECALLED FOR ADDED SCS.

EYEWITNESS

EXTRA TALENT — MUSICIANS, ETC.

No	Rate	Adj. To	O.T.	T.T.	Ward	MPV	No	Rate	Adj. To	O.T.	T.T.	Ward	
59	56		1.4				1	56		.3			
12	56	100	1.4				2	56		.4			
7	56		2.6				1	56		.9			
6	56		2.1				3	56		1.8			
5	56		1.4		11.00		1	56		1.9			
1	56		3.2				3	56	66	1.4			
1	56		2.1		11.00		2	56	66	.4			
1	56		.4		11.00		2	56	66	3.1			
1	56				11.00		NOTE: 10% NITE PREMIUM 8PM TO 1AM					
1	56						20% NITE PREMIUM 1AM TO WRAP					

Staff and Crew

1	Director
2	Asst. Directors
	Asst. Dir. Trainee
1	Script Supervisor
1	Cameraman
3	Operator
5	Assistants
1	Still Man
1	Mixer
	Recorder
1	Mike Boom Man
2	Cable Man
8	VTR Crew
1	Propmaster
2	Asst. Propmaster
1	Key Grip
1	2nd Co. Grip
1	Crab Dolly Grip
	Crane Grip
2	Extra Co. Grips
1	Craft Service
	Greensman
1	S.B. Painter
1	Gaffer
1	Best Boy
6	Lamp Operators
1	Generator Man
	40 Man
1	Special Effects Man

4	Makeup Artist (1 Fonda)
1	Hair Stylist (Fonda)
	Body Makeup Woman
2	Wardrobe Man
2	Wardrobe Woman (1 Fonda)
	Wranglers, Trainers, Handlers
25	Drivers

Miscellaneous Crew

1	1st Aid
	Fireman
2	Police
X	Prod Designer + Dept.
	Art Director
X	Set Decorator + Crew
	Swing Gang
X	Construction crew
2	Watchmen: 1 @ 5P & 1 @ 5A
3	Water truck ops.
1	Helicopter Pilot

Equipment

	Camera/Sound Truck
1	Prod Van — Grip/Elec/Gen
2	Crew Cab
1	FX Trailer
1	Utility Truck
1	Prop Truck
1	M/U Ward Trailer
3	Honey Wagon 19 DR
2	Motor Homes
2	Busses 40 passenger
1	Maxi Van
6	Station Wagon
	Misc Cars
20	Picture Cars (see notes *)
3	Cameras 2 Panaflex, 1 Arri
1	Grab Dolly
	Insert Car
1	Crane Titan
X	Lunches 235 Dinners

REMARKS & EXPLANATION OF DELAYS:

* Vehicles: 1 SWAT Truck, 1 Fire Truck, 1 Fire Rescue, 1 Ambulance, 4 Minicam trucks,
1 Coroner's wagon, 3 TV station wagons, 4 Sheriff & Police cars, 2 motorcycles,
1 helicopter, 1 BMW
10% Nite Premium 8PM to 1AM & 20% Nite Premium 1AM to Wrap

Assoc Prod—
Production Manager Jim Nelson   Assistant Director Kim Kurumada   2nd Asst. Director Barrie Osborne

wherein they all can contribute to the end product. With the help of my staff on *The China Syndrome*—including first assistant Kim Kurumada and executive secretary Debbie Getlin, who helped gather these sample pages—I was free to concentrate on the dramatic telling of the story. Making *The China Syndrome* was a rich and satisfying experience.

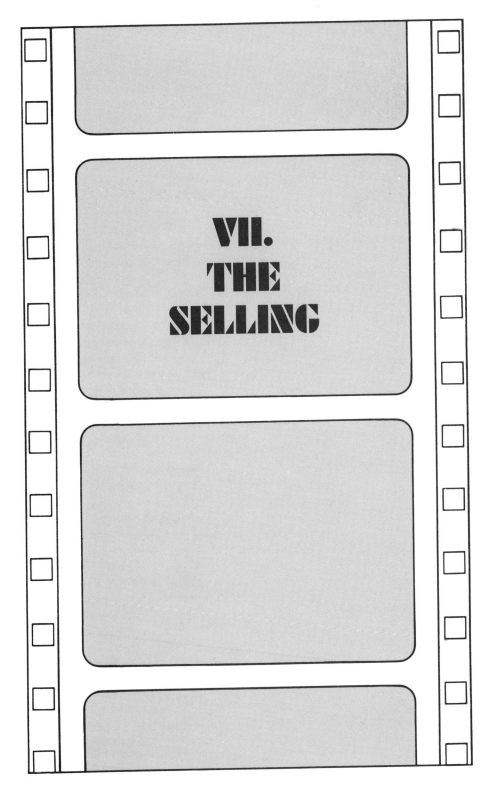

VII.
THE
SELLING

Distribution and Exhibition: An Overview

by **A. D. Murphy,** who was financial editor, film critic, and news reporter for *Daily Variety* and weekly *Variety* from 1965 to 1978. He continues to write for those publications in a special correspondent status, having shifted to a new full-time career teaching in the cinema/television division of the University of Southern California's School of Performing Arts, where he is the founder and director of a new, two-year graduate program in motion picture producing and management.

This article is from the journalism of Mr. Murphy which originally appeared in the *Daily Variety* issues of January 10 and February 14, 1977 and June 14, June 28, August 3, and October 26, 1978; it is included here through the kind permission of Syd Silverman, publisher of *Variety* and *Daily Variety*, as updated and revised by Mr. Murphy expressly for this volume.

In the dawn of the industry, say, before 1910, the earliest films (one-reelers) were sold outright to exhibitors at so much per foot. In time, public demand and selectivity forced production costs higher and led to the introduction of percentage rentals to justify the investment risk.

EARLY PERCENTAGES

The early distribution percentages were under 20%; by the 1920s, they were under 25%. By the mid-1960s, a theatre circuit comprising a mix of first-run, key neighborhood, and lesser theatres wound up at the end of the year paying out to distributors in the aggregate no more than about one third of the related box-office. This overall one-third cost of renting film derived from hundreds, even thousands, of different film play dates, some at high percentages, some at low (25–30%), some at flat (or fixed) rentals.

The realization that an exhibitor's overall film costs are composed of various percentage splits of the box-office with the distributors on thousands of different runs of hundreds of different films is the beginning of wisdom in understanding the film business.

In key first-run dates, the distributor takes 90%. But, as in all such things, one must always ascertain the percentage of *what?* In this case, it is not of the total box-office, but 90% of the box-office minus what is often held to be the theatre's operating costs or "nut."

FIGURING THE NUT

A major New York or Los Angeles first-run house can claim a house expense of, say, $10,000 per week; this, like so much else in the industry, is a *negotiated figure*. It is not arrived at by examination of actual records; the exhibitor announces his claimed costs, and the distributor accepts or rejects. They finally agree.

It is not unheard of for an exhibitor to have, at a given time, and for the same theatre, different allowed house nuts with different distributors. (And is it not now apparent that the paradoxical theatre expansion in the face of a limited film supply is, maybe, just a way to set brand new house nuts?)

But assume for the moment, at least, that house nuts approximate reality. (The old distributor claim that there was a lot of "water" or "air" in house nuts—in other words, a built-in profit—may be set aside by the realization that some house allowances have not changed for years, though everyone is aware of inflation.) An example or two may be of benefit.

Say that a certain key N.Y.–L.A. first-run theatre does, in the first week of a film's premiere run, a box-office of $30,000. Take out the $10,000 house allowance, and the distributor's share is 90% of $20,000 (the adjusted box-office figure), or $18,000. That $18,000 in film rental is, in actuality, 60% of the public's money, not 90%. If the raw box-office figure had been $60,000, the adjusted figure would be $50,000, of which the distrib's $45,000 rental would be 75% of the public's ticket money. The bigger the box-office gross, the bigger the rental percentage; but at bigger numbers, *nobody complains*.

But let's say the film is a dud, and the week's box-office is $15,000. After taking out the house allowance, the distrib would *seem* to get 90% of $5,000, or $4,500, which is 30% of the raw figure, unless floor figures are operative (see below).

Looking at the 90/10 deal another way, the exhibitor's share can be considered a guaranteed covering of costs plus a guaranteed 10% profit. Cost plus 10%—it doesn't sound nearly so bad that way. A lot of businessmen would be glad to know that their expenses would be covered and they would make a 10% profit as well.

FLOORS

But now what about these floor figures? They came into being in the late sixties as a countermove by distributors who questioned the validity of house nuts. The *floor* percentage innovation meant that, however the 90/10 arithmetic went, in no case would the distributor take less than that floor percentage of the raw or actual box-office figure.

Floor figures typically are 70% for the first few weeks of a film's run, 60% for the next leg of the run, then 50%, and then 40%. Once again, when business is torrid, nobody complains; when it is sluggish or bad, the floor figures, ranging from 70% on down, are operative. Floor figures, however, only apply to film ticket revenues, not total theatre receipts, which include concessions and, nowadays, pinball machines, and so on.

It is left for others to assess the righteousness of these licensing terms. An exhibitor may sincerely object to relatively high percentage takeouts by the distributor, but the film supplier points out that high-profit concession income is not divided at all. The distributor can further claim that he has assumed the total up-front risk in making the film, a process that may have taken as long as 18 months before opening day, and has assumed most of the promotional burden as well.

Aha, you say, the distributor has assumed *all* the up-front production risk? What about those (nonrefundable) guarantees and (refundable) advances that exhibitors these days must put up before getting the film delivered? Good question, even though the record is filled with cases of exhibitors offering front money *even when it wasn't asked for* in order to get a film away from a competitor's house. (On that point, 90/10 deals are often requested by an exhibitor, not always imposed by a distributor.) Let's explore this guarantee-advance (front money) situation. Over and above the morality of it all, the mechanics may be interesting.

The bulk of the front money pledged by exhibitors is not due until a couple of weeks before opening day; thus, while the nonrefundable (guarantee) portions of it can be numerically compared to production investment risk, it is not in the distrib's hand until shortly before opening, although the filming may have begun a year or more earlier. And then, after opening, the exhibitor keeps every cent of the box-office money—*all of it*— until the guarantee is earned. With the blockbuster films of recent years, front money has been earned in the first days or week of a run, or at least very early on.

The point is, the exhibitor has not posted his collateral until just before opening; he keeps all the box-office money until the front money is earned, and if he has one of those big pictures, he is inconvenienced for a relatively brief period.

To be sure, some films don't earn their guarantees (though the advances are refundable), and that is certainly a potential burden on an exhibitor who guessed wrong, especially when he made his commitment without even seeing the picture, through blind bidding. (Contrary to uninformed opinion, you can't find any responsible people who actually defend blind bidding as a positive market force, and state legislatures are slowly outlawing the practice, under pressure from exhibitors.)

In the early days, Marcus Loew and William Fox owned theatres, and, then as now, a theatre owner would go berserk not knowing what film to put on the screen when the film showing had ended its run. For Loew and Fox, the solution was to go into direct production to assure enough films for their own houses; since neither had theatres everywhere, they automatically went into *de facto* distribution to market their films when their own first-run preemptions had occurred.

SELF-PROTECTION

Also in that era, Adolph Zukor, a producer and then a producer-distributor, was faced with rising talent costs (spell that Mary Pickford) and decided that if he couldn't dominate the industry through talent, he'd protect himself by owning enough theatres at least to guarantee first-run exposure for Paramount pictures. Thus, from opposite directions, the "vertical integration" emerged, with production, distribution, and exhibition functions consolidated under what became five major corporate roofs.

These companies had it made in the shade, but they were too greedy. Nonaffiliated theatre owners, not permitted to participate in various cozy reciprocal product poolings, began to agitate. It took nearly 40 years, but finally the government acted. After a key Supreme Court opinion, the studio-owned threatre chains were divested; however, the producer-distrib partnerships were left legitimately linked.

The loss of guaranteed key first runs on films, the competition of the new TV medium, and a general expansion of what is now known as the *leisure-time* sector all worked havoc on the industry. As previously documented by *Variety*, the real end of this postwar decline came in 1971, fully 25 years of industry erosion after the peak year 1946. Since 1971 (which climaxed a disastrous industry depression escaped by no major company), there has been a steady improvement in industry health.

It is true that major producer-distribs dominate 85 to 90 percent of the market. It is also true that such concentration occurs in most industries; the definition of a "major" anything presumes the impact. Not fully appreciated is the fact that the film industry's traditional source of production money is not the Bank of America or the First National Bank of Boston; the largest single source is recycled film rentals from the major distribution companies. To be sure, the majors have lines of credit with the big banks, but they properly represent standby money, not unlike one's use of bank credit cards. When many large companies forgot their self-financing responsibilities and drew down all their credit to the limit, the result was the 1969–71 Hollywood depression.

A lot of people—not just exhibitors and their new-found political and populist allies—are wondering more and more why it is that, given the generally improving conditions of the theatrical film industry since 1971, the major American film companies are making fewer and fewer pictures? One answer is that, within the current economic realities of the business, they cannot extend production investment too much without repeating the mistakes of overproduction that helped cause the disastrous Hollywood depression of 1969–71.

In the following analysis, which attempts to explain the proffered answer to the question, a few preliminary ideas are worth stating.

• Neither a film producer-distributor nor an exhibitor can claim some Divine Right of staying in business; staying alive in business is the perpetual problem of every individual company.

• A major diversified film production-distribution company—active in music, recreation parks, telefilming, whatever—cannot be expected to lose money on theatrical filmmaking (in many cases, the primary business of such companies) and make it up on the diversification. Nor can the secondary markets for features—TV, pay TV, and so on—be required to create the overall profit; that's the type of deficit financing nightmare that long prevailed in network TV program production.

• The last preliminary idea to get is the speciousness of citing exhibitor "demand" as a reason for making more films. Retailers of all kinds in all industries always clamor for "more" product (more "successful" product is always meant, but is rarely explicit). This is specious because the only safe "demand" to which a supplier can respond is that of the ultimate consumer—the public.

Thus you have to start with the prevailing public demand (as measured in box-office dollars) and then work back up the system, through the film suppliers' share of that box-office (measured in film rentals); through current and anticipated costs of marketing (prints and advertising); through outlays in creative talent gross and net participations; through actual production costs and actual overhead (that is, people overhead, not the percentage kind); through project development (the industry's R & D expenses); through the annual interest on any outside production borrowings; and so on all the way to a final dollar figure that you sincerely hope is a positive number.

But what of the film projects that, before release, are often largely covered by a television license deal, a soundtrack or book deal, a merchandising deal, or some other deal? That's fine on a case-by-case basis. However, not every film lends itself to such lucrative peripheral and secondary exploitation. In other words, when you find these an-

248

gles, great; but when you *need* them up front, to justify the financial risk, you're already in trouble.

Moving now into some numbers, assume one of the major companies early in 1982 is trying to get a reasonable fix on a feature production program outlay (including pickups from independent producers) that will go to market in 1983–4; this assumption allows for the long lead time in the feature business.

THREE-YEAR AVERAGE

Early in 1982, it would be prudent to see what the three prior years' figures showed. (Why three years? To allow for a stronger data base.)

Looking at the 1979–81 period, the three-year average of domestic *box office* was approximately $2.6 to 2.7-billion, of which the major companies (Motion Picture Association of America members plus Walt Disney Productions and American International Pictures, now Orion) plucked something near $1,200,000,000 in film *rentals.*

Foreign markets averaged over this period about $750,000,000 in rentals, some of which was of course left in those markets for business purposes. In round total, say that the annual average global rental in that time span came to approximately $1,900,000,000.

This industry-wide rental figure could reasonably support direct production investment in the $850,000,000 range. (This number comes from applying a rule of thumb that break-even for a *group* of films is slightly over twice—not as much as 2.5 times—the production costs.) The long way around—taking out the distribution fees (but then applying the excess of such fee income over actual fixed distribution organization costs to various recoupment); subtracting the costs of prints, promotion, and participations; and charging off abandoned development costs, interest, etc.—will produce the same ballpark figure.

Next, divide this "safe" industry-wide production figure by seven; there are six American majors with comparable production levels, so add Disney, Orion, and some smaller companies together to get a sort of composite seventh. The resulting "safe average" of production investment for each studio is therefore in the $120,000,000 range.

Finally, for each of the majors, divide that studio figure by the prevailing $8–10,000,000 average cost per film—the "event" pictures plus the costs of all the rest—and you wind up with the reasonable number (about 15, give or take) of films which that figure can yield, including acquisitions, negative pickups, etc. In other words, the proposed future production investment planning has got to be based on the current and recent public theatrical market, using as a point of departure an "average" expected market share.

This model has so far contemplated the theatrical market as the *sole* market. When you consider additional revenues from TV, pay TV, home video, and so on, another $25–30,000,000 or so in feature production investment per studio becomes feasible.

Why deal in averages? Because one of the overblown film business myths is that the paying audience, having seen one good film, immediately makes a *drastic* change in its film-going habits. Admittedly, since 1971 there has been a real increase in patronage (as well as in admission prices), and demographics portend well for further increases.

But those are long-term considerations in what is, for the year-to-year stability of a major company, a short-term, immediate situation: The increase in patronage this year alone is not going to be that substantial. In any year, the top 10 films will corner around half the business; the higher that ratio goes, the less is available for all the rest of the films in release.

There's just no getting around the fact that the film hits draw the available business like magnets. When there are several strong films, a mediocre picture becomes a box-office dud, and a weak release is a box-office bust.

Since 1971, U.S. theatre-ticket sales have on the average risen about 4% at an annual compounded rate. That's nice, but in any given year that increase does not justify an enormous increased gamble in production investment on an industry-wide basis. Maybe one or two companies will look over the potential competition and take an extra risk, but not everybody.

Over a decade ago, as a matter of fact, most companies put on blinders, thought that their high-budget pictures were going to knock out everybody else's high-budget pictures, and recall what happened. By the end of 1968, the American film industry had more than $1,200,000,000 tied up in feature film inventory—nearly three times what global film rental capacity could bear at the time. (*Daily Variety,* April 15, 1970). Shedding half that inventory figure to reach manageable proportions was the bookkeeping version of the personal and industry horrors that occurred over the following three years.

All right, then, assume that you budget on the averages, enjoy the greater market share if it happens, and don't hurt too badly if another company's greater market share squeezes your own (as it truly will). But now comes the question, why can't a studio get more films for that $120,000,000 annual outlay? It would be nice if it could; it's safe to say that if a studio could get 30 films for the figure, it would make them. However, it's really asking too much for creative and craft talent to sit out an upturn in the business; agents and union leaders would quite properly be sacked for a dereliction of responsibility if they did not try to get more for their people.

OUTSIDE MONEY

Next question: Why not then augment the studio's investment with outside money—overseas tax shelters and so forth? That's being done, too, but remember that an outside partner isn't working for nothing, either; the more partners—fiscal as well as creative—the more outside payments to them from gross and net.

Well then, what about these big new independent production companies that are fully financing the production of their films? A complex question; for one thing, they are competing with major studios for the same talent, which means talent prices won't be going down, all other things being equal. On the other hand, these self-sufficient production companies at least provide more places for film ideas to flourish and develop. Also, ultimate distribution through a major company will enhance the number of released pictures (unless of course the distributor simply allocates more acquisition money at the expense of house production coin, in which case there is no increase in the number of films available to exhibitors from that source).

But isn't there a paradox lurking here? If in a given year there isn't that much of an increase in the public market, won't a significantly larger number of films being released result in more pix fighting for essentially the same business? Yes, that's true. Then won't somebody, or somebody's films, get squeezed in the crush? You better believe it. The surviving suppliers will be those who have the broadest and most diversified base, as well as the least fiscal recklessness.

THE LAST MYTH

The last myth—and maybe the biggest one of all, among the unsophisticated—is worth discussing. There are those who with apparent sincerity believe that if the current major film production-distribution companies weren't so firmly established in their ways, and if filmmakers and exhibitors dealt directly in an Adam Smith–type competitive open marketplace of many suppliers and many buyers, there would be peace and prosperity. "Eliminate the middleman," as the saying goes; "Plain pipe racks, direct to you."

If that happened—and it did happen once, in the dawn of the

film business, when the pioneer producer sold his product direct to his exhibitor customers—there would be no strong industry. Filmmakers would be living hand to mouth, waiting for the last film's payoff to begin the next one; exhibitors would be scrambling for product when the promised film was delayed; and so on. But, in time, there would evolve an idea: a person or company would undertake the risk of financing volume production in some orderly fashion and then assume the added risk of marketing to make it available to theatres concurrent with periods of maximum patronage.

The decisions of this entity or force would frequently become controversial; filmmakers and exhibitors alike, for common and different reasons, would grouse, often bitterly. But the force would be with them, and when business conditions stabilized again, there would be perhaps five to ten of them. Their collective name: *major distributors.*

ROADRUNNER VS. WILE E. COYOTE

If one wanted to make an animated picture out of the film business, the characters of distribution and exhibition already exist: the Roadrunner for distribution and Wile E. Coyote for exhibition. Those two Warner Brothers cartoon personalities fit the situation like a glove, especially Coyote, the clever but frustrated adversary whose best laid plans always blow up in his face.

The soap opera relationship between distribution and exhibition began more than half a century ago, perhaps from the day that theatres no longer could buy film for so many cents per foot. Whatever the initial incident, the drama has been running ever since. The usual episodic climax finds exhibition sandbagged, just like Wile E. Coyote.

A few of the more dramatic episodes come to mind. When Paramount's Adolph Zukor decided that he couldn't keep paying Mary Pickford more money and revised his strategy from controlling the industry through stars to control via ownership of key first-run theatres, a major theatre-acquisition spree ensued. It was marked by the delicacy often associated with waterfront labor practices. Some key regional exhibitors decided to band together to resist. Their brainchild: First National Pictures, which they bankrolled in return for regional first-run preemption and, presumably, lower film costs. But to get established, First National immediately paid Pickford and Charles Chaplin more money than they had ever extracted from anyone else. (So much for lower film costs and rentals.)

252

Then came the outcry in the '20s from exhibitors who, shut out of the various theatre-circuit product-pooling arrangements, complained about restraint of trade. The United States government accumulated a lot of evidence, and many indictments were expected. But along came an unexpected event—the Depression—which diverted attention to more pressing national concerns.

In 1938, when the national recovery was stumbling along, exhibitor complaints again got the ball rolling, and the government finally took action against these distributor miscreants via a *civil* complaint, not a criminal one. The usual legal jockeying took place again only to be interrupted by another event—World War II.

Then, by the late '40s, when the handwriting was on the wall for theatre-circuit separation from major integrated companies, the inroads of television and an enlarged leisure spectrum on theatrical box-office made such separation most attractive for the distributors. Exhibition is a cash business and also a cash drain (the majors, which went into receivership in the Depression, did so because of their theatre subsids); the lights must burn every day, the staff must be paid every week, and so on.

Distributors by 1950 were not unwilling to unload what was in fact a major cash hemorrhage in their overall operations. In the process, by no longer having to supply their own and affiliated houses every week, the studios lopped off their creative contract talent as well.

PADDING THE NUT?

Come the '50s and '60s, and distributors are getting higher percentages to license films to exhibitors. Samuel Goldwyn is often credited with the 90/10 licensing deal, whereby the distributor gets 90% of the box-office *after* a reduction for the exhibitor's house expense. But those house-expense figures were (and still are) negotiated numbers, and there was the lingering suspicion that some of the house nuts had a little built-in profit to the theatre's benefit.

Thus, the next countermove was a minimum floor figure, a percentage of the *actual* box-office total that the distributor would get regardless of the 90/10 house-nut formula.

All this time, mind you, the haggling over settlement of played-off films resulted in many tens of millions of overdue film rentals, held by exhibitors pending settlement of the play-date contracts. This situation has become less severe in recent years through a combination of factors: the final executive upheavals in most major companies, with employee managers succeeding founder managers; the simple march of computer accounting technology; and a new ploy by distribution, the obtaining of guarantees (nonrefundable) and advances (refundable in certain circumstances) on major films.

It should be apparent by now that every trade practice breeds its own countermeasure, which in turn leads to a new gambit. With major distributors now asking for (or receiving) front money, the tables have turned badly on exhibition. It's one thing to play with a distributor's overdue film rentals, but quite another to come up with front money that doesn't even exist in the box-office till.

SHAKY COUNTERMEASURE

But there was one exhibition countermeasure that, in its own small, shaky, and unstable way, occasionally worked out: *splits*. Distributors regularly issue stern letters (in shocked and appalled prose suitable to for-the-record-file correspondence) saying they do not recognize splits. On the other hand, in split situations, the distributor sends out bid letters or otherwise announces the availability of a film, and—surprise!— only one exhibitor shows up. He's the one who got the film through the prearranged local formula by which the local exhibs divided up the product. Splits are very shaky since a couple of bad pictures can get an exhibitor so hungry for a hit that he will torpedo the local detente. Distributors look forward to such an event since, with more than one potential buyer, the terms can easily improve to the distributor's benefit. When most local exhibitors are tired of losing money on overbid films, a split often resumes.

We are now near the present time, with its long (and easily documented) record of sweetheart arrangements (one circuit, amazingly, gets a whole string of films from the same distributor), second looks at bids, and other intrigues. Oddly enough, although it takes two to tango, exhibitors put all the blame for this on distributors. As in marital infidelity, someone else is always the real cause.

The National Association of Theatre Owners and the newer National Independent Theatre Exhibitors (groups that, like Annie & Sandy, Mutt & Jeff, etc., correlate directly with the old Theatre Owners of America and the Allied States gadflies) have lately brought to a head the traditional exhibitor complaints. NATO a few years back was really getting close to hard action (too close perhaps, considering that, if dirty laundry is to be aired, there might be some embarrassment to the allegedly united theatre operators), but retreated into conciliation; NITE moved in at the right time to carry the ball farther. So, off they go, seeking government intervention.

IMPECCABLE TIMING

And what happens? By the perfect timing that exhibition has always managed to achieve, the government seizes upon and declares illegal the one trade practice that, in some places and at some times, alleviates a burden on exhibition—the split.

The lessons of history are obvious. In a reverse of the situation that obtains in the TV and radio industries, where legislators (or their families, or their law firms) are cozy with broadcasters, exhibition (which pretends to grass-roots consciousness and under certain circumstances has it) lacks sufficient friends at the source of the magic federal power it wishes to turn against its natural enemy.

Will Hayes, Eric Johnston, and now Jack Valenti, as successive heads of the Motion Picture Association of America, have a long-standing relationship with Washington. Maybe exhibition can get its act together and rapidly develop a strong lobbying pressure there. But, considering past history, maybe this latest situation is just another example of Wile E. Coyote assembling his Acme-brand Roadrunner kit only to find it's another boomerang. In fact, exhibitors flopped so badly at the federal level that they are lobbying at the local level, with much better success.

BOX-OFFICE VS. FILM RENTAL

Perennial confusion, both in the film trade and in consumer media, centers on the terms *box-office* and *film rental*. Feature magazine writers interchange the terms with abandon, and filmmakers don't help the situation with their careless intermixture of figures. Confusion arises from the premise that, since the paying public buys tickets, the theatre box-office total is therefore the best measure of a film's performance. Right? Wrong!

Every film booking every week generates some box-office coin. But that money is divided between the exhibitor and the distributor according to the terms of the licensing agreement (90/10 with floors, 50%, sliding scale, etc.). The exhibitor's share remains in the theatre to pay the mortgage, staff, and so on and sustains the brick and mortar of the exhibition arm of the industry.

255

The distributor's share of the box-office is what is known as *film rental* (or distributor's gross; the terms are reasonably synonymous). Film rental is the crucial figure because film rentals pay for the production, promotion, and prints of the film as well as for participations in gross when the creative talent is in the superstar echelon.

In short, film rentals are what recycles the industry—the pool of money that is continually reinvested in new production, in addition to sustaining the distribution organization and being allocated to marketing new product.

If this is the case, why do people keep talking about box-office figures? Because, when a new film opens, the box-office results in the first few hundred play dates give an indication of the film's potential strength. There's another reason that, for devious reasons, box-office figures are flung about: Being the larger numbers, they make a conversation more exciting.

In percentage licensing engagements, distributors do in fact get a box-office report that can also yield the number of admissions and other data. But in tail-end play dates (where the exhibitor pays a fixed amount to play an older film), no box-office report is required. Thus, for many films, nobody really knows what the box-office total was. Finally, it's very difficult to extrapolate from rentals to box-office, since a film generates its box-office (and hence rentals) from many different price scales and licensing contract terms.

On a statistical basis (that is, throwing dozens of films of different appeal and performance into one pot for analysis), one might *with care* multiply rentals by 2.5 or 3 to get an idea of the box-office. But that's a largely meaningless exercise, more suitable for cheap puffery and aggrandizement than for really understanding what makes the film business tick.

DISTRIBUTION FEE

There is also some confusion surrounding the concept of the distribution fee.

The distribution fee is a percentage charge on incoming film rentals from theatres, TV, pay-TV systems, and so forth. It is simply a service fee (not unlike the doctor's office-call or house-call fee) designed *solely* to support the existence of the sales organization; it does *not* apply to the recovery of any expenses directly related to releasing a film (such as prints, advertising, etc.). Deductions for direct costs of marketing a film are made after imposition of the fee.

For U.S.-Canadian theatrical distribution, the fee is normally

30%; for the U.K., 35%; elsewhere, 40% or even higher. When doing arithmetic, it's often easy to use a global average of 33⅓%. The fee pays the fixed costs of the marketing organization: salary, office leases, and so on. For a major American production-distribution company operating its own sales arm directly on a global basis, these annual expenses now approach the $20,000,000 mark, slightly less than half being the domestic market component. Since one can use (statistically) an average worldwide distribution fee of approximately one third, this means that when, in a given year, theatrical rentals pass $60,000,000 (depending on the company), the sales department is off its nut. Beyond that incoming rental figure, additional distribution fee income represents . . . what? Call it what you will, except don't call it *profit*, because it isn't, in the sense of free-and-clear money available for stockholder dividends and such.

What this excess fee income (over actual costs of maintaining the distribution organization) does is accumulate a pool of money that is often absolutely essential for use in recovering direct and actual marketing and production costs otherwise unrecouped; this pool of money also gets recycled into new film production.

Film companies have large lines of credit with banks, but these are more or less standby credits for seasonal and occasional use. The idea that film companies are forever running to the bank for more money is ludicrous; there wouldn't even be a film business if that were so.

Excess distribution fee income, and any later distribution profits that it helps augment (or create), is quite literally the blood pressure in the circulatory system that keeps pumping money into new production, thereby keeping the system alive. Reducing this financial equivalent of blood pressure to a minimal life-support level can have the same effect on a company that it would on an individual.

In describing the chronic anemia of the pre-1951 United Artists Corporation to an interviewer a few years ago, Arthur Krim (who certainly knows) put his finger on the matter. He pointed out that the concept of a passive distribution organization—lacking sufficient financial resources for direct and continuing production investment, relying on privately financed producer affiliates to deliver on time, and hoping to make money but nervously praying simply to break even—is a blueprint for disaster.

To the comment that there are many current and potential new markets for feature films besides theatres, one can agree that other sources of revenue and profit exist. But it can be shown easily that theatrical film rentals generate on an annual basis 10 to 15 times more feature rentals than any other market; it will be some time before any emerging market even begins to approach parity. Optimism is fine, but the orders of magnitude will remain staggeringly skewed towards theatrical distribution. Yet these secondary markets can, for a given film and for all films, remain important backup sources of revenue and fee income for a distributor. The current proliferation of independent production companies preselling these secondary markets confronts a major distributor with the dismal spectre of having to make it in the primary market—where the marketing risks are the greatest.

Assume a major American distributor can figure an average of something near $250,000,000 per year in global theatrical film rentals. (The fee income from this is therefore in the $80–85,000,000 range; after covering the fixed costs of the sales department, this leaves excess fee income of about $60–65,000,000.) After deducting the fee from the annual worldwide rental take, this leaves something like $170,000,000 available to pay for four items conveniently remembered as all starting with the letter p: prints, promotion, production, and participation costs.

With reasonable annual production program investment in the $100–110,000,000 range, this leaves $60–70,000,000 available, out of which $40–50,000,000 may, with current soaring media costs, be a fair estimate of the direct distribution costs of the films.

What's left is something like $20,000,000, about 8% of the original average annual rental revenues, and if one (quite easily) imagines the presence of many 10% gross participants scattered throughout the film program, even this pile becomes depleted severely. It could even be wiped out.

But there still are some *unrecovered* costs. What about the company's R & D money—covering the developed film projects that never got off the ground? What about unallocated costs that a production overhead charge doesn't cover? The answer comes in part from that $60–65,000,000 excess distribution fee income noted earlier, which is available to cover these things as well as to provide money for the next production program.

This is not to say that procedures cannot be improved and more equitable arrangements achieved, nor that customary practices are sacrosanct and inviolate. But, before changing an environment, it might be a good idea to understand the existing one a trifle better; that's sound ecological practice.

RESTRUCTURED EXHIBITION

Resurgent American film industry prosperity over much of this past decade derives in part from the obvious factors of rising attendance levels in combination with rising ticket prices. Less apparent, but no less important, is the significant transformation in the exhibition branch of the industry: there has occurred a major increase in the number of theatres that enjoy key or subkey status in the types of runs. This has had the effect of keeping major films at a higher level of release, during which admission prices are higher, for longer periods of time.

From a 10-year analysis of the *Variety* key U.S. city box-office data, it is estimated that the proportion of the nation's theatres that regularly enjoy key or subkey run status has doubled, from less than a quarter of all houses to a level that is steadily approaching half.

This upgrading of theatre run status has been effected by both exhibition and distribution. Exhibition has responded to the related factors of urban decay and suburban sprawl by expanding into shopping centers with multi-screen theatres and subdividing older picture palaces; distribution has played its part by radically changing release patterns so as to bestow key and subkey status to thousands of these smaller houses.

A brief look back may make the current situation clearer. For decades, there was a sort of three-tier exhibition industry. At the highest level were the key first-run presentation houses, charging the top ticket prices and seating thousands; among them were world-famous local landmarks. The next level comprised both very important neighborhood (more precisely, regional) theatres and many more early subsequent-run houses where the ticket scales were lower. At the bottom were those late-run, small, low-priced screens that are accurately, though perhaps crudely, known in the trade as *dumps*.

A feature film in former times would move down through this market structure like clockwork. In fact, before major circuit exhibition was divorced from production-distribution, it *was* a clock, with play-off intervals separated by fixed clearances of 14 days, 28 days, 42 days, and so on, between successive play-off periods. Thus, a major and popular film would play in first-run theatres to audiences willing to pay top prices; next would come the subrun fanning out to less-prestigious (but also lower-priced) theatres for those audiences unwilling or unable to pay top scales; finally would come late-run exposure at the cheapest price with a lower-income audience to support that tail-end market. The merchandising pattern was the same as that of other consumer goods—the exclusive shops, then the general department store, and finally the close-out sale.

ENTER TELEVISION

But over the past 30 years, major social and business upheavals have occurred. The introduction of TV rapidly dried up most of the tail-end theatres (though some shifted to foreign films and thereby became the entering wedge for new film styles from abroad; this important causal influence on the art-house subindustry is rarely discussed). Also, the transformation of metropolitan areas from a wheel-spoke configuration to that of a doughnut with an empty core killed off many of the key presentation houses. At the same time, this change had the positive effect of gradually upgrading the run status of those surviving middle-tier secondary regional and neighborhood theatres, augmented by the post-war drive-in boom and the shopping-center phenomenon in these newly affluent middle-income suburbs.

The 25-year decline (1946–71) in film audiences naturally made many of the older middle-tier theatres into a new bottom rung—the nouveau poor of exhibition. Look at it this way: a lake dries up from the edges, and a consumer market dries up from the fringe; theatres that once were in moderately deep or shallow economic water wound up on the beach.

'70s TURNAROUND

This brings us up to the early '70s and the turnaround in attendance. Rising production costs and, more significantly, soaring costs in advertising and promotion combined to influence distributor marketing decisions so as to launch films from a wider base than the old single-screen exclusive run. Hence, there are the mini-multiples that go by various corny names and involve not one theatre but six or eight or ten strategic houses that fairly well ring, but do not saturate, a metropolitan area. Suddenly, many older suburban houses and many brand new outlying theatres have become first-run situations.

Following the launching of new major films comes the first general release, which automatically elevates many more suburban screens into subkey status. The net result of this transformation has been to upgrade the middle-tier theatre into, as often as not, day-date, first-run, and regionally exclusive status for films that play their preem runs longer in smaller houses, but at top ticket prices.

Thus, (1) rising numbers of patrons (2) willing to pay the highest prices at (3) conveniently accessible theatres (4) for popular films (5) with longer runs at those locations, along with (6) ticket-price inflation throughout the entire exhibition spectrum constitute the more comprehensive explanation for the latter-day revenue boom. That distributors are getting a higher proportion of film rentals from this higher box-office gross is both an effect of stronger licensing terms as well as the fact of life that newer product commands a better price than last-run bookings.

By *Daily Variety* estimate, something near 23–25% of the 13–14,000 U.S. theatres a decade ago were in this key and subkey run status. It is estimated that almost 45% of the recent higher tally of about 18,000 theatres are regularly accorded that top-tier run status. Naturally, with longer early runs of films, there is the likelihood that the audience for these films is almost totally exhausted by the time—many months later in a lot of cases—films reach the bottom tier of theatres. As a matter of fact, this is the underlying reason for a lot of current small-exhibitor agitation.

That old three-tier play off of films is now largely obsolete; it's a two-tier marketplace at best—first run, leftover run, and not much in between.

The enlarging market array for feature films—theatres, pay TV, free TV, home entertainment systems, and so on—accelerates and aggravates this situation. The next shakeout of the lower exhibition tier will be triggered by the supplanting of this leftover market by the new technologies and markets. The top tier of exhibition will shrink but will not likely ever disappear; there is still an enormous amount of money to be made there by all parties.

The improvements have been not just in ticket prices, but also in actual attendance. Also, the population demographics have changed—that onetime post–World War II "baby-boom" which became the college crowd in the sixties is now moving into adulthood and is still turned on to films; through the end of the century those people will be a big factor in both theatre attendance and home entertainment markets.

In distribution, there is a new and higher plateau of annual film rentals; nowadays, it's a slow year when a major's *domestic* film rentals are not over $150,000,000. There was a time when that number was a good *worldwide* figure for a big company. The distribs' involvement in higher-budget "event" pictures has led to the extraction of lots of guarantee front money from exhibitors.

Thus, exhibition is facing a situation where, in 10 to 15 years, there will probably be another reduction in the number of screens from the current 18,000 total to a level of 8,000; the shuttered houses will represent, as always, the fringes that will not be able to survive when pay cable and other new media become the second and third run of a new film. However, the endurance and survival of key first-run and suburban houses seems assured.

The question now arises—who is going to control this remaining core of film houses? Who is going to be listed among the 25 to 30 circuits that will dominate the theatre business in a decade? General Cinema Corp. and United Artists Theatre Circuit are already very large chains; their continued presence in exhibition seems insured by their current moves.

But in a decade the exhibition end of the business would be far more stable if there were half a dozen to a dozen key circuits operating in all or most areas of the country. The long-term costs of current and competing expansion by regional circuits is enormous, and the dangers of two or more consecutive flop films on which high guarantees have been posted are even now threatening too many regional circuits.

One answer to this potential situation is the consolidation of some major regional theatre chains into larger, more financially stable, nationwide operations. Exhibition is filled with many successful entrepreneurs who have built themselves, over the past 30 years or so, into mighty regional businessmen. They are properly proud, properly powerful, and perhaps understandably reluctant to surrender their positions of success.

But that's what has happened over the past decades in the production and distribution ends of the business; the older pioneers and entrepreneurs eventually yielded, sometimes under the force of new business circumstances, to a more contemporary era of economics and management. It may be approaching the time when these regional exhibitor powers ought to begin considering the merits of orderly advance planning and combinations of units into larger chains. The perilous alternatives include localized overbuilding and outbidding, which amount to a deadly game of chicken in which some people do get hurt very badly.

Given the temperaments of some of these regional exhib titans, quite a lot of diplomacy will be needed to effect a combination of business operations. However, a proper long-range look seems to demand that some thinking and action begin to take place now.

Motion Picture Marketing

by **Richard Kahn,** who is executive vice-president, motion picture distribution and marketing, for MGM/UA Entertainment Company, after serving as Metro-Goldwyn-Mayer's senior vice-president in charge of worldwide marketing since 1978. He joined MGM in January, 1975, as vice-president, worldwide advertising, publicity, and exploitation from Columbia Pictures, where he was vice-president in charge of worldwide special marketing projects. Prior to assuming that position, he had served as Columbia's vice-president and national director of advertising, publicity, and exploitation. Kahn had been with Columbia since 1955, following his graduation from the University of Pennsylvania's Wharton School of Finance and Commerce and a tour of active duty as an officer in the United States Navy.

Mr. Kahn's article is based on a talk delivered by him at a University of Southern California marketing seminar co-sponsored by the Film Information Council, a marketing fraternity of working professionals, and the USC Graduate School of Business Administration and the School for Performing Arts.

Trained judgments, intuitive leaps, good guesses, and common sense must remain the hallmarks of motion picture marketing; if we veer away from these criteria, we're going to be in a great deal of trouble. . . .

What are the tools of movie marketing? They are advertising, publicity, promotion, and research. For a long time these were considered merely a basketful of specialties, but today they are the integrated functions of marketing, each having evolved its own general theory, methodology, and practice.

Marketing is no longer a secondary element within the motion picture industry. It has become just as dominant and as costly a force as the movies for which it is employed. The marketing of movies is a unique phenomenon, as unique as the product it sells. It cannot be equated to selling homes, hardware, or hair spray. Motion picture marketing deals with shadows on a screen, the merchandising of emotion. In his book *Mayer and Thalberg*, Sam Marx gave an apt description of movies as merchandise: "Theatres are the stores where customers buy entertainment, but unlike most merchandising outlets, the buyer doesn't take his purchase away. He pays for it and looks at it, then leaves with only the memory of it. When the last customer has paid and looked and left, the material that was bought still belongs to the man who sold it."*

That is why the marketing of motion pictures is a world unto itself, and why the tools of marketing must be specially designed for such a one-of-a-kind commodity.

The following is a breakdown of each of the weapons of the movie marketeer.

ADVERTISING

The marketing tool with the highest profile is advertising. It's a pretty high profile indeed, with over $500,000,000 being spent on movie advertising in the United States and Canada in 1978.

* Samuel Marx, *Mayer and Thalberg: The Make-Believe Saints* (New York: Random House, Inc., 1975), pp. 14–15.

Although advertising, according to Webster's, is any form of public announcement intended to aid directly or indirectly in the sale of a commodity or service, for our purposes the word *paid* should be inserted before the words *public announcement*. A better definition might be an announcement brought to the public's attention via its paid-for appearance in a communications medium such as a newspaper, a radio or television broadcast, or an outdoor poster.

The first movie ads were an outgrowth of the announcements made for such live entertainments as the circus or carnival, the traveling medicine show, or the more permanent music hall variety vaudeville of the nineteenth century. In those days an advance man, the movie marketeer of his time, was assigned to precede a live attraction into town. Via the liberal dispensation of free tickets, he managed to get a lot of posters nailed up around the area.

It soon occurred to the advance man that he could get a lot more "reach" (although he didn't use that word) with his advertising message by placing an announcement in a local newspaper. These became the first advertisements for an amusement attraction. Regrettably, the advance man by definition was just that, and by the time the ad appeared, he was long gone to the next town; woe to the newspaper that didn't collect its money for the ad in advance. Since paper after paper was being stuck for payment, they retaliated not only by demanding payment in advance, but by imposing a higher rate for circus or other amusements to advertise than for any other advertising. Most newspapers today, one-hundred years later, still charge a higher rate for amusement advertising than for other local advertisers.

Newspaper advertising has been the bulwark of the motion picture ad campaign, and up until a few years ago, it was the primary communications medium of motion picture marketing. Magazines were also used, as was radio (in some instances, in heavy doses). Outdoor posting was also employed on certain films, but the concentration at the creative level was always on the development of an advertising concept that would work in black and white in the print medium.

The creation of a motion picture print ad is usually a team endeavor by a copywriter and art director from either an in-house or outside advertising agency and a motion picture studio advertising executive. All are exposed to the film at its earliest stages by reading the shooting script, looking at still photographs taken while the picture is being filmed, and viewing the film itself before it is in its completed form. The objective is always the same: to seize upon the factors (or preferably a single all-powerful one) that stand out as the dominant reasons people have for wanting to see the movie and to communicate the resulting theme via the words and images contained in the ad. In other words, find the reason people have for wanting to see the movie and dramatize it accordingly, whether it be the fact that John Travolta is the star or that the film comes from a popular best seller. Of course, this process holds true for the creation of advertising in the other media—a radio spot, theatre trailer, or television commercial.

Movies began to use radio as an advertising medium early on, but most radio commercials at the outset consisted solely of some words that copywriters supplied to a radio station announcer, who would read them accordingly. By the 1940s it was the motion picture marketeer's brainchild to do better than that on radio by recording those words in advance and adding sound effects, along with music and perhaps even dialogue from the movie. When that happened, radio came of age as a selling tool for motion pictures.

Magazines have been used through the years, but with the demise of general-circulation publications like *Life* and *Look* in the late 1960s and early 1970s, that medium temporarily lost favor with the movie marketeer. Today it's on the rise again.

During this same period, a funny thing happened to motion picture marketing: We discovered television, and a revolution ensued. Today, the creation of an effective television commercial is of primary importance in the marketing of motion pictures.

Advertising is indeed an all-purpose marketing tool, but just as it is pretty difficult to build a house with only a hammer, it is impossible to market films with just advertising. The second tool of marketing—publicity—is of equal importance.

PUBLICITY

What is publicity? Webster's says it is an act or device to attract public interest, and, more specifically, information with news value issued as a means of gaining public attention or support. But Webster's thus equates publicity with advertising, and that is not the case in the motion picture industry. Put quite simply and within the context of marketing, publicity refers to directing public attention to a product in the media of newspapers, magazines, radio, and television using time or space *that has not been purchased,* either directly or indirectly. That sounds like publicity is free, but it isn't. It takes money and skilled manpower to create and place publicity because the competition is fierce for the space and exposure accorded to motion pictures today in the communication media.

The motion picture marketeer strives for a strong and continuous program of publicity that begins with the acquisition of the motion picture property and doesn't end until the film moves from its premiere engagements all the way to its final neighborhood bookings.

In the pre-production period, news and feature stories are prepared to announce the acquisition of the property as well as to give information about the filmmakers, the casting, and the actual filming. If the property has come from another medium, such as a play or a book, the importance of that factor is noted in the publicity. Unique production plans, such as impressive set construction, unusual location sites, or other interesting facts of filming, are dispatched to the press regularly. These announcements cover key city newspapers, radio and TV commentators, the trade press, and even further, a mailing list of exhibitors who will be handling the product at the theatre level. It's very important to whet their interest as early as possible and to maintain their enthusiasm until the film reaches their hands.

A qualified unit publicist is usually assigned to a picture several weeks before filming begins. It is his job to stay with that picture through its entire life and to generate a flow of press material that will continue to call attention to the film during the course of its production, right up to theatrical release. He prepares a voluminous amount of press material, from which is distilled the press kit on the film. In addition, the unit publicist handles the visits to a set by media representatives who are assigned by their publications to cover entertainment news in the making.

Every motion picture has its own personality and its own theme. The unit publicist, along with the studio publicity department, works at developing that theme, that personality, and all of the publicity that grows out from the production center of the motion picture. Publicity is meant to spotlight and emphasize that personality, to make the film appealing and attractive, to give it a "must-see" quality. This is accomplished through several methods: interviews with the stars; the preparation of a documentary film on the behind-the-scenes making of the movie; and the very careful analysis of what ingredients in the script lend themselves to special stories or feature articles usable in selected publications and in a mass send-out to newspapers and TV and radio stations all over the world. The unit publicist seeks the most important breaks possible—a wire service story that encircles the world, a cover story in a major national magazine, a solid news item on network television, a lead story in a nationally syndicated column, a photo and story in a news magazine like *Time* or *Newsweek*. It takes a lot of these breaks to make the general public fully aware of a movie and to give that product a "want-to-see" quality.

During production, the publicist usually operates in a secondary position; the picture comes first. Publicity cannot interfere with or interrupt the main thrust of getting the project on film. The gathering of news and information on the film will continue throughout the course of the production period and then will wane slightly in what is called a "shadow period." This period occurs after the film has closed down production and before the prerelease campaign is stepped up in earnest. During the immediate post-production period, the performers have more free time and are more available for interviews and other publicity projects; special photo sessions can be scheduled. On-film interviews to be incorporated into the documentary film (the featurette) can be arranged. Suddenly, the making of the film is not all-encompassing, and the selling of the film moves into the leading position.

The tools of publicity are sharpened at this time. The film's production notes are updated and finalized. The several thousand black-and-white stills and color photographs taken during shooting are examined closely, and the best of the lot are selected and printed in quantity. The press kit—including feature stories, production notes, and stills—is assembled.

As the film editor is beginning to assemble the movie, the publicity department is also examining the film's content, seeking out the most interesting footage to be made into film clips or to be spliced into the backstage coverage in the featurette.

The publicity campaign in the magazine field is now stepped up. Working against already-established releasing dates and patterns, efforts are made to have important magazine breaks occurring as close to the release date as possible. Many magazines have deadlines months ahead of publication, so the timing of these publicity breaks takes on a special importance.

Thousands of press kits are dispatched to distribution offices for delivery to motion picture editors and critics in newspapers, radio, and television.

A regular mailing of national mailers is begun. Feature stories illustrated by photographs are sent to motion picture editors at major newspapers throughout the country.

Sometimes, even though the motion picture is in a rough-cut state, the film can be screened for a writer if it is necessary to lock up an important publicity break. On other occasions, a promo reel can be put together—an editing of some key scenes that highlight what the movie is all about—to stimulate interest not only among the press but among exhibitors as well.

By this time, if everything has worked out as planned, the press and the public are well aware of the product, and publicity has helped to do the job.

PROMOTION

The third tool of motion picture marketing is promotion, which is a relatively new word in the lexicon of the motion picture marketeer. Promotion used to be called something else, *exploitation.* The word itself as a noun, *exploit,* came to mean a heroic deed or act, and that described the work rather well. The verb *to exploit* meant to utilize for one's own profit; that was okay, too. Today, however, the word *exploitation* has come to mean selfish or unfair utilization, and since nobody wants to go around with a card in his pocket announcing his own venality, exploitation as a motion picture marketing art is no more. But what exactly is promotion or exploitation?

Let's go back to that circus advance man. When he arrived in town, he tacked up his posters and placed his announcement ad in the local paper, performing the work of an advertising man. He then dropped off a news story with the local newspaper editor, which dealt with the wonders of his traveling show and its star attractions. He was now doing two jobs—advertising and publicity. But the advance man was also a promotion man, because on the outskirts of town, a trusty lieutenant stood guard over the final character in the marketing drama . . . an elephant! With the help of a few eager young boys whom he outfitted from a trunkload of uniforms, the advance man was ready to stage a promotion stunt—the oldest in the world—a parade. All those people standing along the line of march seeing that elephant with its conspicuous banner announcing "Big Show Tonight" were being exposed to a promotion for that show. Now suppose that elephant inadvertently crashed through the front door of the local general store and an industrious newspaper editor rushed into print with all the exciting details— "Circus Elephant Runs Amok in Town!" What we have here is a promotion device being transformed into an act of major publicity for the show.

That is promotion at its very simplest and is the direct antecedent of the excitement of motion picture promotion today, whether it be a gala premiere with searchlights traversing the skies, the hoopla of the internationally renowned film festival, or the visit of a film star to a distant city to open a new shopping center. All of these promotion techniques can call attention to a film and are capable of providing marketing's sister tool, publicity, with additional ammunition as well.

Promotion has matured since that elephant and the parade were guided to the front door of the local emporium. Today promotion activity on behalf of a film exists throughout the fabric of our daily lives. A good example is found on the paperback book racks in supermarkets and newsstands, where the titles of films are emblazoned on their literary counterparts, frequently using the same art work and title treatments as the newspaper and magazine advertisements for that particular film. In record stores the promotion tool of soundtrack albums abounds, designed initially to call attention to a film and now possessing the potential to produce as much income as the film itself.

Motion picture promotion extends even further: from the millions of dollars spent on merchandise that takes as its inspiration *Star Wars, Grease, Superman, E.T.*, and other pictures; to promotion with religious groups of films with appropriate themes; to the study guides and materials prepared for schools and colleges, distributed with ample promotion plugs for the picture to be studied; to product tie-ins for which an advertiser (not the film company) highlights a movie in its own advertising to gain the rub-off popularity of the movie for its own product.

MARKET RESEARCH

Motion picture marketing is a lot more complex than it was for our old-time advance man. The stakes are incredibly high. The domestic box-office gross on all films released in 1980 was over $2.7-billion, and the costs of marketing were in excess of $700-million. That marketing-to-revenue ratio of about 25% is high for most industry categories in the United States, perhaps exceeded only by the cosmetics business. The question must therefore be asked: Are we getting our money's worth from the marketing investment? That brings us to the final tool of marketing, market research.

This tool is a relatively recent phenomenon, and its goals and roles are still in an evolutionary state. Beginning in somewhat ignominious fashion as a rubber stamp to provide numerical support for foregone conclusions, market research in its second stage has evolved into a watchdog waiting to evaluate finished newspaper ads, television commercials, or radio spots in an attempt to get some kind of reaction to that material from the public before tons of money are placed behind those marketing tools.

Market research is of real importance not only in evaluating the tools that are created, but in stepping up to a third stage that exists today at several companies where it has become an equal partner in the marketing process.

Our business is constantly changing; it's very dynamic. The trends, preferences, and motivations of the movie-going public are constantly evolving and shifting. Marketing executives have had to create a kind of marketing mentality, or marketing disposition, whereby they are able to manage and juggle the business, science, and art of selling a movie ticket. We do this with the ideas and instincts that we have and with outside information as well. That's where market research is useful. In carefully designed, articulated, and interpreted programs of market-research studies we can increase the effectiveness of our decision making not just in sales and advertising, but also in the very judgments that determine what movies will be made.

However, it must be kept in mind that research is also an art. It cannot make decisions for us; its only value is as input into the decision-making process, and it has proven itself an invaluable tool when regarded as just that. Opening our eyes and ears to the market provides a surer lever on the ticket window at the box office. But a warning must be sounded about this maturing of market research, for the danger exists of elevating its findings to an unassailable pinnacle and misusing, misinterpreting, or overtrusting them. Motion picture marketing is not a computer science and never will be. Trained judgments, intuitive leaps, good guesses, and common sense must remain the hallmarks of motion picture marketing; if we veer away from these criteria, we're going to be in a great deal of trouble.

Webster's definition of a *tool* is anything that serves as a means to an end. The tools of movie marketing readily fit that definition, for they are very much the means to attract an audience into a theatre to view a motion picture. The selection of these tools and the marriage between them and the amounts of money spent for them are the elements that can bring success.

As we use these tools, questions must be asked. What kind of movie is it? Can it be categorized as a comedy, love story, adventure, mystery? Sometimes the movie marketeer is stuck right there because, if the film can't be readily categorized, it's difficult to answer the next question: What is the target audience for the movie—families, young people under 25, women, sci-fi buffs, or some combination thereof? Once these questions have been dealt with, there are many others to consider that blend distribution and sales expertise with marketing: How is the picture being released—slow, fast, exclusive, multiple? What kind of competition is there in the marketplace? If the plan is to release a picture at the end of April, during one of the slow periods, the degree of competition is going to be less than on December 22 or June 29.

There are still more questions. How much missionary work must be done to bring the film to the attention of the public? If it's *The Godfather*, there is a presold element through a book of immense importance. If the film stars Robert Redford or Barbra Streisand, it has po-

271

tent star value. And, of course, not to be overlooked is the quality of the film itself. Simply put, is it any good? Will the word-of-mouth (in a way the strongest of all marketing tools) be favorable?

All this leads to the employment of the marketing tools in a media plan—a strategy. Regardless of what the movie may be, that strategy should have as its basis an optimism that one can successfully bring the film in question to the marketplace by maximizing its positives and by identifying the key roadblocks to success and overcoming them one by one. In so doing, one can successfully circumnavigate the shoals and rocks of the perilous but exciting waters of motion picture marketing.

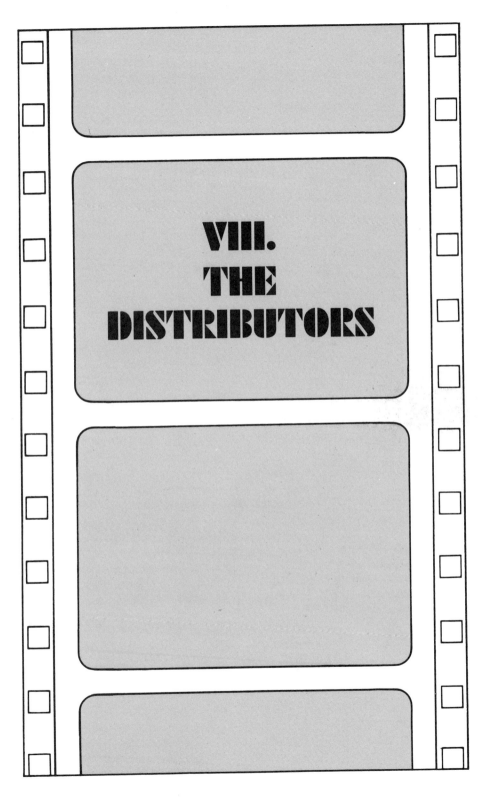

VIII.
THE
DISTRIBUTORS

The Studio as Distributor

by **Peter S. Myers,** who is senior vice-president of Twentieth Century–Fox Entertainment Inc., having served as senior vice-president of domestic distribution for Fox, based at the Fox studio in Los Angeles. Born in Toronto, he was educated at the University of Toronto, spent four years overseas with the Royal Canadian Air Force, and has been in the motion picture business ever since. He began his career as a salesman for Warner Brothers, then became Toronto branch manager for Rank. He joined Twentieth Century–Fox as Toronto branch manager and was promoted to managing director for Canada. In 1968, he was named general sales manager for Fox and, one year later, was made vice-president of domestic distribution.

The role of Twentieth Century–Fox, as a major financier-distributor, is: (a) to finance the negative cost of a picture, which can run from $5-million to over $20-million; (b) to advertise, which can involve costs per picture from $3-million to over $8-million; (c) to secure the proper theatres and terms; (d) to get guarantees from these theatres, thus reducing the financial risk; and (e) to collect the film rentals.

Motion pictures generally are played in theatres on consignment; payment is made when the box-office receipts have been verified and film rental has been calculated. This takes place between 7 and 60 days after a week's engagement.

At present, about 40% of our domestic income from films is derived from the first 50 markets, 20% from the markets rated 51 to 150, 20% from the markets rated 151 to 500, and only 20% from the balance, which could amount to as many as 10,000 bookings. Ten circuits contribute 50% of a major's income in a given year. From these figures, some conclusions are:

1. Revenue for a special film could be skimmed off the top 50 markets by someone well versed in distribution without the use of an expensive major organization;
2. It would be unwise to pass up the last 20% of the potential income, which could represent the actual profit in the play-off of a film;
3. An independent producer shying away from a major distributor may reconsider on the basis that the last 20% of that income could offset most of the 30% distribution fee.

The domestic distribution department of Twentieth Century–Fox comprises twenty-five offices in the United States and six in Canada. These offices are supervised by five division managers—one in Canada; one in New York, covering the Northeast; one in Chicago, handling the central area of the country; and two in Los Angeles, one covering the West and one the South-central and Southeastern states. These division managers report to our home office at the Fox studio in Los Angeles, where there are two general sales managers, responsible for overall selling and booking of pictures, who report to me. I work with the president of the feature film division, and we develop release patterns that complement the advertising and promotion effort of the company.

Each branch is supervised by a branch manager and staffed by a salesman, bookers, and cashier. They are required to extract the greatest film rental for each picture in their area at the most efficient cost. To accomplish this, they study the receipts and demographics of each theatre in their area and make recommendations to the division office and home office as to where a Fox picture should play.

With these recommendations, management at the studio decides how a picture should be released, and the salesmen go into their respective territories and develop the release pattern with their theatre clients through bidding or negotiations. Once agreement is reached, our standard license contract is signed by the exhibitor, stating the terms, playing time, guarantee, holdover, clearance, and cooperative advertising. (See sample, p. 324.) The salesman submits the contract to his branch manager, who approves it and sends it on to the division manager, who forwards it to the home office at the studio.

The staff of each branch includes a head booker and assistant booker who see that the contracts are played off, that the prints are available on agreed-upon dates, and that clearances over specific theatres are observed. The staff is rounded out by a cashier who collects the money from theatres. If an exhibitor pays his bills, Fox will ship one film "open," that is, while the account reflects an unpaid balance, but will not ship a second film until that account is up-to-date. A former function of the branch—shipping and inspecting films—is now handled by National Film Service through local joint warehouses where prints are kept for all the majors.

Basically, there are two release patterns for motion pictures: fast and slow. The fast pattern is for any well-known or easily exploitable subject that lends itself to a massive, national television advertising campaign. The slow pattern is for a more sensitive picture, without presold ingredients, which would require a gradual familiarizing of the public through favorable reviews and articles and the deliberate spreading of word-of-mouth, the single most important element in selling pictures. Obviously, there are variations of each pattern.

In a slow release, Fox may open the picture in New York and Los Angeles only, where reviews and magazine articles will begin to filter out to the rest of the country. In the third week, cities like Toronto, Boston, Philadelphia, Washington, San Francisco, and Chicago may join the pattern, with the picture playing in a handful of theatres in each city, since one theatre cannot generate enough film rental to pay for the advertising campaigns.

With *An Unmarried Woman*, which was released slowly, Fox

played three theatres in Manhattan and five theatres between Long Island, Westchester, and New Jersey—an eight-theatre New York metropolitan area run, which paid for its advertising in the first week. In Boston, this can be accomplished in four theatres; in Washington, six; in Chicago, eight or nine; in Detroit, six. What used to be known as an "exclusive run" has now grown into a run in several theatres as a matter of economics.

Economics also dictates the saturation booking of a fast release pattern. When we saturate a film nationally in the top 40 markets, it costs about the same to buy network television time as to buy local time in those markets. Once we're advertising a picture on the networks, it pays for us to play the picture in the entire country, not just 40 markets, since our message is reaching everyone. This can lead to playing from 400 to 1,300 or more play dates at the same time. *Star Wars* reached a high of nearly 1,800 play dates. Another way of saturating is market by market, buying television time locally and playing all of the theatres within that TV umbrella, thereby limiting the number of prints used.

Print costs vary according to the release pattern. The slow release of a little-known but excellent film that will rely on word-of-mouth would require as few as 50 or 100 prints, which at $1,000 each would cost $100,000. For the saturation booking, between 1,000 and 1,500 prints would be needed, at a minimum cost of $1,000,000.

When we establish a release pattern that works for a picture, it's prudent to drop a similar picture into that same pattern a year later. The *Planet of the Apes* pictures followed a successful release pattern, as did four Gene Wilder pictures. *Young Frankenstein* was released at Christmas, 1974; *Sherlock Holmes' Smarter Brother* followed for Christmas, 1975; and then *Silver Streak*, in 1976. For the fourth Christmas, 1977, we played *The World's Greatest Lover*, for which Fox received over $10-million in guarantees from exhibitors who wanted to be part of our successful release pattern for Gene Wilder.

The most successful picture of all time is *Star Wars*. In 1980, three years after its release, we selected almost the identical pattern for the sequel, *The Empire Strikes Back*. *Star Wars* opened on May 25, 1977, with 43 engagements, remaining at this level until June 17, when the number of runs increased to 157. We further accelerated our release because of the huge box-office success, going up to 362 on June 24; 504 by July 1; 585 on July 8; 628 on July 14; 811 on July 21; 956 on July 29; 1,044 on August 5; and 1,098 by August 19. After Labor Day, 1977, no new engagements were added, but existing runs continued for as long as they could play. Because certain runs terminated, the number reduced to about 750 theatres in October, 650 in November, and just short of 600 through the end of the year. The engagements that continued into 1978 got down to 180 in February, 150 in March, and 100 in April.

Fox then reopened *Star Wars* for a seven-week release to 1,756 theatres during the summer of 1978, resulting in the greatest number of prints ever bought for any picture. Because we wanted to have credibility with the public, we ended these engagements after the seven weeks, with the single exception of the original run in Portland, Oregon, where there was a holdover clause in the contract; the picture never fell below the holdover figure. Portland played the picture through Christmas, 1978, which resulted in a lawsuit because Columbia's *Close Encounters of the Third Kind* was booked in that theatre for Christmas. The judge recognized our contract in Portland, the picture held, and Columbia sued the exhibitor.

On August 15, 1979, we set a second rerelease of *Star Wars* for three weeks, through Labor Day, in 1,350 theatres. *Star Wars* has grossed over $295,000,000 at domestic box offices; Fox as distributor has taken in over $175,000,000 in film rental, or 59.3% of the total domestic gross.

Star Wars opened with 43 engagements; we tripled that to 126 when *The Empire Strikes Back* opened on May 21, 1980. Four weeks later, on June 18, we added another 665 bookings and continued to add runs throughout the summer. *Star Wars* is one example of a fast release pattern.

A good example of a slow release pattern is *Julia*, the extraordinary motion picture directed by Fred Zinnemann and starring Jane Fonda. It was such a sensitive picture that it had to be released slowly in order to sell itself. *Julia* opened in the fall of 1977 in 10 cities, playing one theatre in each, in an effort to create lines around the theatres. Any theatre opening the picture that October had to play through Christmas. A wider release was set for February 2, 1978, at the time of the Academy Award nominations. The pattern grew from 43 theatres through the fall of 1977, to 152 in February of 1978, to 321 in March. Several Oscar nominations were a big help. Ultimately, this long buildup paid off; although it meant a multi-million-dollar advertising investment, the picture returned a good profit. A similar pattern was followed with *Turning Point*, starting small in November, 1977, then adding engagements at Christmas, and more in February, 1978; the result was also very profitable.

At Fox, weekly production-marketing meetings are held at which the production executives cover the progress of scripts in development and the start dates of pictures. The sales executives follow this progress carefully and keep the production people informed of theatre grosses throughout the country and the success or failure of our and competitors' pictures.

When a Fox picture starts principal photography, we begin planning distribution and marketing strategy based on reading the script and knowing the cast and director. This includes evaluating the target audience, visualizing advertising approaches, and slotting in a preliminary release date. Like forecasting in any business, we project sales, profits, and overhead on each picture. Later on, as we learn more about the picture and see dailies, we refine these plans; the marketing staff generates information from the set, and a personality begins to develop for the picture. (See article by Richard Kahn, p. 263.) By the end of shooting, we lock in a marketing plan at one of these Tuesday production-marketing meetings.

Then, at a meeting of division managers, the marketing approach is discussed in detail, including the initial play date, number of cities, numbers of theatres in each city, and the time lag between the first and subsequent play dates. The division managers then return to their territories and confer with the branch managers, who prime the salesmen to prepare for locking in engagements with exhibitors once bids are received.

When bids are returned, if Fox is not satisfied with all aspects of the offers, all bids are rejected, and the picture is either rebid or negotiated with each theatre to achieve the terms and kind of release pattern desired. Negotiations are conducted by the branch managers directly with each interested theatre in his area. The data covering the key 230 towns are submitted to the home office for approval, along with the branch managers' recommendations. All this planning occurs four to six months before the release date, and many times before a print is available.

When the advertising creators are able to view a rough cut of the picture, the ad campaigns are firmed up, both on film and in print. At this time, a picture's advertising budget is forecast, including cooperative advertising, which refers to the 230 towns known as *co-op markets*, where the playing of the picture and its advertising disseminate into surrounding areas. (See list of top 50 co-op markets, p. 284.) Fox usually shares the cost of advertising in these markets because of the potential reach; this cost is known as *cooperative advertising*, and exhibitors are asked in bidding to state to what extent they would share this cost with Fox. Fox has tried various cost-sharing procedures with exhibitors, such as taking advertising off the top of a theatre's gross; sharing advertising in the same percentage as film rental (if Fox gets 70%, we would pay 70% of the advertising); or asking exhibitors to commit a fixed amount. In the summer, 1978, release of *Star Wars*, we paid for a huge network television campaign and required theatres to pay for local newspaper advertising of a specified size.

To review: four months before the projected release date, the sales format is being set through bids that are approved or through negotiations with theatres, advertising in all media is created, and publicity is flowing from the studio; all continuing the link between sales and marketing in the selling of a picture.

At the picture's opening date, the monies spent on those 230 cooperative advertising locations are now on home screens in the form of television commercials and in the local papers as print ads. Money is going out to support the picture, coming, in part, from guarantees from exhibitors. Guarantees must be received two weeks in advance of a booking or the print is not shipped.

Much can be learned from the daily tracking of receipts from the nation's theatres. The first figures to be analyzed are from the opening day and then the opening weekend. After the first weekend, the executives at Fox get a good impression of the strength of a picture; what we don't yet know is its staying power. Confirmation of word-of-mouth occurs on the second weekend. If the second weekend is as strong as the first, it's potentially a big-grossing picture; if it falls off by 20%, it can still be very big; if it falls off 40% or more, there's a real problem.

On the Monday morning after a first weekend, we analyze our advertising spending and second-guess all decisions. If one town is not performing, we may arrange for a personality to visit or use an alternative ad campaign to boost the figures. However, a backup campaign seldom alters the success of a film.

We know we have a problem if a picture opens poorly and declines from there. In that case, we'll play off many engagements quickly and cut back on advertising costs, since the gross can be less than advertising expenses. On a disastrous film, the distributor will not recoup costs of prints and advertising. Some producers criticize the distributor as the first to run from a picture. My criticism of my company is that we tend to support pictures too long. We're very conscious of our partners, the creative participants, and try to salvage a picture whenever possible.

There is a great deal to be learned from test marketing films. Markets such as Phoenix, Arizona and Madison, Wisconsin have demographics that represent the average of the country. With an expenditure of $30,000 in prints and $150,000 in advertising, we can learn how a certain campaign will perform. After all, a national network television buy can cost $3-million or more; if we can cut losses before such an expenditure is made through test marketing, that's helpful.

The relationship between distributor and exhibitor is based on mutual distrust, although the parties are working a little more closely recently. For instance, there is distrust in the awarding of bids. Fox experimented with "open bidding" by inviting exhibitors to be present at the opening of bids, which created more exhibitor uneasiness than it dispelled. One exhibitor bid for a run in a zone, putting up a guarantee of $75,000 and asking for clearance over a certain theatre; he put in a second bid with a $50,000 guarantee with clearance, and a third bid of $25,000 with another clearance. He was present when the bids were opened, saw that the highest bid was $47,500, and withdrew his $75,000 bid. Since bids are not binding until a contract is signed, we were left at a competitive disadvantage. Because of this practice and exhibitor apathy—many failed to show up at all—we abandoned open bidding. Other issues between distributors and exhibitors are blind bidding, product splitting, guarantees, collections, checking, print damage, and screen advertising.

Blind bidding is an issue because many state legislatures have passed laws against the practice. That's a real problem for a distributor planning a national release and spending millions on network television, only to be prevented from including certain states in the run until the picture is screened. It's true that some exhibitors have been hurt by bidding on an unseen picture that later fails at the box office. But there are also pictures that exhibitors *have* seen and bid heavily on that have been unsuccessful. If Fox was forced to delay a release date six months in order to screen the picture for our customers, that would add at least $15-million annually in interest costs, further delaying the return on our investments, and would give television and other media the chance to copy our pictures.

Product splitting deprives the distributor of a certain competitive advantage. Many years ago, a study was done comparing towns where there was a product split with towns with no split but with free competitive bidding. In the split towns, we received 5% less in film rental than in the other towns; that 5% represents millions of dollars. Another problem is that a split may result in a picture playing in an inappropriate house. If a sensitive picture must play in a large "action" theatre because of a product split, revenue may be lost because it's playing in the wrong theatre. Also, splitting reduces the opportunity for us to receive proper terms and guarantees. Although exhibitors claim guarantees are hurting them, as far as Fox is concerned, the total value of unearned guarantees (the figure which is not offset by film rental) is less than 1% of total film rental.

Collections is an important issue considering today's high interest rates. If an exhibitor holds Fox's share of the gross for any length of time, he is using this money to finance his business, instead of borrowing money from the bank. The only pressure that effectively collects money (short of litigation) is the anticipation of our next big picture. In this regard, we have a considerable advantage over smaller distributors.

A box-office statement is due from each theatre seven days after a picture's run. Sometimes, it reflects some cheating; either an exhibitor will skim or an employee will steal. To prevent this, Fox subscribes to a service through Sargoy and Stein in New York, which does blind checking. They go into a town and stand outside or in front of a theatre, counting the number of admissions. If the reported figure shows a discrepancy from the blind check, further investigation is necessary.

A computer system attached to a box-office turnstile would reduce stealing. If exhibitors and distributors cooperated, their sharing arrangement could be fed into a computer before an engagement, and the computer attached to the turnstile could, by the end of an evening, transfer film rental into the distributor's and exhibitor's accounts. The parties could easily punch into the computer to get information in order to make decisions about holdovers and advertising, as well. What's preventing computer use is that exhibitors realize this would speed up their payments so they would not have the usual float.

Print damage in theatres is serious. Years ago, one print could serve 60 to 75 engagements; today, the number is down to 10 or 12. Recently, the majors cooperated in a program of 100% inspection on one picture each. When we compared notes, we found the damage was being done in the same theatres. It would have been worth it to buy new equipment for these theatres, but the others would have complained; now we simply encourage exhibitors to maintain their equipment at high standards by awarding pictures to the theatres with the best performance.

Screen advertising in theatres is a practice we deplore. Business is improving because people are tired of watching commercials on television and want to get out of the house, see other people, and enjoy a movie on a large screen in a comfortable theatre. They don't want that performance interrupted by the commercials they left home to avoid, and Fox has taken a strong stand to discourage the practice. In our bid solicitations, we ask for all information regarding the theatre's use of advertising and state that screen advertising revenue is to be included in the gross receipts.

The motion picture industry is really like any other business in which the middleman promotes orderly manufacture and orderly marketing. The middleman (the distributor) links the manufacture (production) with the marketplace (exhibition). Production is aided by research and development in the form of the creative talent. The motion picture business faces problems much like those encountered in other speculative businesses, such as the oil industry. Huge capital sums are invested in production before any return is realized, and often the investment is never recouped. As a matter of record, only two out of ten motion pictures show a profit or break even. In addition to the production costs, other risk factors include cost of prints, distribution , advertising, and promotion.

Motion pictures is the most democratic of all art forms. Through the purchase of tickets at competing box offices, the public votes its approval or disapproval at every performance. The patron becomes an advocate for the picture.

The Top 50 Cooperative Advertising Markets
in the United States and Canada
(Listed in Approximate Order of Revenue Potential)

1. New York, NY	26. Milwaukee, WI
2. Los Angeles, CA	27. Cincinnati, OH
3. Chicago, IL	28. Indianapolis, ID
4. San Francisco, CA	29. Tampa/St. Petersburg, FL
5. Philadelphia, PA	30. Phoenix, AZ
6. Boston, MA	31. Honolulu, HI
7. Toronto, Canada	32. Vancouver, Canada
8. Detroit, MI	33. Sacramento, CA
9. Dallas, TX	34. Salt Lake City, UT
10. Washington, DC	35. Broward County, FL
11. Houston, TX	36. Buffalo, NY
12. St. Louis, MO	37. Portland, OR
13. Minneapolis/St. Paul, MN	38. Memphis, TN
14. Atlanta, GA	39. Charlotte, NC
15. Pittsburgh, PA	40. Columbus, OH
16. Miami, FL	41. Calgary, Canada
17. Cleveland, OH	42. New Haven, CT
18. Denver, CO	43. Rochester, NY
19. Baltimore, MD	44. Jacksonville, FL
20. Montreal, Canada	45. Louisville, KY
21. Kansas City, MO	46. Winnipeg, Canada
22. San Diego, CA	47. Las Vegas, NV
23. New Orleans, LA	48. Tucson, AZ
24. San Jose, CA	49. Hartford, CT
25. Seattle, WA	50. Toledo, OH

Independent Distribution: New World Pictures

by **Barbara D. Boyle,** who for years was executive vice-president, general counsel, and chief operating officer of New World Pictures, based in Los Angeles. Before joining New World, she practiced entertainment law as a partner in the firm of Cohen and Boyle and served as an attorney in business affairs and as corporate assistant secretary at American International Pictures. A graduate of the University of California at Berkeley (B.A.) and UCLA (J.D.), Mrs. Boyle has served as president of Women in Film and has been active on the advisory committee of the UCLA Law School Entertainment Symposia. After completing this article, Mrs. Boyle was hired from New World Pictures to become senior vice-president of production for Orion Pictures in Los Angeles.

There are two formulas for distribution. . . . One is the "net deal." . . . The second formula is the "adjusted gross deal." . . . Since one point of gross . . . equals 1.8 of net, the producer may end up with the same monies with either formula. . . .

When New World began in 1970, two companies were formed: New World Productions, which produces films, and New World Pictures, which distributes the product of New World Productions and acquires films not produced by New World Productions. The founder and guiding light of New World is Roger Corman. He has long been recognized as one of the most successful low-budget producer-directors, and the first two years of the company's history in distribution and production reflected his style in such pictures as *The Big Doll House* and *Angels Die Hard.*

In 1972, New World acquired Ingmar Bergman's *Cries and Whispers* for distribution in the United States and Canada in a deliberate effort by Corman to avoid the image of New World as a straight exploitation company. The picture was highly successful commercially and won the Academy Award for best foreign film. In the following year, New World acquired *Fantastic Planet* and *The Harder They Come* as well as Fellini's *Amarcord*, which also won best foreign film. During the period that New World was acquiring the films of Bergman, Fellini, and Truffaut, the company continued to finance and distribute such pictures as *Summer School Teachers, Student Nurses,* and *The Night of the Cobra Woman.* Thus began the dichotomy in product that has proven very successful for the company.

In the early years of the company, New World released films primarily to drive-ins because that market traditionally belonged to the so-called independent. Drive-ins would also play product of the majors eight or nine months after initial release in a given territory. Then, two changes occurred. First, the market that was originally New World's was invaded by the majors. As advertising costs increased, a major distributor opening a picture in certain key cities began to orbit the picture to the suburbs of those markets because they needed a sufficient number of theatres to support the enormous advertising campaign. The result was that the majors intruded into the traditional area of the independent, the drive-in. In Los Angeles, for example, it is now common for a major's picture to open "day and date" (simultaneously) in several theatres, including Westwood and a drive-in.

Second, the land on which the drive-ins were located became so valuable that it began (and continues) to be developed into shopping centers. Often, these centers include a multi-screen complex housing several small theatres (with seating of 250–400) to replace the drive-in. (See article by Durwood and Resnick, p. 327.) The net result is more screens needing more product.

New World Pictures releases about fifteen pictures a year. The types of pictures include in-house created and financed pictures, co-produced and co-financed films, and acquired pictures, which are usually financed independently and brought to New World as completed films. In this last category are the "foreign art films" as well as commercial films.

1. *In-House Productions.* The production process of in-house pictures begins with the idea, which can usually be traced to Roger Corman, chairman of the board and president of New World. He will then consult with various New World executives. For instance, he will ask the vice-president of domestic distribution to evaluate the theatrical box-office potential of the idea; he will ask the international vice-president to judge the overseas market potential; he will ask the vice-president of television to assess its television potential; he will then ask the story editor to suggest writers. Depending on the proposed negative cost, Corman will also try to generate some prefinancing through guarantees from such markets as network television, pay television (Home Box Office, etc.), and foreign theatrical.

Avalanche, the highest-budgeted picture ever made by New World before 1979, is a good example. The budget was $2-million—raw cost. New World's budgets differ from the majors' in that a $2-million figure does not include any overhead percentage to New World, any interest on intercompany financing agreements, or any fees to Roger Corman, all proper negative-cost items that are normally included in a studio budget. This $2-million cost, under any other studio's definition, would be $3 to $3.5-million. *Avalanche* was presold to CBS for well over $1-million, presold to HBO, and presold to foreign theatrical markets. Prior to domestic theatrical release, New World had nearly $3-million in contracts.

Interim financing has never been a problem for New World, nor has a completion bond. Usually, when independent producers bring such contracts to a bank, the bank will require delivery of the picture to a guaranteeing distributor as a condition for a picture loan. New World can loan itself the money or borrow money from its bank under a substantial, existing revolving line of credit, and know that the contracts and its own financial position are there to guarantee the necessary funds.

2. *Co-Production/Financing.* A second type of in-house production can be submitted to the company from the outside, perhaps with partial financing. For example, *Piranha* was presented as a script with half the financing (approximately $500,000) attached to it. The financier, United Artists, wanted a completion guarantee and wanted the picture to be produced by New World Productions. New World Productions did produce the picture and financed the other half of the negative cost. New World Pictures retained distribution rights in the United States and Canada, while United Artists, for its $500,000, held distribution rights outside the United States and Canada. Under Corman's guidance the script was rewritten, a budget prepared, all casting done, and the director selected. For their investment of $500,000, United Artists has billed about $10-million in gross film revenue; New World has grossed from its territories approximately $4-million. *Piranha* opened in July of 1978 in hundreds of theatres with the support of much television advertising since the release pattern was so broad. In all, it has had to date 4,300 play dates using 500 prints. That is an example of a fast release pattern. An art picture would be an example of a slow pattern.

3. *Acquisitions.* A third category of film New World Pictures releases is the straight acquisition, which is divided into two areas: first, the "art pictures" or foreign films, and second, the commercial pictures. The potential domestic gross for art pictures is between $1-million and $3.5-million (distributor's gross film revenue). Exceptions are pictures such as *Amarcord* or *Autumn Sonata* that reach a broader audience. New World competes successfully with the majors in this area because a $2.5-million gross means little to a major, barely covering their overhead. That size gross usually means a profit to New World as well as substantial payments to the producer.

The ancillary markets for foreign films are limited. There is little pay-television marketing potential at this time, no prime-time network sale (except PBS), and limited value in syndication. Because there is relatively little revenue from ancillary markets and because the New York opening and other advertising represent large expenditures, New World will generally advance only a limited amount to the owner of an art film. Instead, New World feels it is to the owner's advantage to allow the money to be spent on advertising the film.

As for the commercial pictures New World acquires, they are handled as if they were internally financed pictures, and their domestic gross potential is unlimited.

There are two formulas for distribution that are common in the movie industry. One is the "net deal," in which the first item that is deducted from every dollar of collected film revenue is the distribution fee. The standard distribution fee is 30%. (In discussing distribution terms, references will be to the domestic theatrical gross only.) Second, the cost of prints and advertising is recovered, as well as all other distribution costs. The amount remaining is sometimes referred to as "the producer's share of gross receipts," and it is from these sums that the producer (owner) recovers the negative cost of the picture.

The second formula is the "adjusted gross deal" or "gross deal," in which the first item deducted from every dollar is cooperative advertising. After this "off the top" item is deducted, as well as taxes and other minor charges, the amount of gross receipts remaining is called either *adjusted gross receipts* or *gross receipts*. This amount is then initially divided 70% to distributor and 30% to the producer. All distribution costs other than cooperative advertising (prints, preparation of advertising, shipping, etc.) are borne by the distributor from its share. At agreed-upon escalating levels of adjusted gross, the distributor's share decreases and the producer's share increases.

The advantages many producers find in an adjusted gross formula are:

1. The money flows through faster because all distribution costs are borne by the distributor;
2. There is less chance of erroneous distribution charges;
3. The heavy burden of cooperative advertising is borne in major part by the distributor, who will therefore control advertising costs and other spending.

Since one point of gross theoretically equals 1.8 of net, the producer may end up with the same monies with either formula. Depending upon the negative cost of the picture, the higher the gross, the more favorable the adjusted gross deal is to the distributor. Conversely, the higher the gross, the more the net deal favors the producer; in an adjusted gross deal, the percentages usually have a floor of 50% to the distributor. In the net deal, the fee is fixed at 30% to the distributor.

New World owns distribution branches in Los Angeles, New York, Atlanta, Dallas, New Orleans, Chicago, Detroit, Washington, Memphis, and Oklahoma. New World's first foreign office was opened in Canada in 1978 and its second, in the United Kingdom in 1979. In other domestic areas, such as Kansas City and Cincinnati, New World product is handled effectively by subdistributors.

Technically, the standard domestic theatrical distribution fee of 30% is divided between the regional branch and the national distributor. For both New World branches and those not owned by New World, the subdistribution fee is the same; anywhere from 15 to 20%. Whether it is the Kansas City subdistributor or New World of Chicago, both branches function under the same fee. The wholly owned branches are regarded as independent businesses by New World and are dealt with at arm's length. That is true of almost all domestic distributors. Whatever they pay their branches on their books to evaluate their performance is not in addition to the 30% fee, but is included in the fee. Occasionally, New World will run an incentive for older pictures, where the branches' fee may escalate to 22½% as a bonus after a specific gross is reached. Another incentive plan may find branch managers receiving a profit participation out of the branch if certain goals are reached. The exchanges book the pictures, but distribution strategy, term approvals, and advertising allotments come from the home office in Los Angeles.

Anyone who understands the movie business will agree that grosses are achieved 70% by the film itself and 30% by marketing, sales, and promotion. If New World opens a picture on a Friday, the key executives will have all figures on Saturday, and decisions will be made through the use of comparison figures. For instance, *Grand Theft Auto*, released one year after *Eat My Dust* and in a similar release pattern, was easily charted by comparing grosses and advertising expenditures of the earlier picture. A box-office figure on its own is meaningless. A figure coupled with a comparison or with the number of theatres begins to have meaning. If a picture did $26,000 in one night in 52 theatres, that's terrible; less than $500 per theatre. If it did $52,000 in ten theatres, or over $5,000 per theatre, it may be a winner—the next question to ask is how much was spent on advertising to generate that $52,000.

An interesting illustration is *Rock 'n' Roll High School*, which opened with 250 prints in drive-ins and a traditional exploitation ad campaign. However, the grosses were low. Staff members who believed in the picture concluded that New World was seeking the wrong audience. There are many movie audiences: the art audience, the midnight show audience, the hip audience, the older or younger audience. Two weeks after its opening, *Rock 'n' Roll High School* began to accumulate great reviews from the "underground" press, such as *Rolling Stone*. It was decided that this picture belonged in small theatres in college areas and that it needed to be "discovered," requiring a print campaign rather than a television campaign. This meant a new advertising approach and a new booking strategy. New World pulled the 250 prints, and six weeks after the first release, the picture went out again. This kind of effort required the support of exhibitors, who felt they were taking a gamble on that second wave. They track pictures very closely, comparing grosses earned to advertising dollars spent. They can spot if a gross is being bought by heavy advertising. If real profits are generated by a new release pattern, that news travels fast. *Rock 'n' Roll High School* found its audience and will eventually show impressive film rentals on a negative cost of under $400,000.

In connection with cooperative advertising, New World is similar to the majors, averaging 30% of expected gross spent on cooperative advertising. The more a picture grosses, the lower the percentage of advertising costs. If 30% is spent on the first million dollars of gross, perhaps only 25% is spent on the second million, and so on. Opening a picture in New York costs about $250,000, and the exhibitors contribute nothing to advertising costs.

There are serious issues that independent distributors such as New World are facing. Because the majors are releasing more pictures in broader patterns, it is difficult for an independent to set bookings during peak seasons, such as the summer. The solution is to avoid opening pictures in the summer and to open in March or April instead. If a picture is released early enough to establish strong grosses, but not too early so as to use up all the markets before summer, it will find exhibitors who will play it through the summer. October and November are also emerging as lucrative playing times. As for the issue of blind bidding, New World does not object philosophically to the idea of exhibitors wanting to see a picture before they commit their money to it. The problem at New World is that it cannot afford the time it takes (in this costly money market) to have pictures screened before general release in those states that outlaw blind bidding.

New World has responded to the changing marketplace by making more ambitious and expensive pictures, such as *I Never Promised You a Rose Garden* and *Saint Jack,* in order to control a larger amount of the available domestic theatrical market and to compete with the majors for the hard-tops. Also, the entry of New World into the ancillary markets has been dramatic. In the last few years, New World has licensed 12 films to the networks. Since 1974, the company has moved steadily into the pay-television areas. In the international market, New World has become a viable and important supplier of product, both on the basis of Roger Corman's reputation as a filmmaker and on the strength of the product.

This is a very demanding period for independents. A new and very influential type of producer is emerging: producers powerful enough to gather complete production funding without going to the U.S.-based distribution company. Individuals such as Dino DeLaurentiis, Joseph E. Levine, Melvin Simon, George Lucas, and Robert Stigwood, as well as companies such as Lorimar and Polygram, can offer films to the majors stripped of all rights but those for domestic theatrical distribution. Assuming their pictures perform at the box office, the effect will be that the traditional major studios will have less control and less power.

New World will continue its tradition of training new directors. Ron Howard *(Grand Theft Auto)*, Joe Dante *(Piranha)*, Alan Arkush *(Rock 'n' Roll High School)*, and Lewis Teague *(Guns, Sin and Bathtub Gin)* all came up through the Roger Corman ranks. They started in the editing room (with the exception of Ron Howard), then worked second unit, and later earned opportunities to direct, all in three to four years. That requires a lot of nurturing, and we all enjoy that aspect of the company.

New World will also continue its philosophy of producing and acquiring a wide spectrum of films—from *Big Doll House* to *I Never Promised You a Rose Garden;* from *Student Nurses* to *Cries and Whispers;* from *Big Bad Mama* to *The Story of Adele H.*—a philosophy that recognizes and respects the diversity of the film-going audience.

Independent Distribution: Midwest Films

by **Raphael D. Silver,** president of Midwest Film Productions, Inc., formed in 1973 to produce *Hester Street,* written and directed by his wife, Joan Micklin Silver. When major distribution was not forthcoming, the Silvers were forced to distribute the film independently; the picture became a critical and commercial success. In 1976, Ray Silver produced *Between The Lines,* directed by his wife and distributed by Midwest Films. In 1977, he directed his first picture, *On The Yard,* which was produced by Joan and released by Midwest. Before his entry into the movie business, Silver was president of Midwestern Land Development Corporation, a company involved in urban redevelopment, commercial building, and modular housing. The Silvers live in New York City.

When my wife, Joan, finished writing the screen adaptation of the short story from which *Hester Street* was made in 1973, my only experience in the film business had been as a moviegoer. *Hester Street* was never taken to the studios for financing because we were both convinced that the subject matter was too parochial for them. Instead, I suggested to Joan that I would try to raise the money for the movie from a group of investors. My business experience in the area of real-estate development had included financing a number of projects by putting together pools of money from a series of different investors. The same technique, I found, can be applied to the movie business.

We invested some of our own money in *Hester Street* and asked others who had invested with me in real estate if they would be interested in a very long shot in the film business, without any guarantee of success. I felt confident that the script was excellent, that Joan would do a first-rate job directing her initial feature, and that when the film was finished it would be good enough to secure distribution, perhaps through a major. A number of these.investors ultimately joined us and put up small amounts of money, after I pointed out all the risks and some of the possibilities to them. We organized a limited partnership that raised a budget of about $350,000. *Hester Street* was completed for about $15,000 above that budget figure in a 35-day shooting schedule.

We had decided to make a nonunion film in order to reduce costs, but we were forcibly unionized. We had agreed to hire a crew of experienced union technicians, all of whom were willing to work on a nonunion basis, in order to complete the movie within the budgeted figure. But, when word got out that *Hester Street* was about to be shot on the streets of New York, we were threatened with a shutdown of production unless we unionized. The transition to a union picture was smooth but costly, forcing substantial increases in wages and benefits as well as the hiring of additional personnel. This forced us to make certain budget reductions and was part of the reason the picture was slightly over budget.

Another pressure during the filming was the necessity to finish on schedule because we really had no source of money for the picture beyond our budget. One of the unique aspects of independent film production is the consistent tendency to bring films in on or below budget, since otherwise they may not get finished at all; there is not always the luxury of a completion guarantee. Independent producers become inventive in finding ways to bring pictures in on budget.

When the film was finished, the first question was how to reach the distribution people at the majors. One danger is that a film can be seen by the wrong people at a studio, people whose opinions don't matter. If they turn it down, you have no further recourse at that studio. An agent at the William Morris Agency in New York, Howard Hausman, loved *Hester Street* and was very helpful in arranging for the proper decision makers to see the movie. They all responded with glowing praise but no interest in distributing it, believing it was too small a film, too parochial in its appeal, and too limited in its market. They saw *Hester Street* as a Jewish film that would appeal to Jewish audiences in several key cities, and that was about it.

We then decided to enter the film in some festivals while it was being shown to the studios, in order to prove that it appealed to a broader audience. The film was entered in Cannes, in the Dallas Film Festival, and elsewhere. *Hester Street* was extremely well received in Cannes, and a number of small American distributors as well as exhibitors saw it there and realized that it appealed to a larger market. When we returned from Cannes, we made a final effort to sell the film to one of these smaller distributors, but they felt it should be shown as a "small" film, distributed aggressively only in markets with large Jewish populations. By this time, we knew that *Hester Street* was cutting a much broader swath; it was appealing to younger as well as older audiences, Jews and non-Jews alike. Joan and I both felt that the film should be marketed as a broad-based, popular film. But we couldn't find a distributor who would go along with that, so we were forced to distribute it ourselves.

One of the first things I did was to phone some people who had worked for John Cassavetes, who at that time was also an independent distributor of his own films. They had seen *Hester Street* and loved it, and a couple of them were willing to come to New York to work on its distribution. They became the center of our distribution organization.

We built an ad campaign around presenting the film as a love story dealing with the conflicts brought about by the persistence of tradition and the need for change in a new world. The advertising and publicity made no effort to highlight the ethnicity of the film, since that message would get across easily enough. Because of our success at festivals, we were getting interest from exhibitors who were willing to

295

book the film in cities with large Jewish populations, such as New York and Chicago, but the challenge was to get it beyond those cities to a broad, national market.

We decided to open in four cities more or less simultaneously. We opened at the Plaza Theatre in New York because we needed the New York reviews to carry us nationwide. We opened at the Orson Welles Theatre in Boston because it provided an exposure to the youth market, which we had to test. Washington was selected as the third city because the American Film Institute based there had given us a screening at the Kennedy Center that was so successful it set us up in that city. Finally, we opened in Los Angeles because we wanted the film community to become aware of the movie. Box-office records were broken in three of the four cities, and that type of business opened up a tremendous amount of American distribution potential. Six months later, Carol Kane received an Academy Award nomination as best actress, and that opened up hundreds of smaller communities that would ordinarily not have shown the film. Clearly, we were learning as we went along.

The men and women who came to help us launch our distribution company, Midwest Films, were experienced, having distributed John Cassavetes' *A Woman Under the Influence,* among other films. They had negotiated for that film on a theatre-by-theatre basis; they knew the towns and the theatres that would be right for our picture. The kinds of deals we made were 90/10 deals. We did not four-wall the film, that is, rent the theatre outright and handle it ourselves. In a 90/10 deal, the theatre rent is paid to the theatre owner first, and then profits above that are split 90% to the distributor and 10% to the theatre owner. We received very large guarantees in advance of most theatre showings and were able to recover our total investment through advances and guarantees from about 15 key markets within three weeks of the day the film opened in New York. Key-city theatre owners were so anxious to play the film that they paid large guarantees to us to secure exclusive rights in their area. However, it had taken a full year from the time *Hester Street* was finished to the time it opened.

The challenge with film is that it lives to be seen, so the big problem is proper distribution. There are lots of movies made that deserve to be seen, but because of the complications of securing a distribution pattern (which is becoming more difficult for independent filmmakers), the possibility of smaller films getting seen is being reduced. One reason is that the majors are opening their movies in ever-widening multiples, with more and more theatres sucked into these orbits. For certain peak periods when many movies are released, such as Christmas, Easter, and summer, there are rarely any theatres of quality available for independent product. Majors may open their pictures in

300 to 1,500 theatres during these intense marketing periods, with theatres committed as far as a year in advance. Sometimes, in order to play a studio's blockbuster movies, theatres will commit themselves to a full line of studio product. In this way, through tacit block booking, theatres can be booked solid for a year. They become available to an independent only when a studio picture fails commercially. Even then, the major distributor will attempt to recycle an older picture offered as a fill-in at a very attractive price. The combination of all these factors is making it more difficult for independent films to find those little windows through which they can enter the market and secure public recognition.

Collections are another big problem for the independent distributor. He has no continuity of product, so he has no leverage to use in collecting money due from theatres. Further, he's small and the exhibitor is big, particularly if it's a theatre chain. In the relationship between the exhibitor and the studio, it is just the reverse. The studio can always say, "Listen, we know you took a beating on this picture, but X is coming out, and you're going to rake it in. . . ." The independent distributor may have an occasional picture coming along, but that doesn't give the exhibitor the degree of confidence or continuity that the studio can provide. Another problem is that an exhibitor can say to an independent, "I'll give you the Regal Theatre on June 13," and then call four weeks ahead of time and change the engagement to the Exeter Theatre on July 22. He would never do that to a major. The independent who is trying to construct a careful distribution pattern can suddenly find it evaporating.

On *Between the Lines,* we wanted to open in six to eight theatre multiples in certain cities. We'd book these theatres for a particular day, but then find as we approached our openings that one theatre would drop and another would be switched. We'd be frantically trying to maintain the number of theatres we'd originally booked because we had committed advertising dollars in proportion to the number of theatres. If we couldn't hold on to the theatres after we committed to a TV or radio buy, we would be hurt financially; we would be opening with an ad campaign designed for, say, eight theatres, but would only have four theatres showing the movie. This situation would never be tolerated by a major.

The prerelease and opening weeks' advertising cost is split between distributor and exhibitor on a preagreed formula that can vary greatly. Subsequent weeks' advertising will generally be charged to the respective parties based on the film rental percentage split. If the deal calls for the distributor to get 60% and the theatre 40%, then the distributor gets 60% of the advertising costs attributed to his share of the rental, and the theatre will bear 40%. Generally, if the exhibitor knows the distributor, the theatre will advance the costs of print advertising. If the distributor advertises on television, the exhibitor may be willing to give up a higher percentage of the rentals because TV promotion will generate more business overall. Print advertising has traditionally been fronted by theatres, with the distributor's share of that cost recouped out of their share of film rental.

Hester Street ultimately was shown in close to 1,200 theatres in the United States, grossing over $5-million, and was very successful overseas. Most of the deals made for overseas sales were for substantial guarantees against additional monies if the film was successful. For about nine months, we handled all the foreign sales ourselves. The first sale of any kind on *Hester Street* was to a French distributor, negotiated at Cannes before any American distributor or exhibitor had committed to the movie. After the film opened in the States, there was increased interest from other foreign markets, and we continued to negotiate directly with overseas distributors for various territories. We made the first 20 to 25 foreign sales ourselves and gave the residual sales of smaller countries to a foreign sales rep.

In many countries, television is a major source of income. A foreign sale combining TV along with theatrical can be lucrative. For example, *Between the Lines* was sold to Germany for theatrical exhibition and nontheatrical television for an $80,000 guarantee against 50% of the profits. This meant that if the picture theatrically or through its television sales generated more than $80,000 plus our portion of the cost of promoting it, we would receive 50% of the profits beyond that. The deals vary from country to country. Television sales are not very important in France, but theatrical distribution potential is formidable. In Germany, TV revenue is big and theatrical is not. In England, theatrical and TV revenue can both be quite good. Prices for independent pictures will vary greatly, with one country paying $5,000 to $10,000 for certain rights and another country paying $50,000 to $100,000 for the same rights. The independent distributor is at a disadvantage; he can't package sales as well as the studios since he doesn't have as many pictures to sell. He also can't generate the amount of money in a territory that a major will, because the major usually has some big stars connected with its film who have more box-office value overseas, whereas an independent film may feature lesser-known actors.

As for other exploitable rights, the cable companies will pay much more for studio films than they will for independent films. They want the continuity of product that a studio provides, and because they know the independent cannot sit indefinitely holding his film (since he wants to get his money back as soon as possible), the prices tend to be considerably lower to an independent (perhaps 50% lower) than they are to a major.

When negotiating for domestic distribution as well as for other rights and territories, it's important to deal with responsible people. We tried to contract with theatre chains, foreign sales companies, and independent exhibitors who had a reputation for caring, being responsible, and meeting their professional obligations.

There are a lot of people in the business who are unscrupulous. They look upon the independent distributor as fair game. Many exhibitors get pushed around by the studios. In turn, they push smaller distributors around. We were very direct and tough in our dealings with people who were "doing a job" on us. We demanded compliance with our contract terms. We also developed a reputation for knowing what we were doing. Often, we were confronted with another common problem of small independent distributors—an exhibitor who withholds money or doesn't give a fair accounting. We were willing to sue these companies for collection. With *Hester Street*, exhibitors would often accumulate large amounts of money and hold back payment to us. In one or two instances, we actually went to the cities to recover prints in the middle of a run. Someone from our company would appear at the theatre and say, "I'm here for the print." "Why?" "Well, you're not paying what you owe us, so we want our print." Then, of course, the exhibitor would write a check. By doing this, we quickly established a reputation for firmness; the news got around, improving our collecting ability drastically.

When I read Malcolm Braly's book *On The Yard*, I thought it was a marvelous story. The more I got involved with Malcolm, who wrote the screenplay, and with the project itself, the more excited I became. I don't know at what point I began thinking about directing. I asked Joan whether she'd be willing to work on the production end of the film, and she agreed to. The budget for the picture was just under $1-million in 1977. Our company financed the film, which had a shooting schedule of about 40 days. The independent financing of films is a very hazardous way of operating. In the long run, the odds are against you, and you seldom have the funds to produce enough product to get the averages working in your favor. Films should be financed by film studios because they ultimately control distribution and have the financial staying power to produce enough movies to "beat the odds."

Over the last several years, the options for an independent distributor have been narrowing in terms of access to theatres, and that access is key. For the independent, the cost of making movies goes up and the ability to secure theatres goes down. From the point of view of the studio distributor, while costs are going up, access to theatres is going up as well. Another problem for independents is that movie companies have a lot of money today, so they're making more movies. They're not as dependent on pickup deals as they were a few years ago. Even if the independent makes a good film, the possibilities of securing competitive interest from a major in the form of a pickup deal are limited. When an independent movie is acquired, the studios will not pay as much as they are used to paying for product, and having paid less, they are less likely to stand behind the picture with advertising dollars if it doesn't take off immediately at the box office.

Our operation is an anomaly in this business. I wouldn't consider us a distributor; we're just independent filmmakers who happened to have distributed their movies. Today, seven major motion picture manufacturers and distributors effectively control over 90% of the market. Because of this, I'm not overly optimistic about the future of independent distribution.

Distribution: A Disorderly Dissertation

by **Paul N. Lazarus,** who has served at executive levels in various film advertising, distribution, and production assignments for over four decades. Following an initial stint with Warner Brothers from 1933 to 1942, he served with United Artists and then successively as vice-president of Columbia Pictures, Samuel Bronston Productions, and the Landau Company before accepting the position of executive vice-president of National Screen Service Corporation in 1965. Ten years later he retired to Santa Barbara, California, where he is now a lecturer in the Film Studies Program at the University of California. He also serves as associate publisher of *Film Bulletin,* the trade monthly, and is a member of the Film Information Council of Los Angeles. Portions of this essay have been adapted from articles by Mr. Lazarus in *Film Bulletin* and *American Film* magazine, with permission, and have been revised by the author.

*Is the world filled ... with blind bidding, high-priced neg-
atives, exorbitant marketing costs and ... exhibitor-distributor battles? Haven't we made any headway ... ? Sure we
have. ...*

et us begin by defining the term: *Distribution* is the process that
takes a motion picture after it has been produced and arranges for
its exhibition in a theatre. It refers to the machinery that is geared to
take a finished film, research its market potential, prepare the marketing aids (such as publicity and advertising), negotiate the terms under
which each theatre may play the picture, arrange for the delivery of the
print to the theatre at the proper time, collect the monies due from the
theatre, and with luck forward to the producer that portion of the receipts that is due him as his share of the profits.

Sounds simple, doesn't it?

Each of the major distributors has a network of offices in this
country and abroad. There used to be 32 branch cities in the United
States alone, but economic pressures and improved communications
have reduced that number by half or more. These branches have the
responsibility of offering their company's product to the theatres in
their respective territories and obtaining the highest rental terms possible from each contracting theatre. Each company maintains its own
sales office in each "exchange" city. (These branches are often still referred to as *exchanges*. The term was derived in the nickelodeon days
when exhibitors bought their films outright and, when finished with
them, took the films to the nearest big city and exchanged films with
other exhibitors.)

Basically, there are two kinds of deals between the distributor
and the exhibitor: (1) the theatre agrees to pay a specified sum for the
use of the picture during a prescribed and limited period or (2) the theatre agrees to pay a specified percentage for the dollars taken in at the
box-office during the run of the picture. The former is called *flat rental*
and the latter is called a *percentage deal*. Probably 85% of the contracts
made are percentage deals.

The percentage paid by the exhibitor to the distributor is completely negotiable and can range from a low of 20% to a high of 90%.
There are endless permutations involving sliding scales, guarantees,
advances, extended playing time, four-wall deals, floors, and ceilings.

For present purposes, it will suffice to say that all distribution is divided into these two basic types of deals.

Another immutable fact is that all exhibitors hate all distributors and vice versa.

It all began, I suppose, when the first theatre operator tried to tell the first film distributor that he took in less wampum at his box-office than he actually did. Or maybe it started when the first distributor tried to make the first exhibitor pay a little more than his box-office had grossed. At any rate, since then, it's been dog-eat-dog, catch-as-catch-can, biting and gouging allowed. To determine who's winning depends only on when you happen to look.

THE EXHIBITOR'S SIDE
OF THE ARGUMENT

"These gahdam distributors, they've gone absolutely crazy. Not only are they asking impossible terms on their big pictures, but now they're asking the same kind of terms on their weak pictures. Only difference is that on the big pictures they insist on money up front. Guarantees or advances, it doesn't make much difference. You gotta come up with important front money or you don't get the film. So you come up with it, the flick turns out to be a bomb, and you're left sucking your thumb.

"Let me read you this. Here's a request from a distributor for bids on a picture nobody ever heard of with a cast that couldn't get arrested. So what's the distributor asking? Just two weeks at 70%, two weeks at 60%, and two weeks at 50%, that's all. And advertising costs to be shared in the same percentage as film rental. Of course, they say these are merely *suggested* terms. Suggested, my foot. Just you try to buy the film for anything less.

"What's happened to the deals we used to make at 25% up to whatever the picture earned? What's happened to the companies that used to call themselves 'friendly' . . . and used to boast 'we won't let you get hurt'? Seems to me that they're now run by sadists, not sales managers. They get their jollies out of clobbering the exhibitor and showing their bosses that they can get higher terms than the competitive companies.

"Then they scream about slow collections. We're holding their money, they say. Don't they realize that the only way we can put up the guarantees and advances is to use film rental we've collected or borrow from the bank? Only the big theatre chains have enough cash to handle it any other way.

"I don't know where it's gonna end. I just know it can't keep going the way it is. There are fewer pictures so you have to reach for the good ones in order to have something on your screen. Then the terms are so high that when you play the flick, you go broke.

"Gahdam distributors, they're ruining a good business."

THE DISTRIBUTOR'S SIDE
OF THE ARGUMENT

"Gahdam exhibitors, always crying about something! Not enough pictures, too many pictures, terms too high, no more splitting of product, too much blind bidding—they've got more complaints than my wife!

"Sure, it's a sellers' market today. And maybe the asking prices on some of our pictures are getting pretty high. But remember what those pictures are costing us to make these days. The average cost of an A picture is now over ten million bucks, not to mention the ones that hit costs of fifteen, twenty, or even more. Remember, the exhibitors don't share any of the down-side risk of those investments. When one of these pictures doesn't work—and Lord knows it happens often enough—nobody's around to help us eat that loss.

"You know, no producer sets out to make a bad picture. But things happen, and a company winds up with a bomb when they had expected a winner. With a huge negative cost, plus expensive print and advertising charges, who can blame them for trying to salvage as much as they can out of their sales? Nobody has a gun to any exhibitor's head forcing him to buy. But he's afraid the picture will be a smash and that his competition will get it. So he sticks in his bid, gets the film, opens it and then screams 'I've been had!' if it doesn't do the business he expected or wanted.

"And a lot of these guys do nothing to help themselves—or us. They bid for a picture and then expect us to do all the marketing and merchandising on it. They expect us to spend all the money on television and radio and the newspapers. They don't do anything to move the people into the theatres. And we're talking about *their* people and *their* theatres. We come in like gypsies for a few weeks and then we're gone, but the exhibitor wants us to come into his town and do his job for him.

"Every sales manager in every industry—be it automobiles or real estate or oil or razor blades—tries to get as much for his product as he can. That's his job. And it's the customer's job to buy or not buy. I suppose he's entitled to complain a bit, too. But why do our customers always make it sound as if they're getting murdered? Gahdam exhibitors, you can't win."

304

A HISTORICAL RELATIONSHIP

The present era of ill will between distribution and exhibition dates back more than forty years. At that time, the major motion picture companies—Paramount, MGM, Fox, Warner Bros., and RKO—all were making pictures and selling them preferentially to their own theatres. Universal, United Artists, and Columbia produced and distributed but had no theatres. The five theatre-owning companies, however, made survival a severe problem for the independent theatre operator, who just couldn't get his hands on the films made by those five companies.

In desperation, the independent exhibitor called the cops. In 1948, after ten years of legal maneuvering (with time out for World War II), the U.S. Department of Justice won the historic *U.S. v. Paramount et al.* case, and the film companies grudgingly agreed to sign a Consent Decree under which the industry has been operating ever since.*

The first and most dramatic provision of the Consent Decree called for the divorcement by the major companies of all their theatre holdings. It took until 1954 for the five major companies to divest totally the hundreds of key city theatres they owned. But out of it came the complete separation of production-distribution from exhibition. Paramount's theatres became ABC-Paramount; the MGM theatre interests went to Loew's, Inc.; Warner Theatres became The Stanley-Warner Co.; and so on. Completely separate managements, directors, financial structures, and operations were set up under the close scrutiny of government attorneys. There was no hanky-panky of any kind between the formerly allied interests.

Then the Consent Decree turned its attention to the correction of various discriminatory trade practices. In this area, the non-theatre-owning companies were ordered to become signatories. That brought Universal, United Artists, and Columbia within the purview of the Decree.

Foremost among the trade practices outlawed was *block booking*. This was the technique by which a producer-distributor would sell his total annual lineup of films to a theatre owner or circuit in advance of production. I worked at Warner Brothers in pre-Decree days, and at the start of each selling season, we serfs would prepare a gaudy, colorful, large-sized brochure that would announce for immediate sale — but not delivery—three Errol Flynn–Olivia de Havilland specials, two Paul Munis, three Bette Davis vehicles, maybe three Cagney–O'Brien action films, a couple of Kay Francis–George Brent tearjerkers, and a whole batch of films starring the stock company headed by Dick Pow-

---

* Editor's Note: See footnote, p. 105.

ell, Ruby Keeler, Joan Blondell, Glenda Farrell, Guy Kibbee, Hugh Herbert, Allen Jenkins, and Frank McHugh. Maybe we had titles for half the films. Maybe some of them would actually be made during the year. But the whole program would be sold as a block.

In 1948, the government said, "Enough! In the future, you may not condition the licensing of one film upon the licensing of another." From this point on—the new law said—the studios will sell picture by picture, theatre by theatre, and any theatre shall have the right to bid for any picture.

Further, the Consent Decree provided that there would be no more *blind bidding*, the trade practice that involved the licensing of a picture to an exhibitor without his having the opportunity to see it in advance. All pictures—the new law said—must be screened prior to sale.

Exhibitors became brave and aggressive enough to sue some of the majors for past transgressions, and some of the more flagrant cases resulted in the collection of treble damages. These conspiracy suits became a sort of field day for litigious theatre owners and their lawyers. For a period of time, several of the major companies had more pending in damage suits in the courts than the total worth of their companies.

Fade out, fade in to show the passage of time to the present.

The trade screenings have disappeared because nobody comes to them. Theatre owners have licked the problem of competitive bidding by agreeing among themselves to split the product. *Product splitting* is, in effect, an agreement between competing exhibitors not to bid against each other but rather that, "You take the product of this company and I'll take the product of that one," or "I won't bid on this picture that you want if you don't bid on the one I want." It was a convenient ploy, winked at for many years by the Feds. Then, in 1977, the Justice Department declared product splitting illegal, to the accompaniment of moans from theatre owners everywhere.

However, the so-called blind bidding goes on despite its proscription by the Decree. The very nature of the business makes it difficult to eradicate the practice. The building of hundreds of plush, new, smaller theatres has intensified competition. The studios are making fewer pictures than in the past, and that makes outstanding films even more coveted. Besides, the pictures are usually not completed long enough before their scheduled openings to permit screenings throughout the country.

For example, every exhibitor deserving the name can tell you almost a year in advance what films will be released next Christmas, one of the year's biggest movie-going periods. Of course, nothing is available for screening that early, but every theatre owner begins to fret very early about his next Christmas attraction. As a result, he sticks in his bid for what he hopes will be *the* blockbuster. He may have to guarantee the distributor a large sum of money as film rental for that picture. He may offer to put a chunk of it up as an advance. He guarantees to play the picture for eight, ten, twelve weeks at very high percentage terms. If his blind bid is the highest, he gets the film. If not, he scurries for his second choice.

Now what happens when one of these highly touted, avidly sought after films turns out to be a bust? Well, first the exhibitor cries a lot. Then he screams about the evils of blind bidding. Then he prepares his bid for the Easter release.

The major exhibitor organization—NATO, the National Association of Theatre Owners—has put together a "model bill" outlawing blind bidding. They are trying to coax this bill in various forms through the state legislatures. As this is written, it has been approved and is in effect in 23 states: Pennsylvania, Ohio, Georgia, Virginia, West Virginia, Louisiana, North Carolina, South Carolina, Utah, Washington, Tennessee, Kansas, Oregon, New Mexico, Maine, Alabama, Idaho, Indiana, Kentucky, Massachusetts, Arkansas, Missouri, and Montana (as well as the territory of Puerto Rico). In Ohio, there is pending court action.* Many other states have bills pending in their legislatures to outlaw blind bidding. The MPAA, representing the distributors, is fighting against this on every front.

What does all this mean, you may ask, to the average moviegoer? Is this just an intramural fight, or is the public involved? The answer is, it affects every moviegoer.

First, it keeps admission prices high because Mr. Theatre Owner is anxious to get back the money he has guaranteed or advanced to the distributor. Second, it means fewer pictures in many communities because the exhibitor has had to guarantee playing time in addition to dollars: four, six, perhaps eight weeks of guaranteed playing time for a bid picture. If a theatre does that half a dozen times a year and is successful in its bids, it may wind up playing only six or seven films a year. With Hollywood turning out 250 films a year, good and bad, that leaves quite a few unplayed pictures in Middletown, U.S.A. Third, it means that many communities will only get to see films that loom as big hits. The nervous pictures, the problem pictures, the pictures your impossible neighbor raves about when he returns from New York—these may never play in Middletown.

How will it end? Well, the trend is toward larger circuits of theatres and fewer films to fill their screens. The competition will grow

* Editor's Note: The Motion Picture Association of America, whose members are the major financier-distributors, has challenged Ohio's anti-blind-bidding law in the courts as an unconstitutional restraint of trade. In July, 1980, a U.S. District Court ruling upheld the law eliminating blind bidding in Ohio.

more frenzied, and some exhibitors will be badly hurt by bidding for films that don't succeed at the box-office. The battle to outlaw blind bidding will continue in the legislatures and the courts at great expense to everyone, bringing little resolution to the problem.

Then someone or some group will yell for help from the Justice Department, just as someone did forty years ago, and there will be a protracted attempt to clean up the mess once again.

And life in the great world of distribution will go on.

BUT ALL IS NOT LOST. . . .
OR IS IT?

Before we leave the subject of distribution, is it all bad? Is the world filled only with blind bidding, high-priced negatives, exorbitant marketing costs, and caterwauling exhibitor-distributor battles? Haven't we made any headway over all the years?

Sure we have.

The number of branch offices each company operates, for example, has been sharply reduced because of jet transportation, high-speed freeways, efficiency-minded managements, and, in good part, computerization. It is difficult to understand how the companies could ever have justified the maintenance of four branches within what is today commuting distance of New York City. But there they sat, like the monoliths at Stonehenge, fully staffed branches in Buffalo, New Haven, Albany, and Philadelphia. Today, most companies have eliminated all those offices except Philadelphia—and even brotherly love may not be able to save that vestigial operation.

Branch listings have dropped from the traditional 32 to a figure ranging from 10 to 15, depending upon the individual company's pressures.

Another big step forward has been the combining of foreign operations. The overseas merging of the Paramount, Universal, and MGM/United Artists operations into United International Pictures and the joining together of Warners and Columbia in many foreign territories are indications that the time-worn cliché "We don't want to mix our product with any other company's" is being overridden. The combining of foreign offices is the result of enlightened management.

In domestic distribution, the first breakthrough came when MGM gave up its distribution setup and threw in its lot with United Artists in 1973, followed by MGM's acquisition of UA in 1981. Some of the "instant mini-majors" of the early seventies have left the arena. Another development is the growth of strong production entities, such as Orion, the Ladd Company, and Rastar, which either align themselves with a single distributor (Ladd with Warner Bros.) or scatter their product around the industry wherever they can make the most favorable deal. In any event, the domestic distribution profile has undergone some face lifting.

The growth of independent production generally has also forced some major changes. Ten years or so ago, the major and minor companies made and distributed more than five times as many films as the independents. Today, the balance has swung to the point where major-minor production has shrunk by two thirds and independent production has quadrupled. This means that many smaller distribution outfits are required to handle the available product not snapped up by the traditional major distributors. If some of these pictures are unexpected successes, this will strengthen the power of the small distributor in the marketplace. And the *states righters*—the local distributors who either buy rights to a picture for their area or agree to handle sales in their area and only in their area—have begun to flourish once again.

There have been several abortive efforts to handle the sale of flat rental accounts by mail with computerized billing and collection of film rental. In this day of computers and mail-order buying and credit cards, there is no reason why a salesman should continue to pursue the small, nonlucrative accounts whose few dollars of flat rental often represents more nuisance than it's worth.

For a variety of reasons ranging from ineptness to exhibitor resistance, the direct-mail experiments have not succeeded. Until now, the problems have been principally both parties' fear of the unknown: the small exhibitor's hesitation to pay for his film in advance and to deal wholly by mail, and the distributor's distrust of a computer's ability to sell, book, and bill. But the day will come. And once the small-town exhibitor gets used to ordering and paying for his film in the same manner he orders from the Sears catalogue, that end of the business will function smoothly and profitably.

We're making some gains; all is not lost. But as this is written, a major distributor has announced a new sales policy on one of its big pictures: an unprecedented 70% of the gross for a guaranteed minimum run of eight weeks. And another distributor has announced that he wants up-front guarantees of $1,400,000 from thirty New York City exhibitors who want to play a picture they haven't seen and which won't be ready for at least six months. So the exhibitors are up in arms again, cussing the distributors and threatening them with everything from mayhem to litigation.

The more things change, the more they remain the same.

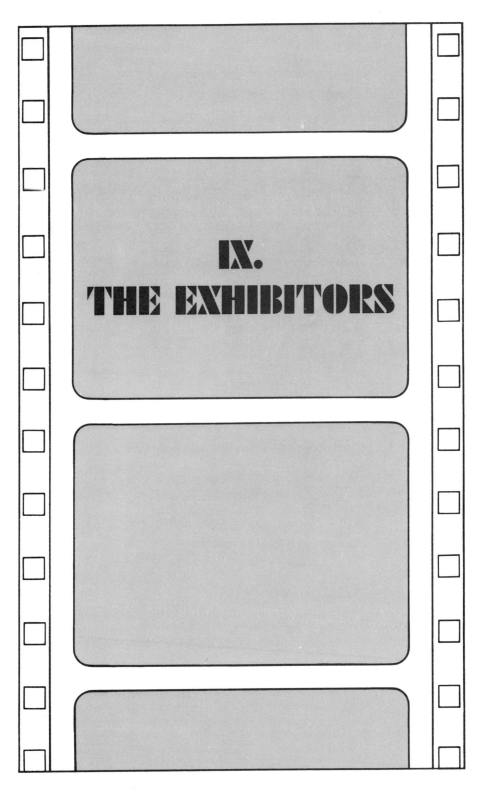

IX.
THE EXHIBITORS

The Exhibitor

by **Nat D. Fellman,** a veteran west coast theatre executive and founder of Exhibitor Relations Company, Inc., a unique consulting firm for the motion picture industry based in Los Angeles. He has served as president of National General Theatres, Inc. (now Mann Theatres) and vice-president of NGT's parent, National General Corporation. Before joining NGC in 1968, he was with Warner Brothers Theatres/Stanley-Warner Theatres, rising from office boy (in 1928) to become vice-president and general manager of Stanley-Warner Theatres, Inc.

*When one considers that a 50¢ increase in admission price
... means that the distributor is receiving 90% of that increase and the exhibitor is left with 10%, or 5¢, that puts
things in perspective. . . .*

Exhibitors are informed of new film releases either directly by distributing companies and producers or by picking up pertinent data
from the various trade magazines and papers. The National Association
of Theatre Owners' monthly newspaper also carries a product schedule, listing releases by month and by distributor. *The Hollywood Reporter* and *Daily Variety* list forthcoming pictures and are good sources
of information. Finally, the distributors' sales organizations or advertising personnel advise exhibitors in writing, by telephone, or by personal
visits about new pictures and their availability and release dates.

Ten years ago, a distributor would launch an important picture
with an *exclusive* run in major cities—a one-theatre run. In New York
or Los Angeles, this run would be the kickoff for nationwide distribution. Today, the national pattern of releases and play-offs for most distributors finds them playing the vast majority of films in *multiple* runs,
getting away from the exclusive run.

The reasons for this change can be found in the shifts in population areas, the growth of shopping centers and multiplex theatres, and
the enormous increase in the cost of production and advertising. Because of the spreading suburban population, a picture can play several
different sections of a town without one theatre interfering with the
business of another. As far as advertising goes, the great expenditures
made by both distributor and exhibitor are relatively reduced by more
theatres playing the same picture *day and date,* or simultaneously.

Another reason is strictly economic. Because of spiraling production costs and interest rates, financier-distributors want to get their
investment back as soon as possible. That translates into playing more
theatres in the broadest possible distribution pattern. In the summer of
1978, during the rerelease of *Star Wars*, Twentieth Century–Fox was
playing that picture in 1,700 theatres, day and date.

A *first multiple run* in Los Angeles will find a picture opening
in a Westwood theatre day and date with a theatre on Hollywood Boulevard and, in many instances, in fifteen or more other theatres, including drive-ins, in outlying areas. Following an opening multiple run in

314

a given city, the picture may play a *second multiple run* in an even wider number of theatres, covering the same territory.

The distributor decides which pattern of run a picture will have (occasionally exclusive but usually multiple) often after consultation with the producer. The film rental deal between the distributor and the exhibitor will be on a percentage basis for all first-run engagements. Percentage deals prevail for most of a picture's run during its exploitable life, while flat fees may be charged for a very late run, or when a picture is played as a second feature.

When a picture opens in its first run, the most film rental is generated, and the usual deal is "90/10." This means, briefly, that the box-office receipts are divided 90% to the distributor and 10% to the exhibitor, after the exhibitor has deducted his *nut,* or house expenses for a given week, from the week's box-office receipts. Against this earned film rental, the exhibitor has probably made a substantial dollar guarantee to the distributor in order to have been awarded the contract on the particular picture for his theatre. The more subsequent runs a picture plays, the lower the financial guarantees, if any. A distributor may still insist on the same percentage terms, but for fewer weeks, with theatres in a small town as compared with a large town. If the company has a policy of 60% on a given film, it may take one or two weeks at 60% in a small town as compared with four or more weeks in a large town at 60%.

There are many instances when an exhibitor, to secure a picture for a theatre, must bid in competition with other theatres. Bidding involves several steps. First, the distributor of a particular picture will send each exhibitor in the same competitive area a bid solicitation announcing that a picture is available for a play date in this given situation, calling for a specific opening date and requesting that each exhibitor make an offer. The distributor may or may not include his minimum terms. He may, for example, offer a picture for a three-week minimum booking and minimum terms. The terms—the actual cost of film rental—will be spelled out in the distributor's letter in this way: First week: 70% of the gross receipts; Second week: 60–70%; Third week: 50–60%. These are minimum terms.

The exhibitor who bids the most will usually get the picture. In bidding, one bids both playing time and terms. If minimum playing time is three weeks, an exhibitor who is anxious to get the picture may bid four to six weeks. He may bid more than 70%, that is, more than the minimum terms. The bid will also ask the *clearance* required by the exhibitor, which means the kind of exclusivity he wants in his area. If he wants to play the picture ahead of theatres A, B, and C, he must make this clear in his response. Obviously, theatres require clearance, as no exhibitor will want to meet high terms to play the picture if it is to open simultaneously with, or shortly after, the scheduled opening in a theatre across the street. Accordingly, he may stipulate in his bid that he expects an exclusive run with so many days' clearance from the conclusion of the run over theatres A, B, and C.

The bid request will specify a return due date. If the bid does not reach the distributor's office by this particular date, it is not considered. There is also a standard bid policy that may state that "distribution reserves the right to reject any and all bids by exhibitors for any reason." If, for example, all exhibitors send in offers considered unacceptable, the distributor will accept none, send them back, and ask for new bids. If the distributor is still not satisfied, he may negotiate with each individual exhibitor and try to secure the terms he wants. An example from a bid invitation reads as follows.

> Dear Exhibitor,
>
> Please be advised that we are soliciting bid offers for the motion picture indicated below. We propose to license this run to one or more theatres, not to exceed 4, which in our judgment will provide the best possible distribution for our picture. We suggest that your bid include proposed terms, including a guarantee; cost of a second feature, if used; the date when the engagement will start, and the amount and method of participation the exhibitor will spend on advertising. We reserve the right to reject all bids received. If your bid is accepted, we will forward to you a contract for your signature.

The picture is named and the availability date is stated. This bid response is due on a specified date. It names the town, and says "First Run." Where no minimum terms are mentioned, the exhibitor simply makes an offer.

Here is a more specific example of a bid in which a number of conditions are set forth.

> We are hereby requesting bids on our feature X for an exclusive or nonexclusive (maximum 3-theatre) first engagement in your city. The availability date is as early as Friday, November 3. No bid will be accepted without a substantial guarantee. Please specify in your bid minimum playing time, minimum terms, number of seats or drive-in capacity; guarantee or advance figure to be paid 14 days

before shipment. If your offer is for a theatre in a multi-screen complex, please designate which auditorium your offer is for, and seating capacity. Clearance desired over any theatres must be specified. In awarding the bids, we will take into consideration the proximity and competitiveness of the theatres submitting bids.

The following minimum terms are suggested:

Playing time: 8 weeks

90%/10% over a reasonable house allowance with the following minimums: half of the specified number of weeks at a minimum floor of 60%; half of the specified number of weeks at a minimum floor of 50%.

If you wish to submit a bid for your theatre, please do so in writing in the enclosed return envelope, to be received in this office no later than August 5 at 12 noon.

If the percentage terms for the above bid are 90/10, it means the distributor receives 90% of the gross receipts after the exhibitor has first deducted and retained his specified house expenses. The *minimum floor* arrangement is rather complex. To review: First, the exhibitor guarantees playing time for a number of weeks, hit or miss. Then, he must gamble on the guarantee in dollars. Against this guarantee, the distributor is asking a minimum offer of 90% over house expenses. If house expense is $3,000, and the exhibitor takes in $10,000 at the box office, he has $7,000 over his house expense. The distributor gets 90% of that $7,000, or $6,300. If $8,000 is taken in, and the house expenses are deducted, only $5,000 is left, of which $4,500 should belong to the distributor. But this bid invitation states that, for half of the specified number of weeks, a minimum floor of 60% is established. This means that the distributor will receive the higher of the "90/10 over house expense" calculation or the "minimum floor percentage" calculation. (Under minimum percentage terms, the house expenses are not deducted.) In the case of an $8,000 gross in this theatre, then, the distributor would receive 60% or $4,800—$300 more than the 90/10 portion of the contract terms. The minimum floor of 60% would prevail over the 90/10 split.

The following are excerpts from an additional bid request. This one involves a blind bid, which means the picture has not been screened; the exhibitor must take a calculated risk based on his experience and business judgment in making a bid offer for the picture.

The following minimum terms are suggested:

Playing time: 12 weeks

90%/10% over a realistic house expense with the following minimums:

First and second week:	70%
Third and fourth week:	60%
Fifth and sixth week:	50%
Seventh and eighth week:	40%
Balance:	35%

Minimum suggested guarantee: $100,000.00

Please include a realistic holdover figure.

We regret not having prints for screening purposes at this time. Because exhibitors are booking now for the important Christmas playing time, we are soliciting offers in advance of screening.

This solicitation for a Christmas holiday attraction was sent out in June. It includes a request for a holdover figure, or a minimum box office at which the exhibitor will agree to continue to play the picture beyond the contracted playing time. If one exhibitor will hold over a picture by doing $3,000 a week, and a competitor puts the figure at $4,000, the first exhibitor has a better holdover figure from the distributor's point of view, since he will continue playing the picture at a lower box-office take.

Since this theatre is being asked to bid on a picture that is not available to be screened, this is an example of *blind bidding*. The exhibitor is being asked to pledge a huge guarantee and commit important playing time to a picture he cannot see. Theatre owners have been fighting this policy in recent years. At one time, there was an understanding that no distributor would blind bid more than two or three pictures a year. That has been expanded in some cases to where nearly all of a distributor's pictures are blind bid. The situation has caused resentment, particularly on certain "blockbuster" pictures for which distributors were able to command millions of dollars in guarantees and commitments for extended playing time. Certain of these big pictures turned out to be box-office failures, resulting in substantial financial losses to the exhibitors.

To combat this, the National Association of Theatre Owners (NATO) has introduced legislation on the state level to eliminate blind bidding by law. At this writing, some 23 states have outlawed blind bidding. This may pose a major problem to distributors spending huge advertising sums on the simultaneous national release of a picture, if they must bypass those states because they cannot make prints available prior to bids being offered. In those states whose legislators have outlawed blind bidding, certain distributors are resorting to negotiating with available theatres immediately after their picture is screened, no matter how close the screening is to the sought-after play date. Many exhibitors are not happy about getting state legislatures involved in the daily operations of exhibition, but they feel they have no alternative if there is to be a change in these objectionable sales policies. The distributor in some cases allows the exhibitor a 48-hour cancellation provision, which means the exhibitor's blind bid may be canceled as late as 48 hours after he has attended a screening of the picture. The problem is that if a print is first available a few weeks or a few days before the exhibition date, there may be nothing else available for the exhibitor to bid for or to play in his theatre—all the desirable pictures having already been bid and/or booked by his competitors.

The following is another bid request.

By this letter, we solicit your offer for the first run showing of picture Y in your city, where we intend to play on an exclusive basis on October 18. We strongly suggest that your offer contain these terms and conditions:

1. A minimum of five weeks playing time.
2. A substantial guarantee.
3. 90/10 over a reasonable house allowance with the following minimums:

> 1 week at 70%
> 1 week at 60%
> 1 week at 50%
> 1 week at 40%
> 1 week at 35%
> Balance at 35%

When an exhibitor guarantees 70% as film rental as in the bid request above, it means he must pay all of his other expenses—rent, light, heat, salaries, advertising, and everything else involved in running his theatre—from the remaining 30%.

Advertising has become more and more expensive for the exhibitor. In many cases, the distributor specifies the share of advertising to be borne by the exhibitor in the bid solicitation.

The Distributor's share on any approved cooperative advertising expense is to be the same percentage as film rental is to gross, computed on a weekly basis.

Another distributor might require a theatre to contribute a specific advertising figure for the first two weeks of a run, stating that the expenditure is a small amount of the total local and national outlay being made by the distributor to enhance attendance. Starting with the third week, such cooperative advertising would be paid in the same ratio as film rental is to gross. Let's say the first two weeks of an engagement require the exhibitor to contribute $2,000 per theatre in cooperative advertising in addition to a substantial guarantee. That could be a big gamble for the exhibitor, considering that, on a 90/10 deal, the theatre will have to do $20,000 in additional business in order to get back the $2,000 contributed for advertising.

In some bid solicitations, the distributor reserves the right to expand an existing run at a later date. This means that an exhibitor bids for a picture believing his will be one of a limited number of local theatres playing the picture, but that the distributor can add other theatres to the run later on, and the exhibitor has no recourse.

Recently, some theatres in Los Angeles have experimented with running commercial advertisements on the screen. These are beautifully produced commercials that play before the feature, for which privilege the advertiser has paid the exhibitor. Some distributors have added language to their bid solicitations asking how many minutes of advertising, excluding feature trailers, are shown at each performance and stipulating that all income from such advertising is considered part of the gross receipts of the theatre, in computing terms.

There's another wrinkle that some distributors have employed. In addition to looking for a minimum percentage for a given week, a bid letter may specify a minimum *per capita* requirement, which means in no event shall the distributor's share be lower than specific figures per adult and per child. For example, a distributor may require film rental of at least $3.00 per adult and $1.25 per child as the minimum per capita requirement. If the theatre is charging $5.00 for adults and $2.00 for children, and the terms for a given week have a minimum floor of 70%, the distributor's share would be $3.50 for each adult and $1.40 for each child, both above the per capita minimums. Should the theatre admission prices be considerably less, the exhibitor is required to calculate the film rental on the basis of the per capita minimums. The distributor doesn't consider this price fixing, for the exhibitor is free to charge whatever he chooses.

Exhibitor *product splitting* is an understanding among theatre owners in competitive areas to divide product without bidding. In one city, for instance, exhibitor A may get first choice of the Christmas pictures by draw of a hat, and exhibitor B may have first choice of the Easter pictures. They would rotate in this manner, depending on the number of exhibitors. Another form of product splitting finds exhibitors assigning certain distributors to certain theatres, done with the tacit approval of the distributors. The exhibitor thus knows far in advance which distributor's pictures he will play, and the distributor knows who his customer is. In 1977, the Justice Department outlawed product splitting, deeming it anticompetitive.

Block booking is an old industry practice that has also been outlawed by the government by which a distributor requires an exhibitor to play all or a number of its pictures, conditioning the sale of one picture on another. Under the Consent Decree, distributors and exhibitors are required to sell and play product on a picture-by-picture and theatre-by-theatre basis.

There is a way for a distributor to rent a theatre outright and avoid the computing of terms. This is known as a *four-wall deal*. Four-walling means that a distributor or producer is renting a theatre by paying the exhibitor a flat fee. This flat fee is intended to cover all theatre expenses and to include a reasonable profit. The distributor pays all advertising expenses. The exhibitor has no gamble since his overhead and profit are covered, and he retains all his concession privileges. Four-walling became popular in recent years with certain independent distributors who spent large amounts of money in blitzkrieg advertising campaigns successfully supporting four-wall theatre deals.

In nonbidding situations, if a theatre's box-office receipts are not commensurate with the terms, it is an industry practice for the distributor to review and adjust the terms of the picture, depending upon the actual gross. He may not hold the exhibitor to the contract unless, in a particular run, the contract specifies that the picture is not subject to any adjustment or review. This does not apply to a bid, however. Once a bid is made, it is binding in every way.

Another important phase of the exhibitor's economic decision making lies in the area of how much to charge. Admission prices generally reflect the size of the community, the type of run, and the economic situation in the area. The inflationary spiral has resulted in an increase in prices generally. However, the exhibitor must be careful that he does not price himself out of business. All organizations are concerned with doing sufficient business to earn reasonable profits on their investments. Admission prices are very flexible. Theatres in certain depressed areas may charge only a $1.00 admission. In such a community, more patrons may attend the theatre at this price, and more patrons means more concession sales. The concession business is a major factor in theatre operations. (See article by Philip M. Lowe, p. 343.) If exhibitors did not have their concession business, there would be far fewer theatres operating today. When one considers that a 50¢ increase in admission price when a theatre is playing pictures on a 90/10 basis means that the distributor is receiving 90% of that increase and the exhibitor is left with 10%, or 5¢, that puts things in perspective.

The examples cited here have covered the earliest runs of a picture. On later runs, an average deal for an exhibitor on a picture would be to pay the distributor between 35% and 50% of the box-office gross, which leaves the balance to take care of expenses and turn a profit. For the very late runs, a picture can be sold on a flat rental basis, with no percentage. If two pictures on a double bill are from different distributors, and if the distributors are both asking for a percentage, each picture could be sold for 15 or 20%, so that an exhibitor would be paying from 30 to 40% total to the distributors for both pictures.

Sample Exhibition Contract

by **Richard P. May,** branch operations manager of Twentieth Century–Fox Film Corporation based at the Fox studio in Los Angeles. This sample exhibition contract is reprinted through the courtesy of Twentieth Century–Fox Film Corporation.

FORM E-1072 STOCK # PF8-REV. 2/76 50M
6 TO SET

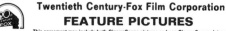

Twentieth Century-Fox Film Corporation
FEATURE PICTURES
This agreement may include both CinemaScope pictures and non-CinemaScope pictures.

EXECUTIVE OFFICES
POST OFFICE BOX 900
BEVERLY HILLS, CA. 90213

Printed in USA

ZONE NO._____

Page Two

SCHEDULE

EXHIBITOR'S COPY

EXCHANGE_____PORTLAND_____ DATE May 22, 1980 SALESMAN_____

THEATRE	CODE	EXHIBITOR	LOCATION OF THEATRE
PALLADIUM	2169	FULL HOUSE THEATRE CO.	MIDDLE AMERICA U.S.A.

PROD. NO.	TITLE OF PICTURES	CONSECUTIVE NO. OF DAYS AND SPECIFIC DAYS OF WEEK, BOTH INCLUSIVE	FILM RENTAL		
			MINIMUM GUARANTEED FILM RENTAL	DISTRIBUTOR'S SHARE OF GROSS RECEIPTS	GROSS RECEIPTS IN EXCESS OF WHICH DISTRIBUTOR'S SHARE IS
	"BLOCK BUSTER"	16 Weeks	$250,000.00	GUARANTEE	
	(70MM Dolby)			90% of gross receipts in excess	
	Opens 5/21/81		4,000.00	HE for length of run	
	GUARANTEE OF $250,000.00 MUST BE IN			vs. 70% minimum weeks 1-4	
	THIS OFFICE 14 DAYS PRIOR TO SHIP-			vs. 60% minimum weeks 5-8	
	MENT OF FILM.			vs. 50% minimum weeks 9-12	
	"SOLD ON COMPETITIVE BID"			vs. 40% minimum weeks 13-16	
	To Play As Single Bill Only			vs. 35% minimum each add'l week	
	This feature shall be exhibited appx.			if held*	
	35 times per week.				

ADDITIONAL TERMS: Payment of film rental is to be made on a weekly basis. Rental will be due on the Monday following the completing of each week's exhibition, at the contract terms for that week, based on "flash" box office receipts, and subject to adjustment upon receipt of the actual box office report.

*Holdover Clause: If gross receipts for the fifteenth week equal or exceed $7,000.00 the feature will hold for seventeenth week, etc.

Advertising to be shared and mutually agreed
Same percentage as film rental earned for run

RUN Exclusive First Run

CLEARANCE All Theatres Greater Metropolitan Area
If TCF chooses to augment run after sixteenth week and guarantee has not been earned, guarantee reverts to film rental earned to date.

Exhibitors "Gross Receipts" shall include all amounts received directly or indirectly by exhibitor for the exhibition of screen advertising at the theatre.

Dist. Share Gross Receipts	SLIDING SCALE IF GROSS BETWEEN		Dist. Share Gross Receipts	SLIDING SCALE IF GROSS BETWEEN
60%	IF GROSS EXCEEDS	$	42%	
59%			41%	
58%			40%	
57%			39%	
56%			38%	
55%			37%	
54%			36%	
53%			35%	
52%			34%	
51%			33%	
50%			32%	
49%			31%	
48%			30%	
47%			29%	
46%			28%	
45%			27%	
44%			26%	
43%			25%	IF GROSS UNDER	$

PASSES AND CUT-RATE ADMISSIONS:—In determining film rental all persons admitted to the theatre must be accounted for at admission prices in effect, except not more than 2% of the number of admissions at any performance may be either free admissions or accounted for at the reduced price actually paid.

UNIT OF PLAYING TIME ALLOCATION

	EACH OTHER	TOTAL PER
SAT._____ SUN._____	DAY_____	WEEK_____

HEATER CHARGES.—THERE SHALL BE INCLUDED IN GROSS RECEIPTS FOR THE PURPOSE OF COMPUTING FILM RENTALS (a) ALL HEATER CHARGES COLLECTED IN RESPECT OF ANY PERIOD FROM MAY 1 THROUGH OCTOBER 31: (b) ALL HEATER CHARGES COLLECTED IN ANY PERIOD FROM NOVEMBER 1 THROUGH APRIL 30 EXCEPT FOR ONE HEATER PER CAR AT NO MORE THAN 25¢ PER HEATER, AND THEN ONLY TO THE EXTENT THAT THE SAME ARE EVIDENCED BY SEPARATE TICKETS AND ARE EXPRESSLY AND CLEARLY PRESENTED AND REPRESENTED TO THE CUSTOMER AS OPTIONAL.

NOTICE TO EXHIBITOR:— If two or more features are included in this contract, it is simply for convenience and this application is a separate application for each picture. The rules of this Company require that each feature should be separately offered to you, the contract therefore separately negotiated, and that the rental of any picture should not be conditioned upon the rental of another.

IN WITNESS WHEREOF, the parties hereto have duly executed these presents including the provisions on the back of this page.

TWENTIETH CENTURY-FOX FILM CORPORATION

By_____
Manager

Exhibitor: FULL HOUSE THEATRE CO.

Signatory: _____

CinemaScope ® is a Registered Trade Mark of Twentieth Century-Fox Film Corporation

Copyright © 1980 by Twentieth-Century Fox Film Corporation.

324

This sample exhibition contract was specifically for the picture *Block Buster*, which had been set to play exclusively at the Palladium Theatre in Middle America, USA, a market that draws from a large population base. The picture had the highest grossing potential of all of the distributor's product and therefore called for the highest terms between distributor and exhibitor. The picture was sold on a competitive bid basis, with Full House Theatre Company winning over other companies. This deal was made one year before the picture was set to open and is broken down as follows.

- *Guarantee:* This represents the minimum amount ($250,000) to be paid to the distributor for this top-of-the-line picture, regardless of theatre gross, payable 14 days before the print is shipped to the theatre.
- *Percentage Terms:* Exhibitor is to pay distributor 90% of gross receipts in excess of $4,000 house expenses ("HE" or "nut") per week. The amount paid is to be no less than the specified percentage of the *total* gross receipts for the week involved. Rental must be calculated both ways—90% over $4,000 and minimum percentage (70% for weeks 1–4, etc.)—and payment is to be greater of the two. No additional money is due until the earnings on a percentage basis exceed the guarantee. Rental in excess of the guarantee is referred to as "overage" and is payable on a weekly basis.
- *"Flash" box-office receipts:* Unaudited daily revenue from ticket sales, generally telephoned to the distributor each day.
- *Holdover clause:* Arrangements establishing grossing levels that require the picture to remain in the theatre beyond the basic play time specified in the contract. As long as the picture equals or exceeds a weekly gross of $7,000, the theatre must continue to play it.
- *Advertising:* Mutually agreed-upon advertising expenditures will be shared between distributor and exhibitor on a week-to-week basis, established after calculation of each week's film rental. The percentage of advertising that the theatre must bear is generally separate from and in addition to the guarantee. When using 90%-over-house-

allowance rental, true net percentage is applied to advertising compu-
tation, as follows:

Gross	$25,000
House Allowance	−4,000
Net Receipts	21,000
90%	18,900
True Net ($18,900 as percentage of $25,000)	75.6%

In this example, the distributor will pay 75.6% of advertising costs for
that week, not 90%, and theatre will pay 24.4%.

• *Clearance:* No other theatre in Greater Metropolitan Area may
play this picture during the engagement in this theatre.

• *Sliding Scale:* Does not apply in example shown.

• *Augmenting of run:* After 16 weeks, if distributor decides to
book the picture in additional theatres in Greater Metropolitan Area,
then the guarantee no longer applies as far as Full House Theatre Company is concerned, even though the picture will continue playing at the
Palladium. In that case, rental is computed based only on the percentage terms of the contract, and the other theatres will make their own
deals with distributor.

The Theatre Chain: American Multi-Cinema

by **Stanley H. Durwood,** president of American Multi-Cinema, Inc., and a director of the Motion Picture Association of America. A 1943 graduate of Harvard (B.A.), Mr. Durwood is an active leader in the civic and cultural affairs of his native Kansas City.

and **Joel H. Resnick,** executive vice-president of American Multi-Cinema, and a graduate of the University of Pennsylvania and New York Law School. After practicing law in New York City, he served as special assistant to the general sales manager of United Artists Corporation before joining AMC in 1970.

... there have been tremendous profits in the motion picture business, but the exhibition industry has not benefited from this. ... Unless this trend is reversed, the effect ... could be disastrous. ...

The past two decades have witnessed the greatest change in the theatre exhibition industry since the golden era of movie palace construction in the 1920s. The motion picture theatre has become an integral part of the suburban shopping center; in every city in the United States, new theatres have been constructed at a tremendously expanding pace.

American Multi-Cinema, formerly known as Durwood Theatres, was founded in 1920 by Edward D. Durwood. It was a small theatre company that operated in Kansas City and other cities in the Missouri-Kansas area. In 1963, American Multi-Cinema opened the Parkway Theatres in the Ward Parkway Shopping Center in Kansas City, which were the first twin theatres in the world, with a common lobby, box office, projection booth, and concession stand. In 1966, the company opened the world's first four-theatre complex, and in 1969, the first six-theatre complex was opened. Even with this new complex, the number of screens in the entire circuit was still less than 30. From 1969 to 1979, however, the circuit grew to over 520 screens in over 25 states. Presently, it has in construction or in architectural planning an additional 200 screens.

Early in its expansion process, American Multi-Cinema established its own marketing department, which analyzed the market potential of all the cities throughout the United States with initial concentration on the potential number of moviegoers within a geographical area. All cities that had a population in excess of 75,000 in their environs were considered as potential locations for a multi-theatre operation. We have tried to concentrate our expansion on those cities that had future growth potential rather than a status quo population, and therefore the bulk of American Multi-Cinema's expansion has taken place in the Sunbelt area of the United States. Our initial expansion thrust was based upon the construction of 4- or 6-screen theatre complexes, but as the success of the multi-screen concept grew, we changed our expansion policy to include up to 12 screens in one location.

The important factor in the change of our expansion policy was the change in the pattern of distribution of motion pictures in major cities. Until a few years ago, the majority of motion pictures were licensed by distributors for first-run exhibition in a major city on either an exclusive one-theatre run or at most on a simultaneous run at three or four theatres. After the initial exhibition of a motion picture, it would then be licensed on a subrun basis to other theatres in the marketplace. The first-run exhibition generally would be in a large theatre with abundant seating; the second-run or subrun exhibition would be in the older suburban theatres or in the new multi-screen shopping-center theatres.

Presently, pictures are licensed in a given market for first-run exhibition on a much broader basis than before, encompassing between 6 and 12 theatres or even more. As part of the license terms, the distributor requires a substantially longer period for exhibition. This requirement has been ideally suited to the smaller multi-screen theatres, which because of their limited number of seats and shared cost of operation, have the potential of exhibiting a picture for a long period of time. As a result, the subrun exhibition of a picture is no longer an important source of revenue, and in many cities the subrun market is now limited to drive-ins and "dollar theatres," which admit all patrons at all times for $1.00.

The risk in establishing any new location for a multi-screen complex has substantially increased over the past decade due to two factors: the increase in space requirements and the increase in construction costs. In the past, when we constructed a four-screen theatre complex, our space requirements were approximately 13,000 square feet. In today's market, when we construct a 6-, 8-, or 12-theatre complex, space requirements increase to a minimum of 22,000 square feet and may go as high as 40,000 square feet, depending upon the number of screens and the size of the individual theatres.

The cost of construction has been spiraling. In 1970, we estimated that, to build a multi-screen theatre, our construction costs would be about $20 a square foot; in today's market, our costs range from $50 to $55 or more a square foot. At the same time, the cost of fixturing a theatre (including seats, projection equipment, concession stands, etc.) has also more than doubled. Therefore, our market evaluations and studies have become more important.

The marketing and real estate departments, in conjunction with the chief operating executives of the corporation, are continually reviewing and analyzing markets and population trends. We attempt to forecast population changes and analyze various economic and demographic considerations, such as average age, income, education, and occupation of residents. We prefer to locate theatres in middle-class areas inhabited by college-educated families and potentially college-educated young people. These groups are the backbone of the existing motion picture audience and of our future audience.

Once we have evaluated the market potential of a city, we locate all of the existing theatres and determine how many additional theatres can be economically supported in that particular city. For example, we may determine that in a city the size of Denver, we would like to erect between four and six multi-cinema locations, or in a city like Toledo, two multi-theatre locations.

After our plans are set, the workload shifts to our real estate department. All of our theatres are located within shopping centers in prime retail space. Since we are constructing only multi-theatres containing 200 or 400 seats in each theatre, the design of our theatres is fairly standard. We do not create a new form for each shopping center, but we construct our theatres to fit in with the shopping center's motif.

The cost of operating theatre chains can be broken down into four basic areas: (1) the rental cost of the motion picture, (2) the advertising cost for the motion picture, (3) the direct cost of operating the theatre itself, and (4) the overhead cost of the entire theatre chain's executive management.

Each picture released by a distributor is licensed to us in each of our theatres on an individual basis. In almost every area, we license pictures on a competitive basis, that is, through bidding with other theatres operated by other exhibitors. All of our pictures are licensed on the basis of a percentage of gross receipts. This might be a straight percentage, such as 60% of the income derived from the exhibition of a picture over a certain number of weeks. Another form of percentage license provides that we keep the first box-office dollars to cover our operating overhead and the distributor receives 90% of the gross receipts in excess thereof while we retain the remaining 10%; this is called a *90/10-over-house-expense* deal. On all first-run exhibitions and at times on subrun exhibitions, the two percentage deals are combined so that the distributor receives as its share of the gross receipts the higher sum between a 90/10 house expense deal and a direct percentage of the gross receipts computed on a weekly basis. Moreover, when licensing a motion picture competitively and as part of the bidding process, we often guarantee a minimum dollar amount that will be paid to the distributor as film rental regardless of the gross of the motion picture and the applicable percentage terms prescribed by the license for the motion picture. Guarantees have become distribution's way of sharing its risk with exhibitors.

The most unfair element in the licensing of motion pictures through the bidding process is the practice of blind bidding, whereby distributors request bids from exhibitors before the picture is available to be screened, which precludes the exhibitor from evaluating its grossing potential. This is analogous to an individual purchasing a home or car by bidding against other persons, none of whom is permitted to see the item before making an offer.

The basic operating cost of a theatre includes such elements as salaries to employees; rent to the shopping-center developer; energy costs; real estate taxes; amortization of the cost of the furnishings and fixtures of the theatre, including cost of seats, projection equipment, screen, and concession equipment; maintenance costs; cost of concession items, supplies, and tickets; and incidental costs. In operating a circuit, we also have management overhead costs, which include the salaries of the film buyers, theatre-operation executives, the accounting and financial departments, and the auditors, as well as legal fees.

For first-run motion pictures, advertising costs are generally split between distributor and exhibitor on a cooperative basis. The exhibitor's share is determined either in accordance with the percentage of film rental earned on a motion picture or is based upon a flat contribution (i.e., $100, $200) to the total campaign by each of the theatres licensing the motion picture within a particular market. The distributor, in turn, will contribute a certain portion to the amount financed by the theatres. Although advertising costs vary with different pictures, we estimate that an average of 6% of the theatres' box-office grosses is expended in advertising dollars.

The general policy of our company is not to use double bills in indoor theatres. They are used only for return engagements of two successful pictures as one show. It is our opinion that people usually want to see just one particular picture, rather than a double bill. The drive-in audience, on the other hand, has come to expect a bargain of two or more pictures for their evening's entertainment. Shorts and cartoons are used only as fill-ins if shows run well under two hours and have become less important as running times of most pictures have increased to two hours or more.

In each area, we attempt to book our theatres to the tastes of the local movie patrons. Thus, in Lansing, Michigan, and Madison, Wisconsin, where we cater to a large number of students from Michigan State University and the University of Wisconsin, respectively, the type of pictures may differ from theatres located in upper-income, conservative, middle-class areas. This distinction seemed quite important to us several years ago; recently, it has diminished in importance due to the great success of many pictures that appeal to a varied audience, spanning all levels of education, income, age, and social background.

Economically, the multiple-theatre operation benefits the distributor. A theatre operator who has one large theatre within an area has a higher overhead than a theatre operated as part of a multiple-theatre complex. With this high overhead, the exhibitor cannot hold a picture for a long period of time. Once the picture falls below a certain gross, the exhibitor must play a new picture. In a multiple-screen operation, the house expense for each screen is much less, so the picture can be held in that theatre at a lower gross. This gives the distributor the benefit of having his picture before the public for a longer period of time.

Although we are the originators of the multi-theatre complex, almost all new theatres being built by exhibitors today are of the multi-screen type. Our concept—that variety is the key to the multiple-theatre operation—has been universally accepted by the motion picture public, and our pattern has been copied by all other exhibitors. In the past, it was our policy to change at least one or two of the pictures in a multiple-theatre complex each week, but with the strong concentration of releases in six or seven periods each year, we have found that often the same movies will be playing for six weeks or longer.

During the past few years, there have been tremendous profits in the motion picture business, but the exhibition industry has not benefited from this upswing. Increased operating costs, especially on the higher terms demanded by distributors for the right to exhibit pictures, have kept exhibitors' profits to a minimum. Unless this trend is reversed, the effect on the exhibition industry in the United States could be disastrous.

The Independent Exhibitor

by **Robert Laemmle,** co-owner of the Laemmle Fine Arts Theatres, a Los Angeles-area theatre chain with 14 screens that specializes in exhibiting first-run foreign language films and quality Hollywood productions. He received a Masters in Business Administration from UCLA.

*... we don't believe in blind bidding for films. ... we could
lose more money on one bad bid ... than we could make
the rest of the year in a particular theatre. ...*

Laemmle Theatres is made up of fourteen screens in eight theatres in Los Angeles, including one twin, one triplex, and one fourplex. The growth of the company since 1964, when we owned one theatre, has occurred by adding screens every two to three years. The organization consists of my dad, Max Laemmle, and myself as partners, and includes my uncle, two secretarial workers who assist with flyer program layout and other jobs, and another person who concentrates on publicity and public relations; in all, an office staff of six people.

Our theatres are broken down as follows: there is neighborhood film programing in the Esquire theatre in Pasadena and on the four Monica screens in Santa Monica; the other six theatres—the Music Hall in Beverly Hills, the Royal in West Los Angeles, the Westland Twins on the border of Westwood, and the Continental and Los Feliz in Hollywood—show foreign films primarily. The Town and Country triplex in Encino shows foreign and fine arts films.

As a company policy, we don't believe in blind bidding for films. Sometimes we might respond to a bid solicitation by sending a letter to the major distributor saying we'd like to negotiate, rather than bid. If they have not received satisfactory bids, they might call us and negotiate with us for a specific picture. Once we've found that our theatre competition has booked itself up by bidding for pictures, that leaves us a free hand to selectively negotiate for whatever other pictures become available. If there's not a "good" Hollywood film to play at those theatres, we have the ability to program them with foreign films. (Most distributors use the term *good* in relation to money-making; I use the term here in relation to quality.) Ninety percent of the pictures we play we screen in advance.

To review our standards of business: we do not blind bid; we have a level or standard of product that we will show; and we don't believe in paying large guarantees. On this third point, we feel that if a film is good, it will find its film rental; we will assist it in making the most money possible through our promotion work. Since we are a small outfit, we could lose more money on one bad bid including a nonrefundable guarantee than we could make the rest of the year in a particular theatre. However, we will pay a refundable advance for a picture, as long as we feel it's a reasonable figure. To determine this, we follow what a foreign film, for example, may be grossing in New York, to judge what size advance is reasonable for a Los Angeles opening.

A sample deal with a distributor for a Hollywood picture on a neighborhood run with no guarantee would call for a minimum number of weeks playing time and minimum percentage terms. For instance, we booked a late theatrical run of *Jaws* as part of a saturation booking all over the city right before its release to local cable television. Universal asked for two weeks at 90/10 over the house expense figure with a minimum floor of 50% the first week and 40% the second week. On first run, of course, these floors would be higher, and there would be a guarantee required. Our competitive edge in this case was that we offered the Monica 1, which has 730 seats. The next largest theatre in Santa Monica available to play the film had fewer than 400 seats.

When booking foreign films, distributors don't establish a release date in the same manner that is used for Hollywood films. A distributor will open a foreign film in New York, get the reviews, develop and test their advertising campaigns, and then set opening dates in other big cities. Opening dates may depend on the availability of certain theatres, since only a limited number of theatres in each city specialize in showing foreign films. At the Royal in West Los Angeles, for example, we have two films waiting behind the current one. The opening dates on these films are not set; they follow in sequence, so the contract on the first film calls for it to follow the current film, as opposed to having a specific opening date. In many cases, distributors negotiate with us specifically for the Royal Theatre because of the tradition and prestige of the house; they will wait for it to become available.

There are a lot of different independent distributors handling foreign films; some handle one film, some handle half a dozen. We get to know them all, and they know us. Sometimes we contact them as soon as we hear that they've acquired a certain film for domestic release; sometimes they call us and ask us to view a new film and consider playing it in one of our theatres. We also discover availability of new foreign films by reading the trades and other papers, attending several film festivals, and going to private screenings, often prior to a picture's securing a distribution deal. In fact, we've been helpful in launching certain films that we've liked.

We generally avoid playing pictures requiring guarantees, but will give advances on occasion. An example is Visconti's last film *The Innocent*, which we very much wanted to play. The deal ultimately involved a five-figure advance plus minimum terms and a minimum playing time. It called for a split of 90/10, with minimum floors for the first two weeks of 60% and for the third and fourth week, 50%. These floors may be slightly lower than for a Hollywood film.

Floors protect the distributor if the film's a disappointment; the 90/10 split also protects the distributor. For instance, let's say a theatre for one week has a $20,000 gross on a 90/10 deal with a 60% floor and a house nut of $5,000. Start with $20,000 as the gross, subtract $5,000, which is the house expense. Then, split the remaining $15,000 90/10; that leaves $1,500 for the theatre and $13,500 for the distributor. How does that compare with the 60% floor figure? 60% of $20,000 is $12,000; 70% of $20,000 is $14,000. Since a net film rental of $13,500 (the distributor's share) is about 67% of $20,000, or about 7% higher than the floor, the 90/10 split will govern, with the theatre paying a higher percentage to the distributor than the straight 60% of gross.

The area of advertising is wide open for negotiation. Sometimes a theatre of ours might agree to contribute $500 to the first-run advertising campaign of a picture or $1,000 to the preopening and first weeks campaign. Generally, the distributor pays for the bulk of advertising because he is keeping the bulk of the generated film rental.

Another type of deal, possible for a small foreign film, would be on a basis of 25 to 50%, using a "sliding scale," with advertising shared on a 50/50 basis with the distributor. If the film grosses $4,000 in a given week, the distributor would receive 25% of the $4,000, or $1,000. A sliding scale adjusts much like an income tax table; if the film grosses $5,000, the scale might peg at 30%, or $1,500 to the distributor. If the box-office gross is $6,000, it might be 40% on a scale, or $2,400 as film rental. The sliding scale is a preestablished and agreed-upon chart of figures that a particular theatre follows, based on its various expenses. Since the scale graduates upward as the gross increases, the film rental increases as well. The distributor would agree to such a sliding scale chart in advance, and the figures naturally take into account the house nut.

The *nut*, or overhead, of one of our theatres includes payroll, rental on the theatre property, maintenance, insurance, utilities, and standard advertising, which is a part of the usual, steady advertising each theatre bears.

Concessions are a much more significant profit center for Hollywood films than for foreign films. We regard concessions as a convenience to the customer, not the primary source of our income. With a Hollywood film, it's often the other way around. Sometimes a theatre showing a Hollywood film would even be willing to give the 70% floor terms and perhaps 80% floors just to get a certain "popcorn movie"; then they make their money at the candy counter. After all, the markup on a bag of popcorn is probably around 75% (which does not, however, take into account the cost of running a concession operation).

Once we make a deal on a film, we put trailers on all our screens announcing the film in advance. In addition, there'll be posters at the theatres and fliers circulating with full reviews or excerpts; telephone calls will be made to certain civic groups, if they would respond to a particular film. For instance, if it's a German film based on Ibsen, we'll go after developing theatre groups and German language groups. We've gained a good reputation for this type of special handling of foreign films.

As for prints, we try to receive a print at least a week before the run begins, for press screenings and to check it thoroughly for damage. There are no protection prints available for foreign films; usually, when a Hollywood film plays in Westwood, however, there's a backup print in case of tearing or other damage. Because a single 35mm print costs $1,000 or more, the small, foreign distributor usually can't afford a backup.

In the day-to-day operation of the theatres, little emergencies arise, such as the breakdown of an air-conditioning system, the need to splice in a print, customer complaints, or employee problems. Otherwise, the day is filled with the routine of planning advance work for future pictures.

Finally, there is one complaint that a theatre owner must voice, and that is with newspaper advertising policies. Newspapers charge higher rates for display advertising than for other forms of advertising. It's wrong that a department store can afford a half-dozen full-page ads in a city while a major film cannot because the same space just costs too much. This practice is discriminatory and should be abolished. It dates back to the days when amusement advertisers would leave town without paying their bills. Local theatres are here to stay, and they make a major contribution to the local economy; it's about time this advertising practice was corrected.

The Exhibition License

by **Michael F. Mayer,** a partner in Mayer & Bucher, the New York theatrical law firm. He has served as executive director of the International Film Importers and Distributors of America, Inc., and is currently secretary of the Film Society of Lincoln Center and a member of the appeals board of the industry Code and Rating Authority. Mr. Mayer teaches courses at The New School on film industry practices and ethical problems in the mass media. He is the author of *Foreign Films on American Screens; What You Should Know About Libel and Slander; Rights of Privacy;* and *The Film Industries: Practical Business/Legal Problems in Production, Distribution and Exhibition.*

> *Contrary to the trade practices of a generation ago, there are now far fewer adjustments of rental terms on major films after the exhibition is concluded. . . .*

Although the trade term is *sold*, practically all theatrical films are licensed, and title to a print rarely passes to another party. This is significant on a number of counts. If a picture were sold outright, copyright protection might be affected by passage of title. Piracy by duplication would be easier if a print remained in the purchaser's hands without an obligation to return. Furthermore, cuts and changes would be more easily made, and these could be objectionable to the producer, director, and author. Ultimately, a film distributor's control of his inventory would be out of his hands.

But films are licensed, not sold. That means the distributor owns the physical property and the theatre operator is merely a licensee. His rights are limited by contractual terms. Under a normal agreement, he cannot duplicate, cut, or alter the print, or damage it beyond fair wear and tear, and he is obliged to return it when the agreed usage is over.

The standard exhibition license (now unstandardized by a growing number of diverse forms) contains a series of significant terms and remains a vital tool of the film distributor's trade. The terms of a run are set—let's say it's first run on a sole or multiple basis in a community. *Clearance* is established, which refers to the time lag between the run granted and subsequent runs. Frequently, the contract establishes the dates of exhibition; a *locked booking* sets firm dates for the extent of a film's run, subject to modification only with both parties' consent. An *open engagement* may run for a prolonged period, as long as the picture continues to perform at the box office. Frequently, a minimum period of engagement is established, subject to a holdover figure if a picture grosses in excess of a particular sum for a week or weekend. In that event, the contract may require that the film continue to play as long as it hits the established holdover figure.

The contract contains a multitude of other terms. It specifies, in accordance with law, that the licensing of one film is not conditioned on the rental of any other film. This conforms to the court rulings, in the Paramount antitrust case and elsewhere, that copyrighted products may not be used to force the leasing of other such works. This barred

339

the pernicious practice of block booking, which remains banned. Human nature being what it is, however, the rule is violated on occasion, and undesirable films have been forced on unwilling exhibitors who are told by distributors, "If you, Mr. Exhibitor, want film *A*, you will have to play the lemon, film *B*." In a recent incident, a major distributor pleaded no contest in court to a judge for precisely this type of conduct. I have no doubt that the practice still exists on a significant scale, law or no law. Nothing, however, prevents a number of films from being licensed on the same exhibition contract, provided that their terms are not conditioned on one another.

While the theatrical film business has prospered in recent years, its strength has been illustrated primarily by a limited group of films. We have gone from a broad market to a powerful but selective one. People choose their film fare with a higher degree of selectivity than in earlier years. Film-going is no longer a matter of habit, but one of pure choice. Consequently, due to this and other competitive factors (television, new home entertainment technology, night sporting events), far fewer films are being made than previously, and only a limited number of them will achieve true box-office success. In the 1940s, for example, about 400 domestic films were released each year. Now, if Hollywood came up with 250 films in any single year, it would be doing amazingly well. From this limited number, there will be a dozen blockbusters, at best. This creates the "product shortage" that exhibitors bewail at length but do very little to cure. (Note the demise of the long-planned Exprodico experiment, which was to be an exhibitor-financed production organization, but whose participants failed to come up with the necessary funds.)

Perhaps ten or fewer films will do 60 to 70% of the business at all theatres at any particular time. The competition for these blockbusters has become highly intense. With this rise in exhibitor anticipation has come an unprecedented increase in film rental terms demanded by the distributor, set forth in the exhibition license.

It is not uncommon to see financial license terms for a first run in New York or other major cities that grant alternative film rentals (whichever is higher) to the distributor. Under formula A, the exhibitor gets back from first box-office receipts his *nut* (presumably house costs of operation but sometimes containing a degree of cushioning in the form of excess charges); thereafter, the distributor receives 90% of the gross. This is a 90/10 split over estimated house costs. Alternatively, the distributor by formula B will insist upon and frequently receive 70% of the gross for the first two weeks of an engagement; 60% for the next two weeks; 50% for the next two weeks, and so on. Whichever formula nets more to the distributor applies.

In practical terms, assume an exhibitor has an agreed-upon house expense of $10,000 per week, and the film gross for the period is $50,000. Under the 90/10 formula, the exhibitor receives back his $10,000 plus 10% of the overage, $40,000, for a total of $14,000. The distributor's share, under formula A, would be $36,000. Under the alternative formula B, 70% of the total gross of $50,000 for this first week would yield a film rental of $35,000 for the distributor, who would then prefer the 90/10 arrangement, which is $1,000 higher for that week. On grosses below that $50,000 figure, the distributor would prefer the 70% formula, at least for the first two weeks of the engagement.

Using another example, if the gross is $30,000 for the second week of the run, the 90/10 formula would see the exhibitor deducting $10,000 as his house nut, then receiving an additional 10% of the remaining $20,000, or $2,000, for a total share of $12,000; the distributor's share would be 90% of $20,000, or $18,000. But under the 70% formula, the distributor's share would be 70% of that $30,000 gross, or $21,000; $3,000 higher than the alternative formula. The distributor would choose the 70% formula in this case.

70% (and don't be surprised if it goes up to 75% before these words are in print) is an unprecedented figure, indicating the ever-increasing spiral of a distributor's share. In fairness, it should be added that the distributor under this arrangement will be paying nearly all advertising costs (and they are very substantial) and that the exhibitor retains the vital candy concession in its entirety. Imagine what the concessions are worth on a run of *Superman II* or *Raiders of the Lost Ark*! Nevertheless, there are many films that fail to generate enough gross even to recoup the theatre's simple operating costs.

The exhibitor's grievance is not limited to the astronomical film rentals he must pay. For major films, he is asked (or compelled) to bid huge sums up front in competition with his fellow exhibitors in the form of guarantees or advances for films he may never have seen. His bid is based on stars, directors, rumor, or hearsay. Legislation has passed in several states, and is pending in many others, to ban this "blind bidding," and the entire subject is likely to be settled in a courtroom.

Distributors frequently require money up front in order to grant the desired film license to a theatre. This can be in the form of a guarantee or an advance. A *guarantee* is dollars that the exhibitor is putting down with no assurance that he will get them back. It is recoupable from the distributor's share only, if and when earned. An *advance* is different, for if the film fails to earn this sum, the distributor owes it to the exhibitor. Nonetheless, both items are cash out-of-pocket on the part of the exhibitor. Of course, the distributor uses the argument that he has put up huge sums out-of-pocket to finance the picture—sums that he is waiting to recoup—and that he needs the cash from the exhibitor to get started on new films and to keep the huge distribution network solvent.

Contrary to the trade practices of a generation ago, there are now far fewer adjustments of rental terms on major films after the exhibition is concluded. Theoretically, when a film has been offered for competitive bidding to exhibitors (a procedure allowed but not compelled by court decrees), changing the rental terms once a high bid is accepted would be a breach of faith and law. But changing rental terms to the exhibitor's benefit was a common practice a few years ago; this is no longer the case. Even where there is no bidding, the major film companies are now strong enough to insist on their terms as agreed, rather than following the ancient practice of permitting modifications to benefit the exhibitors when there was disappointment in a film's box-office performance.

This is not to say that the "look" or modification of terms after a play date is dead. For most minor distributors and an occasional major one, it remains a fact of life, contract or no contract. When an exhibitor cries that business was disappointing and he is losing his shirt, the distributor may adjust the terms of the deal regardless of the binding nature of the written contract. A distributor may feel deep sympathy, or, more likely, a deep desire to license his next epic to the victimized theatre owner. But what was once the rule now has become the exception. The exhibition contract terms on film rental may no longer be characterized, as they once were by this author, as a "scrap of paper."

Refreshment Sales and Theatre Profits

by **Philip M. "Perry" Lowe,** past president of the National Association of Concessionaires, the international trade organization representing food service professionals in the leisure-time industry. A graduate of Harvard College and Columbia Business School, in 1972 he co-founded Theatre Management Services, based in Boston, and Cinema Centers Corporation, which operates over 75 screens in the East and Midwest. Mr. Lowe is also active in New England real estate development and civic affairs.

... refreshment sales range between 10 and 20% of box-office income and ... an indoor theatre's food cost varies between 20 and 30% of sales. ...

During the early years of the movie industry, no food was sold in theatres. The industry was new, and during its infancy of magic-lantern shows, black-and-white silent films, and finally talkies, the emphasis was on technology. As the infant theatre industry grew, refreshments were added, strictly as a convenience. Food was sold to please patrons, not with a profit motive in mind.

In the beginning there was candy, which was easy to sell and stock in large glass cases. No manufacturing was required. Candy bars were individually wrapped and prepriced, so it was easy to control the inventory. Candy was a widely accepted treat for Americans, as statistics on the per capita consumption of candy and sugar attest. The convenience of buying refreshments quickly became an integral and accepted part of the movie-going experience. The theatre owner's initial "good deed" turned into a money machine, without decreasing box-office revenues.

Soon after the acceptance of candy came the breakthrough of ice cream in the mid-1940s, which added another dimension to refreshment sales. Because there was no refrigeration equipment at candy counters, ice cream was sold by hawkers walking up and down the aisles of theatres. Soon, its widespread appeal made ice cream a financial success for theatre owners, who found that it did not cannibalize candy sales. The combined net refreshment profits started to add up.

As the movie industry grew, so did the refreshment portion of exhibition. The expansion of the drive-in market added to this growth. Refreshment stands began to sell popcorn. Its huge success in theatres was due to popcorn's ease of manufacture, broad appeal, high-profit potential, and relative unavailability at other retail outlets. Live popping in theatre lobbies was an added attraction. Popcorn's position as the cornerstone of the movie refreshment business was quickly established and today accounts for about 50% of the refreshment dollar volume. Further, popcorn did not interfere with the sales of sugar-based candies or ice cream.

Cold drinks at refreshment stands were introduced around 1950. Beverage dispensing equipment became readily available, solving the problem of glass bottles rolling and breaking in theatres. Theatres began merchandising popcorn and cold drinks as combination items (drinks satisfying the salt-induced thirst) and offered candy or ice cream as noncompetitive products. Up went unit sales, per capita sales, and grosses. Profits exploded like a kernel of popcorn.

In the early 1950s, the rebirth of the drive-ins was fueled by population growth, the love affair with the automobile, and the return to prosperity. To feed the young parents and children, drive-in theatres adopted full menus with fast take-out service. Refreshment stands turned into multi-laned cafeterias that concentrated on merchandising. Drive-in food went beyond the hot dog. Hamburgers, cheeseburgers, french fries, and cold drinks supplemented the indoor-theatre staples of popcorn, candy, and ice cream. New product development resulted in hero sandwiches, tacos, pizza, chili, cotton candy, milk shakes, and more. Menus, customers, and profits grew until the same demographic trends that brought about the rebirth and success of the drive-in led to its decline and fall. The "baby boom" children who used to be put to sleep in the back of the station wagon grew up to become moviegoers themselves. Drive-in theatre property became more valuable for non-theatre use as the suburbs surrounded previously rural theatre sites.

As drive-in theatres and single-auditorium downtown theatres began to be supplanted by multiple-auditorium indoor theatres, one distinct food service trend evolved: the reliance by theatre owners on refreshment stand profits to support their total theatre operation. In the 1970s, the economics of the movie business placed the distributors in a "sellers' market," and the rental terms of films to theatres skyrocketed. As fewer major films were produced each year and more indoor auditoriums were constructed, the sellers' market became weighted even more heavily against the exhibitor. The multiple-theatre owners were forced to require their refreshment operations to make up for the increased costs of film, energy, labor, and other inflationary operating costs.

How do the economics of refreshment profits operate? A survey sponsored by the National Association of Theatre Owners reported that a theatre's pretax net income runs between 5 and 15% of admissions income; that refreshment sales range between 10 and 20% of box-office income; and that an indoor theatre's food cost varies between 20 and 30% of sales.

Assume that one auditorium in a multiplex theatre located in a middle-American city averages a weekly box-office gross of $3,000. If 15% is added to cover concession income, the total weekly gross would be $3,450. The following chart, showing average weekly deductions from that total gross figure, demonstrates how perilous the exhibition business can be, and how essential to break-even the concession profits are. A straight percentage deal with the distributor is assumed. Each subsequent percentage figure represents allocations made for our hypothetical single auditorium within a larger multiplex operation. The theatre owner in this case employs a management company to buy and book pictures and to oversee bookkeeping, which is a typical arrangement in exhibition around the country.

Box-office gross	$3,000/week
Concession sales @ 15%	+450
Total weekly gross	$3,450
Deduct:	
Distributor's share @ 50% of box-office (typical terms for average city)	$1,500
Advertising @ 10% of box-office	300
Payroll @ 10% of box-office	300
Food cost @ 23% of sales	104
Rent and real estate taxes @ 15% of box-office	450
Utilities @ $150/week (phone, heating, etc.)	150
Management fee @ 10% of total weekly gross	345
Insurance and employee benefits (per screen)	100
Repairs and maintenance	100
Miscellaneous (Includes allocations for equipment rental, checking service, film delivery, ticket supplies, protective service, other supplies.)	100
Total average weekly expenses	$3,449

In this sample, using average distribution terms on a straight percentage basis of 50% (typical of theatres outside New York and Los Angeles), the theatre owner barely breaks even, and concession sales are essential. Profits can be made from a popular picture that attracts weekend patrons lining up around the block.

A recent study of sample theatres compiled by the National Association of Concessionaires in conjunction with Coca-Cola USA has brought more figures to light. The average indoor movie theatre refreshment stand makes 40% of total sales from popcorn, 40% from soft drinks, and 20% from candy. These percentages are based on refreshment stand total dollars, not unit sales. The average theatre's cost of goods is about 25%. This is a weighted average, with candy costing more than 25% (up to 40%) and popcorn costing less than 25%. The theatre industry is very control-oriented, keeping spoilage and shortage to 1% of sales, a highly enviable record when compared with other retailers.

The NAC/Coca-Cola study revealed two critical insights. First, the average indoor movie theatre generates 50¢ per person in refreshment sales. A typical fast-food hamburger unit in a suburb, with much lower pricing and a higher percentage of young customers, will average 2.5 times that amount. The "average theatre" was defined by the study as one that sells only popcorn, soft drinks, and candy, not ice cream or hot foods. It is a twin complex in a middle- to upper-income suburb that does not show double features or X-rated or G-rated films, but rather a mix of films released by the majors.

The second finding is the dismal realization that only one out of every six patrons purchases refreshments. What can be done to improve this? The study endorsed five marketing steps for exhibitors to increase refreshment profits.

1. *Sell large-sized mix of popcorn and soft drinks.* The days of the 9 oz., 12 oz., and 16 oz. sizes at movie theatres are dead. Supermarket trends have dictated serving sizes within the food-service industry. Only a few years ago, 16 oz. was the largest available size; today, the 32 oz. size or one litre size (33.8 oz.) is the fastest growing package in sales. Three sizes are recommended for popcorn and soft drinks today: 14 oz., 24 oz., and one litre. The 14 oz. is for young customers, and the 24 oz. is to satisfy the mid-range. In an analysis of theatres that have gone from offering one size to these three, profits from popcorn and soft drinks increased by 30%.

2. *"Value price" refreshment items.* Theatre owners who run a first-class operation with first-run films and top ticket prices should price refreshments accordingly, as long as there is value. They should establish a price per ounce that decreases with an increase in size. This marketing concept, known as *value pricing*, has proven attractive to the bargain-conscious consumer. An average 14 oz. drink selling at 45¢ represents a cost to the theatre of 9¢, or 20% (not counting overhead); 24 oz. sizes selling at 65¢ cost the theatre 13¢; one litre sizes selling at 80¢ cost 16¢.

3. *Achieve the proper merchandise mix by limiting selections at the stand.* It is recommended that refreshment stands not carry more

347

than 15 selections of candy because it takes too long to decide between more than 15 choices. Furthermore, the top 15 brands contribute over 75% of total candy sales.

4. *Promote popcorn and soft drinks during peak attendance periods.* These are the two highest profit items of all refreshments. Promotions such as coupons, price-offs, and free premiums should be used during the 13–15 week period at Christmas and during the summer (when over 50% of the year's business can be generated) in order to emphasize sales of large-sized sodas and popcorn.

5. *Prevent lost profits by controlling spoilage, slippage, and yields.* An experienced exhibitor knows how much spoilage should occur and how much cash or inventory shortage to expect. Problems of spoilage and shortages don't solve themselves; nine out of ten times, an employee is the thief, and he doesn't stop until management intervenes.

A further study of the NAC/Coca-Cola findings reveals these added facts.

a. G-rated pictures generate 27% more refreshment sales than PG- or R-rated films;

b. Although 65% of total box-office dollars are generated on Friday, Saturday, and Sunday, only 50% of weekly refreshment sales occur on those days;

c. Refreshment sales are 1,000% higher when an adult accompanies children to a family film than when children go alone;

d. Pictures that generate the same box-office gross produce different refreshment sales. For example, both *Hot Stuff* and *Airport 79: The Concorde* generated the same box-office gross, but *Hot Stuff* produced double the refreshment volume of *Airport 79;*

e. The five top refreshment-grossing films of 1979 based upon per capita consumption were *Hot Stuff, Sleeping Beauty* (rerelease), *Sunburn, The Muppet Movie,* and *The Amityville Horror;*

f. The five worst-grossing films in terms of refreshments in 1979 on a per capita basis were *Airport 79: The Concorde, Escape from Alcatraz, Breaking Away, North Dallas Forty,* and *Dracula.*

The NAC/Coca-Cola market research study enabled exhibitors to focus on two key questions: Who are the frequent moviegoers and why aren't they buying refreshments? 82% of all theatre customers are frequent moviegoers, that is, patrons who attend once a month or more. These customers can be described as young, single, active, and upscale. What are they buying at refreshment stands? *Nothing.* Why? The research finds three reasons.

1. *Price.* Prices are very high in theatres, and exhibitors are turning off some customers because of pricing.

2. *Availability.* Theatre owners build refreshment stands in every new theatre, but with space at a premium, they concentrate on maximizing seating, not lobby space. The result has been a traffic-control nightmare at refreshment stands, and crowded refreshment stands turn customers off and away.
3. *Image.* Theatre concessions have such a bad reputation for poor quality and high prices that patrons consciously bypass the refreshment stand or bring in their own refreshments.

These are the issues that confront exhibitors in the area of refreshment profits. The solutions will not be easily found, but here are three proposals.

1. *Solve the pricing problem.* Exhibitors should move to value pricing (where the cost per ounce goes down as the cup size goes up) so that the customer finds value in buying larger sizes.

2. *Solve the availability problem.* Implement hawker trays in theatres during weekends and other periods of high attendance. Hawker trays have generated 20–25% more sales in test marketing.

3. *Solve the image problem.* Exhibitors should use promotions designed to appeal to moviegoers. Promotions fall into two categories, those that attack the current customer base and those that reach the nonbuyer. The Coca-Cola Company, as well as other suppliers, has developed promotions that encourage buying customers, such as "the free refill." The nonpurchaser might be attracted to premiums such as the "*Star Trek* plastic cup and poster." Market research found that theatres running refreshment promotions increased their refreshment business by 17.3%.

The concession industry and exhibitors are working together to continue marketing studies in an effort to maximize profits for the theatre owner who has initiative and to increase the potential purchasing of moviegoers nationally.

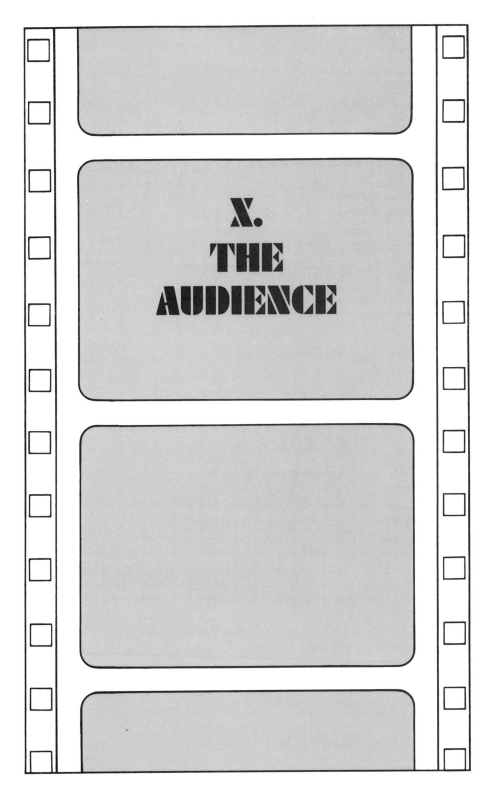

X.
THE
AUDIENCE

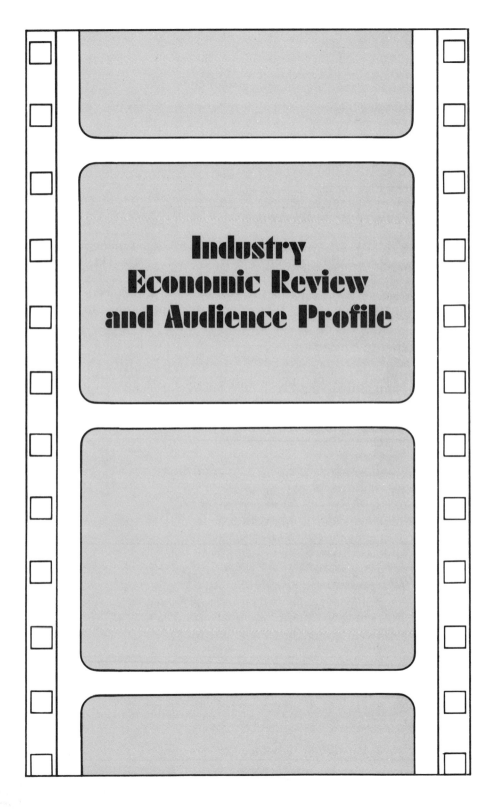

Industry
Economic Review
and Audience Profile

INDUSTRY ECONOMIC REVIEW

The following data are provided by the research department of the Motion Picture Association of America, Inc., Washington, D.C., through the courtesy of Jack Valenti, president. An economic review of the American motion picture industry covering 1981 is followed by a motion picture audience survey conducted in the summer of 1981.

United States Box-Office Gross

American motion picture theatres grossed $2,965,600,000 in 1981, an all-time record, surpassing the 1980 total by 7.9% and eclipsing 1979 (the previous record year) by $144,300,000. Here is how the 1981 total compares with yearly figures from 1977 to 1980:

	BOX-OFFICE GROSS	1981 PERCENT CHANGE
1981	$2,965,600,000	—
1980	$2,748,500,000	+ 7.9%
1979	$2,821,300,000	+ 5.1%
1978	$2,643,400,000	+12.2%
1977	$2,372,300,000	+25.0%

Admissions

Theatre admissions reached a total of 1,067,000,000 in 1981, an increase of 45,500,000 (or 4.5%) over 1980. Here is how the 1981 figure compares with yearly totals from 1977 to 1980:

	TOTAL ADMISSIONS	1981 PERCENT CHANGE
1981	1,067,000,000	—
1980	1,021,500,000	+4.5%
1979	1,120,900,000	−4.8%
1978	1,128,200,000	−5.4%
1977	1,063,200,000	+0.4%

Admission Prices

The overall average admission price for 1981 was $2.779, an increase of 3.3% over the 1980 average of $2.691. However, this 3.3% increase was well below the 1981 increase in the All Items Consumer Price Index of 10.3%.

High Rental Features

Feature films earning $8,000,000 or more in domestic rentals numbered 45 in 1981, two more than in the previous year, and only five fewer than the high water mark reached in 1979, when 50 films reached this plateau. In the category of $10,000,000 or more, the 1981 count of 31 was five fewer than in 1980. Here is a five-year comparison:

	$8,000,000 & OVER	$10,000,000 & OVER
1981	45	31
1980	43	36
1979	50	37
1978	40	30
1977	33	28

Negative Costs

In 1981, the average negative cost (including studio overhead but excluding interest) of new features financed in whole or in part by MPAA member companies advanced substantially to $11,335,600, an increase of almost $2,000,000 (+21%) over 1980. The MPAA companies include Columbia Pictures, Walt Disney Productions, Embassy, Orion (Filmways), MCA-Universal, Metro-Goldwyn-Mayer/United Artists, Paramount Pictures, Twentieth Century–Fox, and Warner Bros. The following chart compares average negative costs over a ten-year period:

INITIAL U.S. RELEASE	AVERAGE PRODUCTION COST PER FEATURE	INCREASE OVER PRIOR YEAR	INCREASE 1981 COMPARED TO
1981	$11,335,600	20.8%	—
1980	9,382,500	5.3%	1980: 5.3%
1979	8,913,700	55.8%	1979: 27.2%
1978	5,722,900	2.0%	1978: 98.1%
1977	5,609,100	35.1%	1977: 102.1%
1976	4,150,600	33.2%	1976: 173.1%
1975	3,115,100	18.6%	1975: 263.9%
1974	2,626,100	13.5%	1974: 331.7%
1973	2,313,400	17.4%	1973: 390.0%
1972	1,970,800	—	1972: 475.2%

Releases

Here is a breakdown of features released by the majority of American distributors for 1978–81. The figures include MPAA member companies along with American Cinema, Associated Film Distribution, Cannon, Cinema 5, Compass, Crown, Dimension, Group I, Lone Star, New World, Pacific International, Sunn Classic, Taft, and Jensen Farley.

	NEW	REISSUES	TOTAL
1981	200	40	240
1980	191	42	233
1979	189	26	215
1978	171	20	191

Advertising

Using 1980, industry-wide advertising expenses totaled $708,400,000, representing an increase of 10% over the 1979 figure of $644,000,000. Significantly, expenditures for network television advertising rose by 61% compared with 1979, while newspaper advertising outlays increased by 12%. The following table illustrates the changes that have taken place from 1976 to 1980 in the distribution of the movie industry's advertising dollars in prime media, and the percent increase in dollars spent in such media over that five-year period.

	SHARE OF ADVERTISING		PERCENT DOLLAR INCREASE
	1980	1976	
Newspapers	69%	71%	+ 66.6%
Network TV	15%	3%	+598.0%
Local TV	15%	19%	+ 41.2%
Radio	1%	7%	− 65.5%

Theatre Screens

As of the end of 1981, the estimated number of theatre screens was 18,040, an increase of 3% over the June, 1980, total of 17,590 screens (excluding military). The following comparison between the number of screens in December, 1981, and June, 1980, indicates a 7% decline in the number of drive-in screens, continuing a trend of recent years. However, hardtops, which represent 82% of all screens, increased in number by 703 screens, or 5%.

SCREENS	1981	1980	PERCENT CHANGE
Hardtops	14,732	14,029	+5%
Drive-ins	3,308	3,561	−7%
Total	18,040	17,590	+3%

Employment

In 1981, employment for all branches of motion-picture activity dropped moderately by 3% to a monthly average of 214,000, compared to an average of 220,000 in 1980.

Demographics

The rapid growth of nonfamily households in the United States would appear to favor the rate of theatrical movie-going. However, the expected continuing decline in the teenage population and the slight rises in marriage and birth rates can be interpreted as signs for caution.

	1980 HOUSEHOLDS		Percent Change 1970–80
	Number	Percent	
Total households	79,080,000	100.0	+24.7
Family households	58,385,000	73.8	+13.2
Nonfamily households	20,695,000	26.2	+73.3

The 1985 projections indicate a 12% increase in total households, an 8% increase in family households, and a 23% increase in nonfamily households.

The average population per household continues to decline:

	ALL AGES	UNDER 18	18 YEARS & OVER
1980	2.75	0.78	1.97
Projection 1985	2.58	0.70	1.88

With 103,420,000 people from ages 12 to 39 in 1981 (46% of the total population), and a projected 105,895,000 in 1985 (45.5% of the total population), movie theatre business is expected to hold up.

AUDIENCE PROFILE

According to a survey of the American motion picture audience conducted during the summer of 1981 by the Opinion Research Corporation (ORC) of Princeton, New Jersey, for the Motion Picture Association of America:

- Audience members aged 12 to 39 accounted for 85% of admissions.
- Frequent moviegoers aged 12 and over (those who attend once a month or more) represented 84% of admissions.
- Those aged 12 to 29 represented 68% of admissions.
- The 12 to 20 age group, which makes up only 19% of the U.S. resident civilian population, accounted for 40% of the movie audience. The 21 to 29 age group, which makes up another 19% of the population, accounted for 28% of the movie audience.

Comparisons can be made to a similar survey conducted by Opinion Research one year earlier, in the summer of 1980.

In the area of frequency of attendance, there was little change in the 1981 figures, compared with the earlier survey. Frequent (at least once a month) moviegoers aged 12 and over, as noted, represented 84% of theatre admissions, though they constitute only 25% of the public. In the category of occasional attendance (once in two to six months), teenagers aged 12 to 17 decreased by 4 points to 32%, while teenage frequent attendance remained at the same level as in 1980.

As in the past, single persons continued to be more frequent moviegoers than married persons, leading the married in frequent attendance in 1981 by 14 points, while singles trailed marrieds as occasional moviegoers by one point. Adults with children under 18 tended to be occasional (once in two to six months) moviegoers. This group accounted for 35% against 24% for the frequent group. Some 31% never attended. For adults without children, 25% went occasionally and 21% attended frequently, but 44% reported they never attend.

In the category of education, every survey since 1969 has found that movie-going increases with higher educational levels. The 1981 survey reported that 66% of those with college educations are frequent (34%) or occasional (32%) moviegoers, compared to a combined total of 34% for those with less than a high school education and 51% combined for those who completed high school.

The tendency toward more frequent attendance by males was more pronounced in 1981, registering for those 18 and over 27% compared with 19% for females. The male no-shows, aged 12 and over, increased 3 points to 34% from 1980. The survey, conducted by ORC in July and August, 1981, was based on the following national probability sample. A more detailed summary of the survey is on p. 359.

2,006	adults, 18 and over
312	teenagers, 12 to 17
2,318	total

Admissions by Age Groups

Age	PERCENT OF TOTAL YEARLY ADMISSIONS			PERCENT OF RESIDENT CIVILIAN POPULATION AS OF JAN. 81
	1981	1980	1979	
12–15 yrs.	16%	16%	20%	8%
16–20	24	26	29	11
21–24	15	17	14	9
25–29	13	14	13	10
30–39	17	14	11	17
40–49	6	7	6	12
50–59	5	3	5	13
60 and over	4	3	2	19
	100%	100%	100%	100%
12–17	26%	26%	31%	13%
18 and over	74%	74%	69%	87%

The bulk of motion picture admissions continues to be generated by those moviegoers under age 40, accounting for 85% of total yearly admissions.

Age groups showing the greatest discrepancy between proportion of yearly admissions and proportion in the population are as follows:

AGE GROUP	PERCENT OF TOTAL YEARLY ADMISSIONS		PERCENT OF POPULATION
	1981	1980	
12–29 years	68%	73%	39%
12–39 years	85	87	56
16–39 years	69	71	48
40 and over	15	13	44

Moviegoers (Aged 12 and Over)

The total number of moviegoers increased from 118,900,000 in 1980 to 119,900,000 in 1981. Since 1969, moviegoers have increased by 27% while the resident civilian population, on which these surveys are based, went up by slightly more than 15%.

Overall, frequent attendance among both the adult public and teenagers is essentially the same as in 1980. A decline in frequent attendance among teenagers evidenced from 1979 to 1980 has leveled off. Frequent moviegoers constitute only 25% of the public aged 12 and over, but account for 84% of admissions, as noted earlier.

Frequency of Attendance

	TOTAL PUBLIC AGED 12 AND OVER			ADULT PUBLIC AGED 18 AND OVER			TEENAGERS AGED 12 TO 17		
	1981	1980	1979	1981	1980	1979	1981	1980	1979
Frequent (at least once a month)	25%	26%	23%	22%	21%	19%	50%	50%	56%
Occasional (once in 2 to 6 months)	29	27	26	30	26	26	32	36	24
Infrequent (less than once in 6 months)	10	13	14	10	14	14	5	9	11
Never	36	34	36	38	39	40	12	5	8
Not reported	*	*	1	*	*	1	1	0	1

*less than ½%

Total Movie-going Public Frequency

	1981	1980	1979
Frequent	39%	39%	37%
Occasional	45	41	41
Infrequent	16	20	22

Movie-going Adults

	1981	1980	1979
Frequent	36%	34%	32%
Occasional	48	43	44
Infrequent	16	23	24

Movie-going Teenagers

	1981	1980	1979
Frequent	57%	53%	62%
Occasional	37	38	26
Infrequent	6	9	12

When limited to moviegoers, an increase in occasional movie going is found in the adult segment of the market.

Marital Status—Adults

	MARRIED			SINGLES		
	1981	1980	1979	1981	1980	1979
Frequent	17%	14%	13%	31%	32%	30%
Occasional	30	25	28	29	26	23
Infrequent	12	16	15	7	11	12
Never	41	44	44	33	31	35

Single persons continue to be more frequent moviegoers than married persons.

Adults With Children Under 18			
	1981	1980	1979
Frequent	24%	22%	19%
Occasional	35	31	36
Infrequent	10	19	18
Never	31	28	27

Adults Without Children			
	1981	1980	1979
Frequent	21%	20%	18%
Occasional	25	21	21
Infrequent	1U	10	11
Never	44	48	50

Movie-going continues to increase with higher educational levels among adults.

Education

	LESS THAN HIGH SCHOOL			HIGH SCHOOL COMPLETED			COLLEGE		
	1981	1980	1979	1981	1980	1979	1981	1980	1979
Frequent	12%	13%	10%	19%	21%	20%	34%	29%	27%
Occasional	22	13	16	32	26	28	32	36	37
Infrequent	11	12	11	11	16	17	8	14	13
Never	55	61	63	38	37	35	26	21	23

As in previous years, males more than females tend to be frequent moviegoers.

Sex

	AGED 12 AND OVER					
	Male			Female		
	1981	1980	1979	1981	1980	1979
Frequent	27%	28%	25%	21%	23%	23%
Occasional	30	27	26	28	26	26
Infrequent	9	13	13	10	14	14
Never	34	31	36	38	36	37
	AGED 18 AND OVER					
	Male			Female		
	1981	1980	1979	1981	1980	1979
Frequent	27%	25%	21%	19%	18%	18%
Occasional	29	26	26	29	25	27
Infrequent	10	13	13	11	15	14
Never	34	36	40	41	42	41

The Movie Rating System

by **Jack Valenti,** president of the Motion Picture Association of America, Inc., who is the spokesman for the organized American film production and distribution industry in the United States and around the world. As president of the Motion Picture Export Association, Valenti travels the globe negotiating film treaties and settling marketing issues with foreign governments on behalf of the member companies. An author and teacher, Mr. Valenti was named president of the MPAA in 1966, after serving as special assistant to President Lyndon B. Johnson.

Should a producer . . . be displeased with his film's rating he could appeal the decision to the Rating Appeals Board, which sits as the final arbiter of ratings. . . .

By the summer of 1966, it had become clear to knowledgeable observers that the U.S. film industry was in radical change. Where the change specifically started and why are obscured by a mix of social and economic upheaval. But change there was.

Perhaps it started in the early 1950s when the Department of Justice, following a U.S. Supreme Court decision, finalized the divorcement of studio and theatre ownership. When the big studios relinquished their theatres, the power that existed in my predecessors, Will H. Hays and Eric Johnston, and in the Hollywood establishment was forever broken. From that collapse of authority came, slowly, the onward thrust of the filmmaker to garner a larger share in the creative command decisions.

When I became president of the Motion Picture Association of America (MPAA)* and the Association of Motion Picture and Television Producers (AMPTP)** in May 1966, the slippage of Hollywood studio authority over the content of films collided with an avalanching revision of American mores and customs.

The national scene was marked by insurrection on campuses, riots in the streets, calls for women's liberation, protest among the young, questioning of church, doubts about the institution of marriage, abandonment of old guiding slogans, and the crumbling of social traditions. It would have been foolish to believe that movies, that most creative of art forms, could have remained unaffected by the change and torment in our society.

---

* Member companies of MPAA include Embassy, Columbia Pictures, Walt Disney Productions, MGM/UA, Orion (Filmways), Twentieth Century–Fox, Paramount Pictures, MCA-Universal, Warner Brothers.
** Member companies include 79 organizations producing theatrical motion pictures and television material.

A NEW KIND
OF AMERICAN MOVIE

The result of all this was the emergence of a new kind of American movie—frank and open, and made by filmmakers subject to very few self-imposed restraints.

Almost within weeks of taking on my new duties I was confronted with controversy neither amiable nor fixable. The first issue was the film *Who's Afraid of Virginia Woolf?*, in which for the first time on the screen the word *screw* and the phrase *hump the hostess* were heard. In company with the MPAA's general counsel, Louis Nizer, I met with Jack Warner, the legendary chieftain of Warner Brothers, and his top aide, Ben Kalmenson. We talked for three hours, and the result was deletion of *screw* and retention of *hump the hostess*, but I was uneasy over the meeting.

It seemed wrong that grown men should be sitting around discussing such matters. Moreover, I was uncomfortable with the thought that this was just the beginning of an unsettling new era in film, in which we would lurch from crisis to crisis without any suitable solutions in sight.

The second issue surfaced only a few months later. This time it was Metro-Goldwyn-Mayer and the Antonioni film *Blow-Up*. I met with the company head, Bob O'Brien, for this movie also represented a first—the first time a major distributor was marketing a film with nudity in it. The Production Code Administration in California had denied the seal. I backed the decision, whereupon MGM distributed the film through a subsidiary company, thereby flouting the voluntary agreement of MPAA member companies that none would distribute a film without a Code seal.

Finally, in April, 1968, the U.S. Supreme Court upheld the constitutional power of states and cities to prevent the exposure of children to books and films that could not be denied to adults.

It was plain that the old system, begun with the formulation of MPAA in 1922, had broken down. The few threads holding together the structure created by Will H. Hays had now snapped.

I knew that the mix of new social currents, the irresistible force of creators determined to make "their" films (full of wild candor, groused some social critics), and the possible intrusion of government into the movie arena demanded my immediate action.

Within weeks, discussions of my plan for a movie rating system began with the president of the National Association of Theatre Owners (NATO) and with the governing committee of the International

Film Importers & Distributors of America (IFIDA), an assembly of independent producers and distributors.

Over the next five months, I held more than 100 hours of meetings with these two organizations, as well as with guilds of actors, writers, directors, and producers; with craft unions, critics, and religious organizations; and with the heads of MPAA member companies.

THE BIRTH OF THE RATINGS

By early fall, the plan was designed and approved. On November 1, 1968, the voluntary film-rating system of the motion picture industry became a fact, with three organizations, NATO, IFIDA, and MPAA, as partners in the enterprise.

That initial plan was, in essence, the same as the program now in effect. Few changes of substance have occurred. There were four rating categories: G for general audiences—all ages admitted; M* for mature audiences—parental guidance suggested; R for restricted—those under 16** must be accompanied by parent or guardian; and X—no one under 16** admitted.

My original intent had been to use only three rating categories, ending in R. It was my view that a parent ought to have the right to accompany children to any movie the parent chose, without the movie industry or the government denying that right. But the exhibitor organization (NATO) urged the creation of the X category, fearful of possible legal redress under local or state law. I acquiesced to NATO's reasoning and the four-category system was installed.

The rating system meant the dismantling of the Production Code Administration and its rigid restrictions, which had been in effect since the 1930s. Our rating concept was a totally new approach.

We would no longer "approve or disapprove" the content of a film, but rather would rate movies for parents who could then make an informed decision on whether their children should attend. This turnabout was not easy to achieve. My predecessors, Will Hays and Eric Johnston, had been opposed to changing the stern Seal of Approval test to a system of rating for children.

But it was a turn in philosophy and action that social change demanded we make, and in the light of a new social environment, we made the turn.

---

* Because this label was misunderstood by the public, it was finally changed to PG—parental guidance suggested.
** Later raised to under 17 years of age.

DUAL RESPONSIBILITIES

From the very beginning of my tenure at the Association, I had sought a way to assure freedom of the screen, to underbrace the right of the filmmaker to say what he chose in the way and form he determined, without anyone forcing him to cut one millimeter of film or threatening to refuse him exhibition.

Yet, at the same time, there had to be some framework of self-discipline, some manner of restraint, in order to fulfill a public obligation. Parents needed to know *in advance* what kind of movie was being exhibited at the local theatre. It was because of this juxtaposition of ideals and goals that the voluntary film-rating system seemed to be the sanest and most practical design to achieve both objectives, despite obvious frailties and inevitable public disagreements over specific ratings.

Under the rating program, the filmmaker became free to tell his story in his way without anyone thwarting him. The price he would pay for that freedom was the possible restriction on viewing by children. I held the view that freedom of the screen was not defined by whether children should see everything a filmmaker conceives.

I would hope it is fair to say that today the screen has never been more free from the standpoint of the filmmaker's right to create any story he wants to tell. And, at the same time, the public is better advised in advance by the ratings about the content of films than ever before, and parents can be confident their children are restricted from viewing certain films. No other entertainment communications medium turns away business to fulfill its pledge to the public.

THE PURPOSE
OF THE RATING SYSTEM

From the outset the purpose of the rating system was to provide *advance information to enable parents* to make judgments on which movies they wanted their children to see and not to see. Basic to the program was and is *the responsibility of the parent to make the decision.*

The Rating Board does not rate for quality or the lack of it. That role is left to the movie critic and the audience. We would have destroyed the rating program in its infancy if we had become arbiters of how "good" or how "bad" a movie was creatively.

Inherent in the rating system is the fact that to those 17 and over, and to those married without children, the ratings have little if any meaning.

Among the Rating Board's criteria are theme, language, nudity

366

and sex, and violence; part of the rating comes from the assessment of how each of these elements is treated in each individual film.

There is no special emphasis on any of the elements. All are considered and all are examined before a rating is given.

Contrary to popular but uninformed notions, violence has from the outset been a key factor in ratings. (Many violent films would have been given X ratings, but most of the directors chose, on their own, to revise the extremely violent sequences in order to receive an R rating.)

HOW THE RATINGS
ARE ARRIVED AT

The ratings are decided by a Rating Board located in Hollywood. It is a full-time Board, composed of seven persons, and headed by a chairman. There are no special qualifications for Board membership, except that a member must love movies, must possess an intelligent maturity of judgment, and must have the capacity to put himself in the role of an average parent and view a film as most parents might—parents trying to decide whether their children ought to see a specific film.

In my role as MPAA president, I do not take part in rating discussions, do not interfere in rating decisions, and do not overrule the Board or its chairman or dissuade them from any decisions they make.

During the long period of the rating system's existence, its critics have been vocal about many things, but I can say this: the Board has never deliberately fudged a decision, bowed to pressure, or done anything that would be inconsistent with its integrity.

No one is forced to submit a film to the Board for rating, but I would judge some 99% of the producers creating entertaining, seriously intended, responsible films (*not* hard-core pornography) do in fact submit their films for ratings. Most makers of pornographic movies do not submit their films but instead, within the rules of the rating system, self-apply an X rating and go to market. The other symbols, G, PG, and R, are registered with the U.S. Patent and Trademark office as certification marks of the MPAA and cannot be used on a film in advertising by any company that has not officially submitted its film and received a rating. They may *not* be self-applied.

NATO estimates that about 95% of the exhibitors in the nation participate in the rating program and enforce its admission restrictions.

THE BOARD VOTES ON RATINGS

The Board views each film and, after group discussion, votes on the rating. Each Board member completes a rating form spelling out his reason for the rating in each of several categories of concern and then gives the film an overall rating based on the category assessments.

The rating is decided by majority vote.

The producer of a film has a right under the rules to inquire as to the "why" of the rating. The producer also has the right, based on the reasons for his film's rating, to edit it if he chooses to try for a less severe rating. The reedited film is brought back to the Rating Board, and the process of rating goes forward again.

ADVERTISING CODE AND TRAILER POLICY

Film advertising is also part of the film industry's self-regulatory mechanism.

All advertising for rated motion pictures must be submitted to the Advertising Code Administration for approval prior to release of the film to the public. This includes, but is not limited to, print ads, radio and TV spots, pressbooks, and theatrical trailers.

Trailers are an important aspect of the program. Trailers are either designated G, which means they may be shown with all feature films, or R, which limits their use to feature films rated R or X. There will be in G-designated trailers no scenes that caused the feature to be rated PG, R, or X.

Each trailer carries at the front a tag that tells two things: (1) the audience for which the trailer has been approved, and (2) the rating of the picture being advertised. The tag for G-rated trailers will have a green background; the tag for R-rated trailers will have a red background. The color is to alert the projectionist against mismatching trailers with the film being shown on the theatre screen.

APPEAL OF RATINGS

Should a producer for any reason be displeased with his film's rating, he can appeal the decision to the Rating Appeals Board, which sits as the final arbiter of ratings.

The Appeals Board comprises 22 members, men and women from MPAA, NATO, and IFIDA.

They gather as a quasi-judicial body to view the film and hear the appeal. After the screening, the producer whose film is being appealed explains why he believes the rating was wrongly decided. The chairman of the Rating Board states the reason for the film's rating. Both the producer and the Rating Board representative have an opportunity for rebuttal. In addition, the producer, if he desires, may submit a written presentation to the Board prior to the oral hearing.

After Appeals Board members question the two opposing representatives, they are excused from the room. The Board discusses the appeal and then takes a secret ballot. It requires a two-thirds vote of those present to overturn a Rating Board decision.

By this method of appeal, controversial decisions of the Rating Board can be examined, and any rating deemed a mistake set right.

The decision of the Appeals Board is final and cannot be appealed, although the Appeals Board has the authority to grant a rehearing at the request of the producer.

WHAT THE RATINGS MEAN

Essentially, the ratings mean the following:

G: *"General Audiences—All ages admitted."*

This is a film that contains nothing in the categories of theme, language, nudity and sex, or violence that would, in the view of the Rating Board, be offensive to parents whose younger children view the film. The G rating is *not* a "certificate of approval," nor does it signify a children's film. Some profoundly significant films are rated G (for example, *A Man For All Seasons*).

Some snippets of language may go beyond polite conversation, but they are common, everyday expressions. No words with sexual connotations are present in G-rated films. The violence is at a minimum. Nudity and sex scenes are not present.

PG: *"Parental Guidance Suggested—some material may not be suitable for children."*

This is a film that clearly needs to be examined or inquired about by parents before they let their younger children attend. The label PG plainly states that parents *may* consider some material unsuitable for their children; however, the parent must make this decision.

Parents are warned against sending their children to PG-rated movies without seeing or inquiring about them.

There may be profanity in these films, but not sexually derived words, which will vault a film into the R category. There may be violence, but it is not deemed so strong that everyone under 17 need be restricted unless accompanied by a parent. Nor is there the cumulative horror or violence that may take a film into the R category.

There is no explicit sex on the screen, although there may be some indication of sensuality. Brief nudity may occur in PG-rated films, but anything beyond that puts the film into R.

The PG rating, suggesting parental guidance, is thus an alert for special examination of a film by parents before deciding on its viewing by their children.

Obviously the line is difficult to draw, and the PG-rated film is the category most susceptible to criticism. In our pluralistic society, it is not easy to make subjective judgments for more than 215 million persons without some disagreement. So long as the parent knows he must exercise his parental responsibility, the PG rating serves as a meaningful guide and as a warning.

R: *"Restricted—under 17s require accompanying parent or guardian."*

This is an adult film in some of its aspects and treatment so far as language, violence, nudity, sexuality, or other content is concerned. The parent is advised in advance that the film contains adult material, and he takes his children with him with this advisory clearly in mind.

The language may be rough, the violence may be hard, and while explicit sex is not to be found in R-rated films, nudity and lovemaking may be involved.

Therefore, the R rating is strong in its advance advisory to parents as to the adult content of the film.

X: *"No one under 17 admitted."*

This is patently an adult film and no children are allowed to attend. It should be noted, however, that X does *not* necessarily mean obscene or pornographic in terms of sex or violence. Serious films by lauded and skilled filmmakers may be rated X. The Rating Board does not attempt to mark films as obscene or pornographic; that is for the courts to decide legally. The reason for not admitting children to X-rated films can relate to the accumulation of brutal or sexually connected language or of explicit sex or excessive and sadistic violence.

APPRAISAL

In any appraisal, what is "too much" becomes a controversial issue. How much is too much violence? Are classic war-type films, with marines storming the beaches of Iwo Jima killing and wounding the enemy, too violent? Is the dirt street duel between the cattle rustler and the sheriff too violent, or does it require the spilling of blood to draw a more severe rating? How does one handle a fist fight on the screen? Where is the dividing line between "all right" and "too much" for a particular classification?

The same vexing doubts occur in sex scenes or those where language rises on the Richter scale. The result is controversy—inevitably, inexorably—and that is what the rating system has to endure.

The raters try to estimate what most American parents would think about the appropriateness of a film's content, so that parents at the very least are cautioned to think seriously about what films they may wish their children to see or not to see.

HOW THE CRITERIA
ARE CONSTRUCTED

To oversee the Rating Board, the film industry has set up a Policy Review Committee consisting of officials of MPAA, NATO, and IFIDA. These men and women gather quarterly to monitor past ratings, to set guidelines for the Rating Board to follow, and to make certain that the Rating Board carries out its duties reasonably and appropriately.

Because the rating program is a self-regulatory apparatus of the film industry, it is important that no single element of the industry take on the authority of a "czar" beyond any discipline or self-restraint.

THE PUBLIC REACTION

We count it crucial to take public soundings annually to find out how the public reacts to the rating program and to measure the public's approval or disapproval of what we are doing.

Each year the Opinion Research Corporation of Princeton, New Jersey, conducts a scientifically sampled nationwide survey of more than 2,500 persons.

A basic question is asked:

"How useful do you think the motion picture industry's rating system—with the symbols G, PG, R, and X—is in helping parents decide what movies their children should see—very useful, fairly useful, not very useful, or have you not heard of the rating system?"

Highlights of the 1979 survey are as follows:

• The usefulness of the voluntary movie ratings to parents in guiding the attendance of children soared to a five-year high in 1979.

• All parents with children under 18 years of age reported by 65% they found the ratings to be very or fairly useful. This was an increase of a significant five percentage points over 1978 and was the highest in five years. Twenty-six percent found the ratings not very useful.

• Parents with children under 13 years of age attested by an even higher figure, 66%, to the usefulness of the classifications for children.

371

This figure exceeded 1978 by seven significant percentage points and also marked a five-year high. The not-very-useful response was 27%.

The motion picture industry began the voluntary ratings in 1968 for the primary purpose of assisting parents in the not-always-easy task of forming the movie-going habits of their children.

It is pleasing to know that parents with children, after the program's many years in the marketplace, are increasing their approval of how we are trying to help them decide what films their children should see or not see. The rating system isn't perfect, but in an imperfect world, it seems each year to match the expectations of those at whom it is directed—the parents of movie-going children.

National Screen Service

by **Martin Michel,** who has served in various film advertising and promotional capacities since 1951, beginning as a writer in the publicity department of Twentieth Century–Fox, then becoming director of radio and television advertising and publicity, and later advertising manager for the same company. After a stint as director of advertising for the Landau Company, he joined National Screen Service Corporation as director of advertising and publicity in 1965.

For the past 60 years, National Screen Service's principal function has been the distribution of trailers (coming attractions) and accessories (lobby displays and posters) for the majority of feature films distributed in the English-speaking markets. It is a publicly held company that grosses approximately $25,000,000 annually for its services. It is the only such national distributor, with a network of nine branch offices in the United States as well as an office in London that services exhibitors throughout England.

Each week, NSS ships a minimum of 8,000 trailers (coming attractions and cross-plugs) to theatres in the United States. Accordingly, each week 7,000 play dates must be recorded, trailer prints shipped in time to arrive an agreed-upon number of weeks prior to play date, and returned prints checked in and reshipped to meet new dates.

Similarly, each week National Screen services about 12,000 one-sheets (27 x 41 inches) at $2.00 each to theatres throughout the nation. These, too, must be delivered to theatres in coordination with their film-booking schedules. In addition to one-sheets, on major pictures, NSS ships larger posters measuring 30×40 inches at about $7.50 each (prices vary in special circumstances); 40×60 inches at about $10.00 and up; 14×36 inch posters at $2.40 and 22×28 inch posters at $2.65; plus 8×10 inch stills at 70¢ each and 11×14 inch stills (photos) sold in a package of eight for $5.00; as well as teaser/cross-plug trailers, radio spots, television spots, press books, and so on. NSS pays all freight costs to its branches. An exhibitor pays freight only from the NSS branch to the theatre and back.

National Screen originally became the distributor of trailers for the major motion picture distribution companies in 1919. At that time, the majors conceived the concept of showing sample scenes of forthcoming feature films to a captive audience and realized that the cost and problems of distribution would be a distraction from the companies' principal job of selling feature films. These advertising film clips came to be known as *trailers* because they always trailed after the theatre's on-screen current feature.

Trailers are leased to theatre owners from nine strategically located NSS service branches at rates that are negotiated, based on the theatre's capacity, location, and intended usage. No trailer is sold outright; it is leased, and the print is returned to NSS on the opening day of the feature or, when used as a current cross-plug on a secondary screen, at the conclusion of the feature's engagement.

In recent years, great emphasis has been placed on the importance of advance 60-second to 90-second *teaser trailers* (shorter than standard trailers and available far in advance of the feature film's play date) and *cross-plug trailers* (teasers used by a theatre chain in one or more theatres to announce the advent of a major film in another of their theatres). National Screen has established a special program to intensify the saturation potential of these trailers and to follow through with individual theatre managers in order to insure maximum usage.

National Screen Service entered into the standard accessory business in 1940 under franchises with two of the major film producers, Paramount Pictures Corporation and RKO Radio Pictures. Shortly thereafter, it acquired through purchase other poster-renting businesses then in the field. Over the years, the majority of the major feature film distributors, as well as most independents, have committed themselves to National Screen's accessory distribution. These companies prepare an advertising campaign on each feature film and deliver the finished artwork to NSS for the full line of accessories. This artwork is sent to a majority-owned subsidiary of National Screen, Continental Lithograph Company in Cleveland, where it is printed and then distributed through the NSS service branches around the country. Technically, all accessories are the property of NSS and are licensed to theatres for use only in connection with the exhibition of the pictures for which they were designed. The licensee (theatre owner) agrees not to trade, sell, or give them away, or permit others to use them, nor is the licensee entitled to any credit upon returning accessories.

Although distribution of trailers and accessories continues to be the mainstay of National Screen's service to motion picture exhibitors, over the years NSS has also become a reliable source for additional services through its subsidiary companies: National Theatre Supply, the country's only national distributor of theatre equipment (projectors, sound systems, amplification systems, automation systems, etc.) and the proprietary manufacturer of Simplex equipment, all of which is sold from branches in eleven key cities throughout the country; Advertising Industries, with manufacturing facilities in Cleveland, the creator and manufacturer of wall-poster frames, free-standing frames, counter frames, display cases (illuminated and nonilluminated), multi-sided, motorized, revolving carousel frames, and indoor mini-marquees for auditorium identification; Continental Lithograph Company, a completely equipped graphic arts plant that prints all posters and lobby displays for most American-made films, now extending its lithograph business beyond the motion picture field; and National Screen Service Ltd., the British subsidiary that distributes trailers and accessories to theatres throughout the United Kingdom. NSS also operates a modern studio outside London, which uses the latest equipment to produce trailers, television spots, main titles, and foreign versions of trailers for use in non-English-speaking countries.

National Screen Service is directed from its home office in a company-owned building at 1600 Broadway in Manhattan. From these executive offices come the policy decisions, direction, and corporate planning that guide this industrial complex. The home office is constantly in touch with its nine service branches, ranging from Seattle to Atlanta and from Los Angeles to Boston, as well as the eleven National Theatre Supply offices, the warehouse in Kansas City, and the offices of the subsidiary companies.

Each fully staffed NSS service branch is headed by a regional sales manager and a branch manager. The regional sales manager (usually aided by additional sales personnel) is committed to contacting every theatre manager within his territory in order to service each theatre's complete promotion-advertising needs. Likewise, the National Theatre Supply sales force in each of its branches is responsible for similar contact to supply each theatre's equipment needs. Backing up sales personnel in each branch is the branch manager, whose primary function is the operation of the branch, seeing that the front office (bookers and clerks) and the back room (shippers) are coordinated to handle all materials with the utmost speed and accuracy.

The NSS Distribution Center in Cleveland serves as the central shipping depot to all of the NSS service branches, as well as the NTS branches, and the repository of all the reserve material on films in current distribution. From there, shipments are sent to each branch every day, filling out shortages that have developed in both film and accessory departments. In the NSS Kansas City warehouse, all available materials are stored on pictures more than five years old. In rural and remote areas of the country, many films continue to play for years. For these play dates, the Kansas City warehouse has material going back to 1950.

Recently, NSS has added an entirely new area of operation, offering theatres a potentially new source of revenue: "Movie Madness Merchandise." On certain selected pictures, NSS offers a researched, premarketed, and tested selection of novelty merchandise items geared to the specific audience for that film: T-shirts, posters, buttons, pins, rings, and so on. NSS offers individual theatres a complete program for

376

selling these items, together with a merchandise display unit for in-theatre retailing. Each theatre has the opportunity to double its cost outlays to NSS, with actual retail pricing at the discretion of theatre management. This represents another expansion of National Screen's continuing effort to supply the nation's 18,000 theatres with all possible material for on-the-spot advertising and exploitation of their films.

Merchandising

by **Stanford Blum,** who was president of The Image Factory, Inc., and Image Factory Sports, Inc., before establishing Stanford Blum Enterprises, based in Sherman Oaks, California. A graduate of the University of Baltimore Law School, he enjoyed an active career directing commercials and short films before turning to the infant industry of exploiting merchandising rights of motion pictures and sports events. His success in licensing items for *Rocky* in 1976 drew attention to the revenue potential of this new area.

> *... the cost of a poster ... might be as low as 25¢ each, on which the producer receives a 10% royalty. ... But ... for 300,000 posters, that 10% royalty equals $7,500. ...*

Merchandising rights are potentially among the most valuable of the ancillary rights that flow from a motion picture, second only to book-publishing rights in revenue potential. But the merchandising of a motion picture was largely ignored until a few years ago. It took the huge success of *Star Wars*, licensed by Twentieth Century–Fox, to awaken the movie business to the great wealth to be derived from merchandising characters or the logo from a picture in the areas of posters, iron-ons, clothing, jewelry, toys, watches, and other products. To date, *Star Wars* products have grossed at the retail level over $1-billion from merchandising rights worldwide.

Star Wars is a phenomenon that produced revenue from sources such as toys, which ordinarily do not yield merchandising dollars from movies. On an average picture, posters and T-shirts are the two most lucrative items, unless a film has characters who can be made into toys, as in *Star Wars, Star Trek, The Empire Strikes Back*, and *E.T.*

The essential elements of merchandising a picture are the rights to the title and logo (or artwork) of the picture; these rights must be licensed from the owner (usually the financier-distributor) in order to exploit them on a poster, T-shirt, or iron-on. Certainly, copyright and trademark protection must be obtained by the owner to protect not only the exhibition of the movie itself, but also to cover the use of the artwork title, created for advertising, in its adaptation to various items of merchandise. Further, if a performer's likeness as a character in the film is to appear on such merchandise, the rights to such likeness must be obtained from the performer, usually in the form of a deal that includes a percentage share to that performer of everything that is licensed or merchandised bearing his likeness.

If a picture is developed and fully financed by a financier-distributor (studio), that company will retain all merchandising rights and the rights to all characters and actors' likenesses as those characters. The studio will have its own merchandising licensing company make the appropriate licensing deals. If the producer realizes there is merchandising potential in his movie, he'll try to negotiate for a percentage (usually 25–50%) of that revenue as part of his deal with the

379

studio. However, the studio will probably cross-collateralize expenses such as advertising against what the merchandising revenue would be.

In order to secure merchandising for *Rocky II,* UA began putting out feelers to major manufacturers a full year before the scheduled release of the picture. UA's merchandising executive contacted, say, an iron-on manufacturer who would be interested in the merchandising rights for T-shirts for *Rocky II.* A sample deal for such a transaction would find the iron-on manufacturer (licensee) putting up a $25,000 guarantee, payable $10,000 up front, with a 10% royalty for the rights for T-shirts. Ten percent of the wholesale price is the royalty rate that would be paid to the financier-distributor after $250,000 of revenue comes in (which would meet the $25,000 guarantee obligation). The manufacturer of the iron-on heat transfers then sells the transfers to a preprinter, who applies them to T-shirts.

Four preprinters supply Sears, J.C. Penney, K-Mart, Montgomery Ward, and Woolworth, the country's main mass-merchandising stores. These stores are the prime outlets for the nation's retail merchandising market, rather than Bullock's, Sak's Fifth Avenue, or Bloomingdale's. One Sears store can buy ten times more goods than any Bullock's or Bloomingdale's. Their strength is in volume. J.C. Penney runs 2,100 stores nationwide; K-Mart has around 2,000; Sears-Roebuck operates 866 retail outlets; and Montgomery Ward has about 480. One chain's opening order could total 100,000 pieces.

The store will buy a shirt from a preprinter for around $2.50 and sell it for $5.00. Of the remaining $2.50, the preprinter's profit is around 25¢ a shirt, after paying for the raw shirts, which he buys from a mill, and deducting his overhead and other costs. On an order of 100,000 shirts, 25¢ a shirt is $25,000. The iron-on manufacturer has sold those transfers for, say, 33¢ each to the preprinter. Then, he has to pay a royalty to the financier-distributor (rights holder), which is 10¢ a transfer, or $10,000 for 100,000 units. (If a star's likeness is involved, half of that royalty would be shared with the star.) When the iron-on manufacturer deducts his overhead and the cost of making the product, his profit would be 10–12¢ per transfer. If one million transfers are sold, that's $100,000–$120,000. Heat transfers can also be sold to the makers of pajamas and tote bags and to individual iron-on shops where a selection is displayed.

The arithmetic for a poster is similar, involving one transaction with a printer. Assume that Stanford Blum Enterprises is the entity that owns the poster and transfer rights to the motion picture *Running* starring Michael Douglas. We arrange for the printing and then sell the posters to distributors at 45¢ each, who mark them up and sell them to department stores, which charge the consumer $2.50 or $3.00. Of that 45¢ per poster, about 15–20¢ covers our printing costs. The rights holders (the producers of *Running*) would receive 10% of our price to the distributors, or 4.5¢, and the balance represents our overhead and profit.

My company is a licensing agency that licenses properties, such as Bo Derek, the actress in *10*, *Running*, and *The Legend of Paul Bunyon*, to national companies that manufacture T-shirts, jewelry, clothing, accessories, or toys. Toys are a special case because toy manufacturers require at least a year to gear up to supply newly created toys to stores nationally. Most toys are manufactured in the Orient, and it takes about six months to perfect the tooling required. When Kenner Toys was licensed by Twentieth Century Fox for *Star Wars*, neither party knew it would be the landmark picture for merchandising. Because of the necessary lead time in creating toys, Kenner didn't have the merchandise ready for stores by the Christmas after the picture's summer release. Rather, they sold a nonrefundable certificate for customers to return in April to pick up the merchandise, and the response was enormous.

A typical deal with a licensee-manufacturer requires three key elements: front money, a royalty, and a guarantee. Front money is good-faith money that can range anywhere from $2,500 to $500,000, depending on the deal. It is really an advance against the royalty. The royalty covers everything sold at the wholesale price and is based on 10% of net sales. *Net sales* refers to gross sales less quantity discounts and returns. If the company's also going to agree to a guarantee beyond the front money, they will sell aggressively because a guarantee is nonrefundable. For example, a deal with a jewelry manufacturing company to make a *Running* pendant may call for $10,000 up front, a 10% royalty, and a $25,000 guarantee. The guarantee is due one year after the contract is signed. However, there's no standard deal. Most toy manufacturers won't step up to a 10% royalty rate; they would settle for a royalty between 5 and 7½%. In that case, all planning and designing is done by the toy company, with approval of samples vesting in the licensor and producer.

There are two further elements in a manufacturing deal: approvals and exclusivity. If an item contains an actor's likeness, a sample contractually must be shown to the actor for his approval. Many companies that license don't give exclusivities; that is, they give out licenses to more than one company for the same product, such as a tote bag. It could be argued that this increases competition, but I believe it only creates unnecessary tension in the marketplace if more than one national manufacturer is licensed for a certain item. Every licensing deal I make is exclusive.

Now let's turn to an independent producer, who may be gathering financing for a picture partially from a distributor and partially through other sources. Assuming he retains merchandising rights, this producer can try to sell licenses to his picture on his own, but he would be at a competitive disadvantage in an unknown market. My advice would be for him to make an overall deal with one of the licensing companies experienced in movie marketing to handle all merchandising exploitation of his picture.

The producer and the licensing agent would enter into a representation agreement, in which the agent would agree to solicit and enter into agreements with manufacturers for merchandising, subject to the approval of the producer. There is usually no difference between basic terms of a studio-negotiated license agreement and one negotiated by an independent licensing agent. For its services, the licensing agent would receive a fee ranging from 40 to 50% of all monies due from the manufacturing companies under all license agreements negotiated by the agent. Licensing agreements usually provide for a royalty payment to the producer's company of between 5 and 10% of all net sales by the licensee, which generally is accompanied by a cash advance against royalties, as mentioned.

When a producer approaches my company to handle merchandising for a picture, I first determine that he and his project are valid and ongoing. Then, the essential questions in determining whether the picture qualifies for a merchandising effort are: How does the screenplay read? Who are the lead actors? Who will be advertising and distributing the picture? If the screenplay content is violent, downbeat, or heavily sexual, it is probably not a picture for merchandising because the vital chain stores would not carry items relating to such subject matter. If the picture is heroic, family-oriented, or youth-oriented, it has a better chance at successfully licensing products. Suggestions can be made in the screenplay stage that would enhance the merchandising potential of the movie.

Next, who's starring in the picture? The mass-merchandising stores want to know if the lead actors have wide appeal or are up-and-coming stars because that will influence how they sell the products in their stores. They easily advertised Sylvester Stallone as Rocky into a merchandising bonanza that included posters, iron-ons, and clothing. The *Rocky* robe was particularly successful around Father's Day. *Star Wars* and *The Empire Strikes Back* not only featured the lead actors, but also Darth Vader, R2-D2, C-3PO, the Wookie, and other characters that kids could identify with. This fed the merchandising success in areas such as dolls and other toys. The producer's obligation is to tie up all merchandising rights from the actors in the very first stage of negotiating their employment agreements.

The next important issue is who is distributing the picture because the essential advertising that will be used in merchandising flows from the distributor. As mentioned, the royalty payment to the distributor on every merchandised item covers the use of the recognized title and artwork (logo) of the picture, which has been created by the distributor for advertising. Planning a product campaign is so sophisticated now that Sears and J.C. Penney want to know where and when a picture is breaking so their stores can be prepared and stocked. When a picture opens with 600 prints, a release schedule detailing theatres and opening dates will help them sell posters in each city.

A producer should not assume that a potential licensee will come to him. Rather, buyers from the key mass-merchandising and retail chains should be invited to an early screening of the picture, along with manufacturers who want to obtain merchandising rights. Product ideas and merchandising angles should be solicited from them. If the retailers are excited over the market potential, the manufacturers will be eager to make deals. The producer should review those manufacturers whose products enjoy screen coverage in the movie. With stills of such coverage, steps can be taken that might lead to a promotional or premium tie-in with companies such as Coca-Cola, McDonald's, or Ford; there are substantial royalties in this area. Again, a separate screening of the movie for such company representatives can lead to generating tie-in ideas. Publicity kits on the picture mailed to manufacturers can also solicit merchandising interest.

Where does the producer make the profits in merchandising? If a financier-distributor is doing the licensing, the producer's deal may call for 25–50% of all revenue from merchandising. If the producer is free to deal with an independent licensor, the producer would receive 50–60% of all front monies, guarantees, or royalties negotiated by the licensor, who would receive the balance, 40 to 50%.

This discussion has centered upon retail merchandising, which is one market. A separate market is the product tie-in or premium market. The *premium market* can equal or exceed profits from the retail market because a single order for a tie-in can range from 1 to 12-million items (posters and other giveaways). An example of a premium deal could center around the Nike shoes Michael Douglas wore in the picture *Running*. If Nike decided to run a promotion, making an initial order of perhaps 300,000 *Running* posters to give away at stores selling their shoes, and to promote this in print ads, the foot traffic to those stores would increase substantially as a result.

Because premiums deal in such volume, the cost of a poster to a shoe company or beer company might be as low as 25¢ each, on which the producer receives a 10% royalty, or 2½¢ per poster. But if a single transaction is for 300,000 posters, that 10% royalty equals $7,500.

Another type of merchandising deal is the sweepstakes deal. There was a lot of *Lite* beer drinking on camera in *Running*, which was shot in Montreal. Anheuser-Busch, makers of *Lite*, might want to run a sweepstakes whereby their customers could win a trip to the Olympic site in Montreal where the picture was shot. This type of promotion would appear in all grocery stores selling *Budweiser* or *Natural Lite* beer. A sweepstakes deal would be a flat deal involving perhaps a $100,000 payment from Anheuser-Busch to the licensor for rights to use the name and artwork of the picture in their contest. Then, they would make a deal with a company that would organize the contest.

Finally, there is the deal wherein manufacturers may simply want to use a picture logo in their advertising. This would also be a flat deal. If, for example, Procter & Gamble wanted to use the *Running* logo in their advertising for a product, the cost for that license would depend on the media involved. If such advertising were to include radio, television, and print, the fee could range from $25,000 to $500,000.

If an unauthorized company uses a picture logo in advertising or on retail goods, it's a federal offense, a violation of copyright law. One response is to send "cease and desist" letters, which have little practical power. A stronger strategy is to sue the company and report them to the FBI. The offending company would have to pay a royalty on everything sold, and all remaining items would be confiscated.

Motion pictures are harder to merchandise than television shows. A TV show can reach 40-million people in one night, whereas a motion picture could take six months to reach the same size audience. Also, a motion picture is widely available for only six months, while a hit TV series stays on a network for perhaps five years and lives on in syndication.

The merchandising industry is in its infancy, and people are learning more about it every year. It's important for a producer to understand the value of this potential market in order to protect this ancillary right.

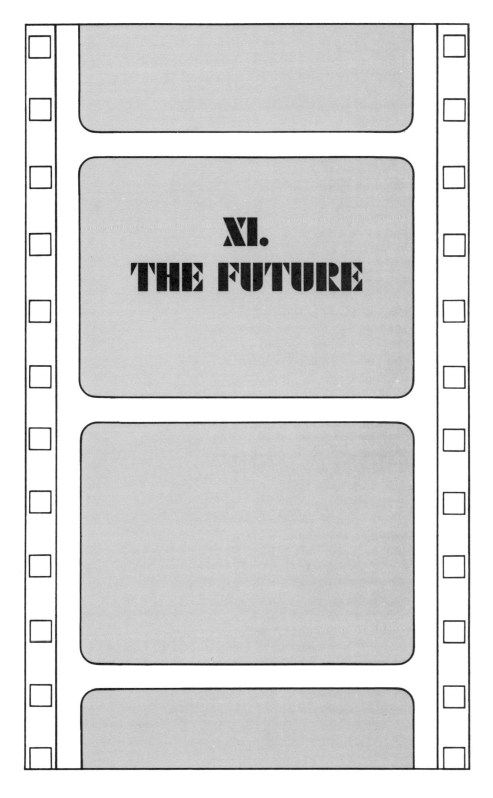

XI.
THE FUTURE

Future Technologies
in Motion Pictures

by **Martin Polon,** a futurist and consultant in the technology of electronic entertainment. He is technical editor for *Computer Merchandising,* columnist for *Billboard,* and consulting editor to *Recording Engineer Producer* magazine. In addition to his writing, Polon is a governor of the Audio Engineering Society and teaches at UCLA about the impact of future technologies on the electronic communications media. He has served as moderator and speaker for such diverse organizations as the Society of Motion Picture and Television Engineers (SMPTE), the Audio Engineering Society (AES), the Aspen Institute, the U.S. Department of Labor, and at conferences on video music, personal computers, electronic mail, and stereo television. Polon is widely published and has presented a technical paper to the American Film Institute on the future of film and television. He is also doing biomedical research concerning how audio and visual inputs are perceived.

The scenario for the theatre of the future relies heavily on space-age technology to provide maximum experience for the audience. . . .

The creative world of the theatrical motion picture has always had an element of fantasy about it. The "Big Screen" holds a special feeling of magic for many people. Weaving a story from the diverse elements of production and film craft has a sense of unreality about it, as though it can't really be happening in front of your own eyes. For the more than fifty years of the sound motion picture, the technology of movie making has been suspended in a genre of its own making. Progress has been for the sake of the craft rather than for the sake of technology. There are examples of aerospace-type "state-of-the-art" technology in the everyday process of making movies. But, there is a feeling of patient quality about the tools of the cinema. It is as though each camera, lens, light source, and microphone—and even the film itself—has been patiently evolved to be the best there is for making a movie. And it shows. Other forms of visual communication lack the total impact of a well-projected theatrical motion picture with its extraordinary resolution.

The only thing constant in the field of communication technology is change. It is this change, as wave after wave of state-of-the-art electronics moves down from aerospace and defense-related systems into commercial applications, that has brought motion pictures and television into the 1980s. The challenge of home TV includes large-screen video playback, video cassette recorders, and satellites. The first time film was impugned by its brash, upstart cousin was during the late 1940s, when television was a very unpolished system with crude resolution of picture on a 10-inch screen. This assault on the movie audience brought chaos to the film studios. Order returned only when the television industry had to turn to the motion picture studios for product. The impact of that confrontation of technologies almost broke the back of theatrical exhibition. The relationship between film and video went through a different confrontation in the 1970s, with the advent of electronic home-entertainment devices. However, home video technology was being perfected at that time. The theatrical motion picture retained primacy in visual presentation, but at the expense of technical expansion.

An electronic crossroad faces the entire entertainment industry in the last two decades of the twentieth century. Motion pictures use as much electronics as any other medium. Yesterday's science fiction is becoming today's science fact. The U.S. Air Force is improving charged particle beam weapons for outer space—the death ray. Anyone in the world can reserve room to ship materials into space on a space bus—the shuttle. Three-dimensional color images can be laser projected from flat pictures—the holograph. The future is the present.

That future will come to electronic entertainment by evolution, given the changing pattern of the worldwide audience. No longer does the U.S. film industry hold all the cards dealt in entertainment. In years past, a decision in Hollywood such as the adoption of 70mm film would be followed quickly by all users of theatrical product. Now, such a decision could as well be made in Tokyo or Eindhoven, Holland, as in Hollywood. The standard for a new medium such as the video disc will indeed come from a merging of international industry. No purely domestic decisions can survive in the future marketplace of global entertainment technology.

The motion picture industry faces its greatest challenge from the highly developed technology that has reached the consumer entertainment marketplace. Film will survive either as the consequence of a reasoned turn in direction of the new technologies or else will be absorbed by an alien force that will reshape film without historic restraint. Change is inevitable, and the shape of today in the film industry suggests that there is room for new technology in the creation and reproduction of the theatrical motion picture.

CURRENT USES
OF TECHNOLOGY

For Production

The making of a theatrical motion picture in the early 1980s encompasses a good deal of modern technique, but by adaptation more often than invention. The spiral of inflation in filmmaking has not left a comfortable margin for large-scale research and development. The industry has found it easier to borrow and adapt existing technology, with some notable exceptions. All production companies make extensive use of radio equipment, for example. Radio provides the synchronism between camera and audio tape recorder. Wireless microphones are commonplace. In both studio and location production, two-way radios are used to cue all the interrelated elements, replacing the old-style bullhorn. The technology to accomplish these tasks came from military communications, television broadcasting, and law enforcement, respectively. Filmmakers adopted existing products.

The tools of the trade have progressed into better instruments to transfer a creative performance to film. Cameras have become smaller and quieter, lenses have shrunk in size with less optical distortion, and all viewing is reflexed directly through the taking lens. The sound-recording process uses very few constraining cables since the link to the camera and microphone is by radio, not wire. The tape recorder and mixer are slightly smaller than a comparable setup of ten years ago; the equipment is quieter electronically and may have further noise reduction built in. The sound recorded is truly high fidelity, with a minimum of noise or distortion. Lighting equipment is smaller and produces less heat through the use of new lamps containing exotic filaments and gases. Editing systems have shifted from the vertical to the horizontal plane, with TV screen-like viewing.

Several innovations have been notable for releasing the act of filming from previous physical restrictions. The gyroscopic back-supported camera mount (Steadicam, etc.) with video viewfinder allows a cameraman to move about rapidly along with the action of a scene, while the camera captures the moment without any image vibration. The stabilizing system transforms any form of transportation into an effective camera platform. The development of new film stocks has allowed more latitude of exposure within varying light conditions. Recycling of the silver-based emulsion after film processing has also been enhanced. Special effects have benefited from computer-assisted effects generation. Laboratory processing of exposed film offers more opportunities for creative development control when governed by computer systems.

Another improvement has been to reduce the size and weight of production equipment, allowing location shooting to be done from specially configured trucks (such as Cinemobiles) with a minimum of difficulty. More time is then available for creative aspects, since the equipment setup is simplified by the reduction in bulk. Current industry practice has brought theatrical film production technology to a point of polish; then, that gloss is sometimes allowed to rub off in exhibition.

For Theatrical Exhibition

It is difficult to discuss current technical practices in theatrical exhibition and not comment on the growth of the automated mini-theatre. In theory, the automated "mini" allows an exhibitor to show more movies to more patrons. The equipment for three, four, or even eight screens can be serviced under one roof by one operator. The fiscal impact is obvious, both in terms of operator utilization and an increase in audience turnover possible within a given time frame. What is not so obvious is that the concept destroys the advantage that the motion picture could have over other technologies. For reasons that are economic rather than aesthetic, screen size is often reduced, in some cases to a seven-foot high image. Sound quality is similarly scaled down to the picture dimensions. Worse still, the automated mode has led to projection machine-induced print mutilation. For the distributor, the continuing spiral in petrochemical and silver inflation has increased release print lab and film costs enormously, so that damaged prints are not readily replaced. The problem is compounded when film exchanges ship prints mangled at mini-theatres to exhibitors with quality, large-screen projection systems. The exhibitor who wants a perfect picture may not be able to achieve that goal, short of demanding a new print. The mini-theatre is not the only culprit in print abuse. Theatres of all kinds are involved, if they use old or poorly maintained projectors or rewinds. In an emerging technology marketplace, audience tolerance for scratched prints is going to evaporate.

There are many positive aspects of the technique of exhibition today. The troublesome arc lamps—burning rods of carbon with variable light output—have been replaced with xenon lamp systems using a lamp filled with xenon gas. This provides a superior projection light source, with no flicker or variance, requiring little or no maintenance. Screens have been developed that are more efficient in returning light to the audience. These two improvements mean that most theatres today have a brighter picture than was possible twenty years ago.

To take advantage of this bright picture, there have been improvements in the wide-screen anamorphic process, both in cameras and taking lenses, as well as in projection. The whole range of Panavision and Panaflex cameras, for example, has evolved to the point where wide-screen production is no different from using a normal aspect ratio. The cumbersome nature of anamorphic equipment has now been simplified.

The improvement of sound reproduction in theatres has been a dramatic implementation noticed by patrons internationally. The most spectacular effect on sound is the application of the Dolby system to film recording and reproduction. Working with developmental efforts at RCA and Eastman Kodak, the Dolby Laboratories have taken their system of reducing film noise and applied it to improve the frequency response of movie sound and provide a stereophonic effect in theatres. The Dolby system reduces high-frequency noise present in optical film sound by recording the noise-susceptible high frequencies with accentuated volume. In projection, this accentuation is removed, leaving a clean signal up to 12,000 Hertz. Dolby also enables a stereophonic sound track to be used on standard optical release prints. This has brought stereophonic sound with good fidelity to thousands of theatres around the world. The conversion equipment is simple to add to current theatre projection systems and does not affect existing films that are non-Dolby. The success of the Dolby format can be gauged by the fact that many directors have insisted on it for their film product. One of the key rules of entertainment technology is that there must be enough entertainment software available for the hardware to succeed. The Dolby system has met this test, and the availability of Dolby-encoded pictures is an ideal compromise for all exhibitors. Dolby films will perform normally on projectors that are not equipped to handle the process.

What distinguishes the theatrical motion picture in exhibition from any other visual communications medium is the quality of resolution, which is the equivalent of thousands of lines of scanned information. The challenge of the future is whether the film industry can use this quality as a base for further technical improvement. Whether theatrical exhibition can continue to attract an audience will partly answer this challenge. The serious problem of print and negative color fading after several years will also have to be addressed.

In-Home Viewing

The home market for electronic entertainment has shown the greatest expansion over the past decade. The 1980s have begun with a whole range of equipment to record, play, and display video software for home entertainment. The world has standardized on three systems of video transmission. The U.S. system, known as *NTSC* (National Television Systems Committee) uses 525 scanning lines to identify a single image. The NTSC system is used in Canada, Japan, Mexico, and 23 other countries. The SECAM system (Sequential and Memory) originated in France and is now used in over 20 countries around the globe. The third system is PAL (Phase Alternation Line), used in 37 countries. Both SECAM and PAL scan at a 625 line rate, affording better resolution than the 525 line system.

The arrival of home video cassette recorders (VCR) in the entertainment marketplace has taken two forms. The Beta system, introduced by Sony Corporation, uses omega-wrap tape cartridges (so named because the tape resembles the Greek letter *omega* when it is wrapped around the video head drum). Machines using this format are manufactured by or for Sanyo, Sony, Toshiba, Zenith, and Sears. The competing system is known as the Video Home System or VHS. Originated by the Victor Company of Japan (JVC), the system uses an M-wrap cartridge and is being made by or for Akai, General Electric, Hitachi, JVC, Magnavox, MGA/Mitsubishi, Panasonic, Quasar, RCA, and Sharp. The M-wrap cartridge is not compatible with the cartridge used for the Beta format.

Projection or large-screen systems for video viewing have also arrived in the home. Several formats have been developed to produce the large pictures. The *picture tube system* uses a screen-type picture tube similar to that found on a conventional color TV. This tube has extra brightness that, when focused through at least one lens (usually fresnel) and reflected through a mirror (or electronically reversed to "read right"), will project a picture onto a screen. Another format uses projection tubes, usually three tubes for the primary red, blue, and green signals that make up a video color signal. The tubes are focused to converge the three colors on a screen, combining to form a complete color picture on the light-intensifying surface.

It is obvious that these emerging home technologies have great potential for the future. Less obvious is the interrelation between these and other emerging technologies for home use such as video disc, interactive cable, direct broadcast satellite, and film. The appetite for home video software has seen legal actions (Disney and Universal/ MCA versus Sony, et al.), and drive-through photo developing services providing video cassette film rentals (Fotomat, etc.). The paradox of the emerging technologies is that some portions of the theatrical movie business will switch or be absorbed into different markets already extant if public interest in theatrically exhibited product wanes. Film is being challenged, and the defiance is just beginning.

DEFINING THE FUTURE
IN THEATRICAL PRODUCTION

Production Advances in the Eighties

The production of entertainment on film will continue beyond the decade of the '80s. Whatever the direction of the public's taste for electronic home entertainment, the need for both film and video product will be greater than at any time in the history of the entertainment industry. There is, however, one codicil to this prophecy. The catastrophic disruption of world petroleum and associated petrochemical distribution would render the use of film a mortal blow. Film production is certainly energy intensive and uses primarily petrochemicals. That reliance could be fatal in an energy crisis. Producing raw film stock would be difficult to justify if transportation systems, hospitals, household heating, and pharmaceuticals were threatened. Videotape, although to some extent petro-dependent, would have a big edge with its capacity for reuse and its nonreliance on silver.

Of course, a doomsday scenario is a drastic one, but the use of energy sufficient systems is going to be one potential direction in which the technology of film production can turn. Solar power assemblies could be used for location filming and remote video setups. This would begin to replace dependence on gas-powered electric generators. Solar power packs are already in use to power military communications systems. The high level of reliability shown is well suited to location film production. The technology of solar cell assemblies and associated power systems is such that weather conditions too severe for filming would still allow energy draw.

Inflation touches all segments of the economy, and an industry as complex as the motion picture business is squeezed by each ripple of energy constriction. As the film industry operates through the 1980s, waves of inflation will see many film production budgets exceed the $15-million level. Of the 25 most expensive films ever budgeted, with an average cost of $27,000,000, 17 of these were budgeted during the last half of the 1970s. This factor of high cost comes at a time when the competitive technologies of video production offer substantial economies. These technologies allow video to be interchanged with film in production. There are three *C*'s of visual entertainment imagery: creation, control, and communication of a particular narrative. As a production tool, video assumes a role approaching unity since all of these three elements can be handled with instantaneous response, electronically. Video systems can capture, balance, and edit instantly. Post-production, especially as video shifts into the realm of digital electronics, will provide many effects not available on film.

The drawback to the use of video, historically, has been poor resolution. At the beginning of the 1920s, 35mm film possessed such high image resolution that projection merely needed the arrival of a relatively reliable light source (the carbon arc) and improved lenses to fully capitalize on image quality. Television started out at about that time with 24 electronic lines scanned. World standards established via electronic improvements after World War II increased resolving ability to 500 lines or better. These postwar standards have remained in use because millions of television sets have been built to operate on them. While there is no way to increase picture fidelity without casting aside all of the world's TV receivers, video production systems do not have to conform to a 525 or 625 line limit.

High-definition video systems are now a reality, spun off from aerospace and video research, where high resolution is vital to visual accuracy. In any situation where the final video image can be transferred, as in production, the image-producing system should resolve at the highest rate technically feasible. Scanning rates over 1,000 lines have proven reliable for on-board systems designed under Air Force contract. NHK (the Japanese Broadcasting Corporation) with CBS and Sony, has demonstrated an entire video production system operating at 1,125 lines. Since the resolving power of the human eye operates logarithmically, rather than in a linear mode, the difference between, say, 525 lines and 1,125 lines scanned is a perceptive doubling in clarity of image. A system operating above 1,000 lines provides significant visual advantages in picture fidelity and definition. Video equipment operating to the end of the century will offer a whole range of production hardware in high-resolution systems. The emerging bubble storage technology and microcomputer systems could allow the scan rate to go higher still. 1,500 line or 2,000 line resolution systems will become switchable quality options, allowing for creative use of various scanning rates, just as film qualities are varied in the lab.

With a high rate of visual definition, a production video system can be exchanged for a film camera, laboratory, and editing facility. The rapid response via VTR playback allows confirmation of any given scene, eliminating the need for costly retakes upon viewing work prints or dailies. For example, directors such as Mel Brooks and Alan Alda refer to video playbacks while shooting on film. Many cameras can be used at once, with the director having an instant edit capability. Alternatively, a single video camera, with computer assistance, can provide the editing convenience of film. Francis Coppola's Zoetrope Studios in Hollywood was a forerunner in experimenting with combining computer and video technology in an effort to reduce costs and the lag time between the first day of shooting and delivery of a completed picture. Post-production video editing has the advantages of preview and of speed. Since video will edit electronically by storing image information in a memory and then transferring the visual images, there will be less danger of destroying original material inadvertently. Various shots can be viewed, stored, and compared prior to the actual edit. The transition can be done via electronics with cuts, fades, wipes, and literally hundreds of other effects that would require lab processing if on film. In addition, complex special effects can be generated directly by computer to videotape. The development of sophisticated multi-dimensional digital graphics computers for further enhancement of program video suggests the direction of special effects capability in the future.

The 1980s and 1990s will see these and other innovations improving the competitive position of video vis-à-vis film. For example, an advanced Japanese video camera contains a built-in videotape recorder. The speed, resolution, and production logistics when video is supported by a computer system with a creative production package (camera, recorder, etc.) will provide alternatives to filmed entertainment. There are examples of the theatrical use of video during the late 1970s such as *Norman, Is That You?*, *Bully*, and *Give 'em Hell, Harry*.

It is impossible to view these and not feel the sense of immediate contact. As the technology of high-resolution video expands, so will the creative comprehension of its use.

The future would seem to include a mix between film and video in production. The economy of video, especially when programing will be direct to the home, is going to be an important factor. The burgeoning home video marketplace will increase the demand for new product to satisfy viewer needs, but film will continue to service the theatrical filmmakers because of its very high resolution and artistic definitions. Video will become the medium of choice for immediacy; film will capture intimacy.

Of course, there are no absolutes in the future technologies of visual communications. There will be a cross-pollination between film and video. It will be commonplace to see film transferred to videotape for editing, utilizing the SMPTE time code. In this way, frame-by-frame reference is possible on the tape. Using the instant effect capability of video, the whole pattern of edits in a film could be rapidly evaluated. The transfer of video to film will reach a quality comparable to film, assuming high-resolution video is used to begin with. Transfers in both directions between film and video will be done by computer control, utilizing such techniques as digital frame storage and laser tracing during the decade of the 1980s. The ultimate transfer capability will come when video makes the transition into digital signal processing. With all video signals encoded in computer language, the use of bubble memory to hold a frame and redistribute it will give flawless transfer capability for any production use.

The future of film as a production tool will be further enhanced by the refinement of film stocks that began in the latter part of the 1970s. The speed of original negative film stock will be boosted without any loss of detail or of resolving power. The match of production color rendition from original negative to internegative to color positive for release prints will continue to improve to a point where the statement "what you see is what you get" will be an absolute. Release prints could also have longer-term color stability due to enhanced cyan dye dark-keeping characteristics (resistant to color fading). These advances will be available to cure the problem of poor release prints not delivering the creators' perceived rendition due to poor color match or color shift in older prints. The only question is whether the film industry will pay the price for print quality.

The trend in audio equipment to digitalize the recording and reproduction of sound will enable movie recording to be virtually distortion-free. This technique, coupled with computerized mixdown consoles for rerecording film audio, will provide the highest quality sound tracks. This will come at a time when concurrent advances in audio technology in exhibition will allow film sound to match the inherent resolving quality of the picture. Computerized audio mixdown will allow the combining of the many voice, effects, and music tracks with fewer trial mixes. The computer will remember the volume settings for each track so that a correct trial mix volume may be locked in. Then on subsequent mixes, more tracks are locked in. In this way, the mixdown session can be considerably shortened.

DEFINING THE FUTURE IN THEATRICAL EXHIBITION

Exhibition Advances in the Eighties

The projection system of the large theatre will be honed to perfection during the course of the 1980s. Utilizing advances in release-print quality, picture brightness will be increased via faster projection lenses and improved light return from screens. Coupling these features with the current trend of xenon light sources, the next logical step will be to further enhance the anamorphic projection process. The use of wider-screen processes will be adopted. The net result of wider, brighter pictures will be combined with advances in film sound. The synergy is expected to provide a motion picture viewing experience heretofore unrealized.

The sound portion of the exhibited motion picture will continue to increase the quality perceived by the audience, to a point equal to the visual excellence. The digitalization of audio will allow film sound to finally escape the frequency response limitations of the optical film-projection system. The nonstable movement of the film through the sound gate of a projector has always limited sonic response due to low-frequency noise, while the high frequencies have been limited by the use of the optical sound process itself, which generates high-frequency noise. Until the Dolby system devised a technique for reducing the noise through electronic treatment, film sound was limited to a frequency response of 100 Hertz (or cycles) to 6,500 Hertz, with some sound reproduced as high as 8,000 Hertz. The Dolby system for film sound allows a high-end response of up to 12,000 Hertz. This all has to be compared with the 20 Hertz to 20,000 Hertz or better frequency response of the modern home stereophonic phonograph system. The Dolby system has greatly improved film sound fidelity, and the promise of further enhanced sound from four to fourteen channels will match the expectations of the audience. The film-viewing public has a very sophisticated appreciation of high fidelity because of what they hear at home on records, tape, and FM radio.

Digital sound recording can be likened to a fine reproduction of a painting by an old master. If that reproduction is run over by a truck (low-frequency noise) or pierced with an ice pick several times (high-frequency noise), it is seriously degraded. The film sound track likewise suffers from the medium of recording and the movement of the film itself. To continue the analogy with digital, in order to create the fine reproduction, the original painting would be copiously logged by computer so that each color and brush stroke would be recorded on paper as a series of numbers, allowing the painting to be reproduced at will following the detailed instructions. So it will be with film, where the sound track will be recorded as a series of binary numbers (0's and 1's). These numbers are retrieved in playback, and the sound track is re-created from the detailed instructions. The use of digital technology allows existing methods of recording and projection to be used, since it is the sound signal itself that is encoded and decoded, totally unaffected by the flutter of the projection movement or the high-frequency noise of optical recording. The resulting digital sound will be exceptional.

There will be an emergence of theatres that are equipped for satellite reception, videotape, or film. The advantages of videotape as an exhibition medium are immediacy, the reuse of the tape, and the tape's imperviousness to scratching or gouging by a defective player. Large-scale projection systems for video have very good quality, such as the Eidophor projector, which uses a viscous oil surface as a reflecting medium to pick up a very high-powered beam of light. The future will see improved versions of this, or more advanced systems employing red, blue, and green lasers modulated to converge an intense picture on a screen. Coupled with satellites and a six-foot receiving dish on the roof of the theatre, special events networking of major attractions such as sports will become commonplace. Again, we will see video augmenting and enhancing the use of film.

The Theatre of the Future

As we shall see, the home will develop an electronic entertainment room with significant capability to display theatrical product on video cartridge, cassette, or video disc. The exhibitor of motion pictures is going to have to offer far more than a small screen and speaker in a mini-complex of eight theatres, because a similar capability will be in the home. The home can provide a show without the need of using scarce and expensive gasoline to get there or paying for parking or having to eat an undercooked hot dog. The movie theatre will have to become an arena; a palace to experience the full grandeur and potential of the theatrical motion picture. The film audience will have to be able to get more in a theatre than anywhere else.

The scenario for the theatre of the future relies heavily on space-age technology to provide maximum experience for the audience. In this arena, visuals will utilize the widest screen technology possible without the optical distortion at the edges of the picture that currently limits the dimensions of anamorphic projection. New developments in lightweight plastic lenses will allow extreme wide-screen projection onto special wrap-around screens. The sound will be cued by the optical track of the film, which will contain two sets of digital information: a stereophonic sound track will be available for conventional theatres, and a second cue track will contain information to operate computer memory disc drives feeding a computer system. The discs will be able to synthesize sound effects while the computer will move sound around the theatre to enhance the stereo effect. The cue track will also instruct the computer to provide other effects: seating would be capable of sustained vibration by being mounted on a platform or shaker-table; air in the theatre would be climatized by a system capable of controlling temperature and water-vapor content very rapidly based on instructions from the computer. The computer would also be able to activate elements capable of producing scent by electrical current flow. These "scent sensors" would be able to provide trace aromas, yet have a rapid dissipation, in contrast to the earlier "smell-o-vision," which could not readily differentiate between aromas.

The result would be to experience a motion picture. If the movie has a scene on the docks of London, the seating would move just perceptibly, while the sound supplies suitable creaks. The smell of ocean and a cool touch of water vapor would complete the illusion given by the multi-channel sound and wide picture. This potential has to be handled with care, but it provides a powerful extension of the creative tools available to filmmakers. The motion picture will add resolution of sound and sensation to the already formidable resolving power of the visual. With this kind of innovation, the film can co-exist indefinitely with home entertainment.

DEFINING THE FUTURE
IN HOME ENTERTAINMENT

Home Entertainment Advances in the Eighties

The home will be the focal point for the development of technologies heretofore reserved for professional television and telecommunications. The technology of video and the computer will reach the home as a system for displaying information and as a method for creating, controlling, and capturing entertainment. The home will have all of the elements necessary to provide complete entertainment and information retrieval.

The television set will change form. It will exist on several levels. The existing box-like apparatus, though downsized, will be used for portable color viewing. Consoles will increase the size of the television picture. Projection television systems will drop in price and size as technologies stimulate production. Industrial and aerospace display technologies will yield the flat screen television. Hanging on the wall, the TV will have a 3 by 4 foot screen composed of liquid crystal elements in a matrix or may be composed of gas discharge display materials. Within the gas display, fluorescent cells of red, blue, and green materials will be arranged in a pattern.

The sound produced by this television system will be greatly enhanced. TV audio will be digitally transmitted on satellite (or within the video signal) to eliminate the distortion of audio transmission via telephone lines. Using techniques currently in use with FM radio stations, the TV audio signal (which is FM) will utilize a subcarrier allowing full stereo transmission into the home. At the end of the 1970s, the transmission of stereo television into the home was an accomplished fact in Japan, both in terms of transmission over the air and the availability of stereo-compatible TV sets. All units capable of television reception and display in the future will have full-frequency audio capability, both to internal speakers and to feed home stereo systems.

The recording and reproduction of video entertainment will be enhanced by the standardization of hardware taking place during the 1980s. In the 1970s, professional video recording used two-inch videotape. One-inch videotape has emerged as a new professional alternative, with better audio quality using smaller tape on a smaller machine. Three-quarter-inch U-matic cartridge video recorders service the industrial video market. The half-inch video cassette is used as the standard for home recording. In the 1980s, the advent of digital video recording will change this substantially. The advantages of digital recording, that is, laying down and picking up video information from the tape independent of the mechanical or electronic negatives inherent in the recorder, will offer substantial quality improvements regardless of format. The two-inch professional machines will give way to a one-inch standard, based on improved audio, video, and reduced machine size. Below that point, there will only be the half-inch VCR system as standard. Once digitalized, the signal-to-noise picture improvements will offer flawless recording of video.

It is important to look at the past when reaching out to the future. At the onset of videotape recording in the late 1950s, the video signal-to-noise ratio (how much picture over the internal electronic interference) was in the middle of the 40 decibel range for network television use. At the end of the 1970s, half-inch machines matched that level. The improvements to come will allow studio quality recording in the home as an everyday reality.

The future holds other technologies for the recording and reproduction of video besides magnetic tape. Spectacular growth in the 1980s could be in video discs, initially for playback, but eventually for recording as well. The initial involvement of MCA, IBM, N. V. Phillips Gloeilampen Fabrieken (Eindhoven), Pioneer Electronic Corporation, and Magnavox in the laser-read DiscoVision system suggests the future potential for video (or digital) discs. There are similar systems (though not compatible) by RCA, Matsushita, G.E., and Thorn-EMI. By the mid-1980s, this disc market is expected to be multi-million dollar in size. The future of the video disc will also be directly related to the development of the digital audio disc (replacing phonograph records), with the ultimate goal of one player in the home reproducing both audio and video discs, and even home computer programming.

The home computer will grow into a billion dollar industry for home entertainment and information control. A video link will allow computer information display on the video system in the home. In addition, the television signal will carry encoded data that can be retrieved as pages of information on the TV screen. This electronic newspaper concept, known as *teletext*, is already well developed and in use around the world. In England, there are two such systems. The British Broadcasting Corporation (BBC) has developed a system known as *Ceefax* ("see the facts"). A second system used by the Independent Broadcasting Authority (IBA) is known as *Oracle*. In France, a competing system is called Antiope and has been tested in the United States. The Canadians have devised Telidon. All of these systems use a modified television receiver with a small remote control the size of a pocket calculator. The systems allow the calling up of any one of several hundred pages of data, everything from recipes and the daily stocks to bus and airline schedules.

The Home Entertainment Center of the Future

The home will be linked via video cable and/or telephone company fiber-optic link and/or direct satellite broadcasting to the broadest base of entertainment and information sources imaginable. Some of the linkages will allow for interactive communications, so that an audience can be polled after a Presidential speech, for example (such as the Warner Qube system, where interactive response exists on several levels). Prerecorded entertainment software, including but not limited to theatrical motion pictures, will be bought the same way a record is acquired today. Tape and disc will both be used for this packaged entertainment.

Playback will take place on a sophisticated linkage of the home computer, video projector, tape and/or disc player, and the stereo sound system. The computer can be programmed to operate such accessories as the audio delay. For instance, a broadcast of the London Philharmonic playing from the Royal Festival Hall in London will be available live via satellite. The home computer could be instructed to present the program for viewing on the projector screen with the stereo TV sound enhanced via audio delay by the exact delay time one senses when sitting inside the hall itself. In the same operation, the computer can also activate the audio tape unit to record the program while the videotape recorder is transcribing a screening of *Casablanca* from a local TV channel without the commercials (which the computer senses and removes). The gathering and interconnection of all the technology tools for home entertainment will yield the most powerful mechanism for consumer control. This technology of the electronic consumer will be a strong barrier facing exhibitors of theatrical films in the future.

CONCLUSIONS

The motion picture industry can dominate the very technologies that seem to menace it. The historic need is there, as when the fledgling television industry turned to film in the 1950s. So can the expanding home software marketplace draw from the industry that has the experience and track record in product development. But film has to change on all levels. The making of motion pictures has to be done with the latest equipment even if that equipment is so technology-intensive that it reduces the number of tasks necessary. The law of supply and demand is one of the few immutable forces in the economy. The enormous potential of home entertainment will not be fulfilled solely by the theatrical motion picture. Software needs will go far beyong the level of old movies, network series episodes, and recent theatrical films. The number of channels available (new cable TV systems are going in with an average of 42 channels) will require new, creative production at reasonable prices. Video can and does meet the software challenge, especially with high-resolution systems and rapid, enhanced edit and modification capability.

Perhaps one way to best consider the future of film is to look at the research and development (R & D) budgets of any major technology user, including television networks, broadcasters, and manufacturers. Communicators such as the telephone companies and computer companies also share the mantle of R & D. The amount spent at each company may approach 10% of gross profits or better. The motion picture industry, however, does not expend enough to sustain an industry-wide research program.

One hopes that the film industry will meets its challenges. These visions of the future should provide motivation to enter a new era of production, distribution (perhaps via satellite to the theatres), and exhibition. Industry concern over fewer jobs will change when there is recognition that the number of productions could quadruple to meet the needs of the new home marketplace. Exhibition of film could become a special experience, capable of competing with the home under any format or technology. This would be especially true if film was to embrace an innovative technology of its own, providing the audience with creative experiences unavailable in the home.

The future will be decided, in the technological world of entertainment, by corporate political discussions among telecommunications multinationals with global standards set for future system growth and by the timeless attraction an audience feels for an entertainment. Theatrical motion pictures can be entering a new age of production and exhibition if the industry looks forward, not back.

Index

409